Conceptualizing Plant-Based Nutrition

Ramesh S. V. • Shelly Praveen
Editors

Conceptualizing Plant-Based Nutrition

Bioresources, Nutrients Repertoire and Bioavailability

Springer

Editors
Ramesh S. V.
Physiology, Biochemistry and
Post-Harvest Technology Division
ICAR-Central Plantation Crops
Research Institute
Kasaragod, Kerala, India

Shelly Praveen
Division of Biochemistry
ICAR-Indian Agricultural Research Institute
New Delhi, Delhi, India

ISBN 978-981-19-4592-2 ISBN 978-981-19-4590-8 (eBook)
https://doi.org/10.1007/978-981-19-4590-8

This Springer imprint is published by the registered company Springer Nature Singapore Pte Ltd.
The registered company address is: 152 Beach Road, #21-01/04 Gateway East, Singapore 189721, Singapore

Preface

Plant-based nutrition has gained popularity in recent years due to its potential health benefits. Plant-based foods are low in calories and high in nutrient density and satiety, and nutrient supplementation makes them wholesome diets. Over the last decade, research efforts have aimed at developing nutrient-dense crops. Further, exploring the biodiversity and caring for soil health and their implications for plant-derived human nutrition have attracted greater interest. Researchers have investigated the ways and means of enrichment of micronutrients in grains through biofortification, fortification, and supplementation. Recent findings have improved our understanding of the role of food matrix and nutrient bioavailability, including the utilization of prebiotic and probiotic microbes in enhancing the nutrient profile of foods. Demand for functional foods (nutraceuticals), phytochemicals, and bio-actives has witnessed a massive fillip led by the consumer awareness and the efforts of researchers alike. An upward rise in consumer preference for nutritious food derived from non-conventional and under-utilized crops has been observed. Furthermore, it is pertinent to acknowledge the fact that food and health are influenced by anti-nutritional factors, metabolic fate of the food, and genomics. Finally, on the regulatory front, food safety issues are imperative to define the concept of safe nutrition.

This book offers a comprehensive coverage on plant-based nutrition, starting with the importance of biodiversity contributing towards nutrition and then delving into the strategy of biofortification, food matrix and its implications for human nutrition. Concepts such as plant-based nutraceuticals, inclusion of prebiotics and probiotics, ways and means to utilize legumes to enhance the protein quality of the diet, and the welcome addition of microgreens are presented thereafter. In addition, a chapter has been dedicated to discussing the importance of anti-nutritional factors. Following the repertoire of nutritional benefits of plant diet, a discussion on the metabolic fate of food and its bioavailability along with the nutrigenomics and its implications for human nutrition takes centre stage. As a follow-up, glimpses of developments in the field of plant biotechnology in devising next-gen crops for human nutrition and the importance of food safety regulations are presented. To conclude, a chapter was dedicated to providing a perspective view on the prospects of plant-based nutrition.

It has been a great privilege to collaborate with experts in the field of plant biochemistry, nutrition science, plant and human genomics, policy makers, and food regulatory authorities among others while crafting this book. We are greatly indebted to the authors and peer reviewers who have contributed in shaping up this compilation, and we are thankful for their time and expertise. We hope that this book serves a one-stop reference for plant scientists, food technologists, and nutritionists looking forward to understanding the concept of plant-based nutrition and its linkage with human health.

Kasaragod, Kerala, India Ramesh S. V.
New Delhi, Delhi, India Shelly Praveen

Contents

Editors and Contributors

About the Editors

Ramesh S. V. is presently serving ICAR-Central Plantation Crops Research Institute (ICARCPCRI), Kasaragod, Kerala, India, as a Senior Scientist (Biotechnology). His field of specialization is plant biochemistry and molecular biology having obtained his master's and doctorate degrees in plant biochemistry. His current research focus includes nutritional biochemistry and bioactives of nutraceutical potential in plantation crops. He is a recipient of DBT-CTEP Travel Award and AABSc-sponsored Young Plant Biotechnologist Award. His postdoctoral research in the field of plant and viral small non-coding RNAs at Washington State University, USA, was sponsored under DBT-CREST Fellowship. He has published many scholarly articles—spread over diverse fields, viz., plantation biology, nutrition biochemistry and plant–virus interactions—in journals of international and national repute and presented his research findings in several international scientific fora. He also features in the editorial boards of international journals PLOS ONE and Measurement: Food.

Shelly Praveen has an illustrious career in research, teaching, program management, and research policy development at ICAR-Indian Agricultural Research Institute, India, leading to the publication of over 100 research articles. Dr. Praveen's contributions as a Head of the Division of Biochemistry at ICAR-IARI, New Delhi, and Director of the Centre for Advanced Faculty Training are immense. She bolstered the industry-academia synergy and launched a portfolio of developing millet-based fortified foods. Earlier, Dr. Praveen led a multidisciplinary team in the development of virus-resistant transgenic tomato and collaborated with international academia including Universidad Politécnica de Madrid, Spain; King Saud University; Scottish Crop Research Institute; CIB, CSIC, Spain; and CREC, Florida, USA. Dr. Praveen has been honored with coveted Awards and Fellowships including Fellow of NASI, Fellow of NAAS, Associate of The World Academy of Sciences, and Panjabrao Deshmukh Outstanding Woman Scientist Award, ICAR, to name a few. Currently, she is engaged in nutrition for health management through service in nutritionally important foods across globe.

Contributors

Steve W. Adkins School of Agriculture and Food Sciences, The University of Queensland, Gatton, QLD, Australia

Ali Ahmad Department of Plant Physiology, Faculty of Sciences, University of Granada, Granada, Spain

Muraleedhar Aski Division of Genetics, ICAR-Indian Agricultural Research Institute, New Delhi, India

Navita Bansal Division of Biochemistry, ICAR-Indian Agricultural Research Institute, New Delhi, India

P. P. Shameena Beegum Physiology, Biochemistry and Post-Harvest Technology Division, ICAR-Central Plantation Crops Research Institute, Kasaragod, Kerala, India

Fernanda Caro Beveridge School of Agriculture and Food Sciences, The University of Queensland, Gatton, QLD, Australia

Chellapilla Bharadwaj Division of Genetics, ICAR-Indian Agricultural Research Institute, New Delhi, India

Begoña Blasco Department of Plant Physiology, Faculty of Sciences, University of Granada, Granada, Spain

Tejpal Dhewa Department of Nutrition Biology, Central University of Haryana, Mahendergarh, Haryana, India

H. K. Dikshit Division of Genetics, ICAR-Indian Agricultural Research Institute, New Delhi, India

Suneha Goswami Division of Biochemistry, ICAR-Indian Agricultural Research Institute, New Delhi, India

K. B. Hebbar Physiology, Biochemistry and Post-Harvest Technology Division, ICAR-Central Plantation Crops Research Institute, Kasaragod, Kerala, India

Kathleen L. Hefferon Department of Microbiology, Cornell University, Ithaca, NY, USA

Sundaravel Pandian Kalaipandian School of Agriculture and Food Sciences, The University of Queensland, Gatton, QLD, Australia

Vinod Kotwal National Pharmaceutical Pricing Authority (NPPA), Government of India, New Delhi, India

Veda Krishnan Division of Biochemistry, ICAR-Indian Agricultural Research Institute, New Delhi, India

Ranjeet Ranjan Kumar Division of Biochemistry, ICAR-Indian Agricultural Research Institute, New Delhi, India

Francisco Javier López-Moreno IFAPA, Institute of Research and Training in Agriculture and Fisheries, Granada, Spain

Lovemore N. Malunga Agriculture and Agri-Food Canada, Department of Food and Human Nutritional Sciences, University of Manitoba, Winnipeg, MB, Canada

M. R. Manikantan Physiology, Biochemistry and Post-Harvest Technology Division, ICAR-Central Plantation Crops Research Institute, Kasaragod, Kerala, India

Gyan P. Mishra Division of Genetics, ICAR-Indian Agricultural Research Institute, New Delhi, India

Zhihua Mu School of Agriculture and Food Sciences, The University of Queensland, Gatton, QLD, Australia

Eloy Navarro-León Department of Plant Physiology, Faculty of Sciences, University of Granada, Granada, Spain

R. Pandiselvam Physiology, Biochemistry and Post-Harvest Technology Division, ICAR-Central Plantation Crops Research Institute, Kasaragod, Kerala, India

G. Rama Prashat Division of Genetics, ICAR-Indian Agricultural Research Institute, New Delhi, India

Shelly Praveen Division of Biochemistry, ICAR-Indian Agricultural Research Institute, New Delhi, Delhi, India

Priti Division of Genetics, ICAR-Indian Agricultural Research Institute, New Delhi, India

S. Rajesh Department of Plant Biotechnology, Centre for Plant Molecular Biology and Biotechnology, Tamil Nadu Agricultural University, Coimbatore, Tamil Nadu, India

Juan Manuel Ruiz Department of Plant Physiology, Faculty of Sciences, University of Granada, Granada, Spain

Ramesh S. V. Physiology, Biochemistry and Post-Harvest Technology Division, ICAR-Central Plantation Crops Research Institute, Kasaragod, Kerala, India

Mrinal Samtiya Department of Nutrition Biology, Central University of Haryana, Mahendergarh, Haryana, India

Seema Sangwan Division of Microbiology, ICAR-Indian Agricultural Research Institute, New Delhi, India

Ajeet Singh Division of Biochemistry, ICAR-Indian Agricultural Research Institute, New Delhi, India

R. Sivaranjani ICAR-Indian Institute of Spices Research, Kozhikode, Kerala, India

Komal Soni Department of Nutrition Biology, Central University of Haryana, Mahendergarh, Haryana, India

Tsering Stobdan Defence Institute of High Altitude Research, DRDO, Leh, Ladakh, India

Sijo Joseph Thandapilly Agriculture and Agri-Food Canada, Department of Food and Human Nutritional Sciences, University of Manitoba, Winnipeg, MB, Canada

Maharishi Tomar Division of Biochemistry, ICAR-Indian Agricultural Research Institute, New Delhi, India

S. Varanavasiappan Department of Plant Biotechnology, Centre for Plant Molecular Biology and Biotechnology, Tamil Nadu Agricultural University, Coimbatore, Tamil Nadu, India

T. Vinutha Division of Biochemistry, ICAR-Indian Agricultural Research Institute, New Delhi, India

Abbreviations

AACC	American Association of Cereal Chemists
AAS	Amino acid score
ADME	Absorption, distribution, metabolism, and elimination
AEBP1	Adipocyte enhancer binding protein 1
AEEP	Aqueous enzymatic extraction process
Akt/PKB	Protein kinase B
ALA	α-linolenic acid
AMPK	AMP-activated protein kinase
ANF	Anti-nutritional factor
ANGPTL4	Angiopoietin-like 4
AoA	Anti-oxidant activity
APOBR	Apolipoprotein b receptor
AQP7	Aquaporin 7
ATF4	Gcn2/activating transcription factor 4
ATP	Adenosine tri-phosphate
BAT	Brown adipose tissue
BBB	Blood-brain barrier
BCAAs	Branched-chain amino acids
BFN	Biodiversity for Food and Nutrition
bHLH	Basic helix–loop–helix
BLs	Bioactive lipids
BPs	Bioactive peptides
BV	Biological value
BZR1	Brassinazole-resistant 1
CAC	Codex Alimentarius Commission
CAGR	Compound annual growth rate
CAM	Calmodulin
CAX	CAtion eXchangers
CBD	Convention on Biological Diversity
CCFA	Codex Committee on Food Additives

CCFH	Codex Committee on Food Hygiene
CCPR	Codex Committee on Pesticide Residues
CCRVDF	Codex Committee on Residues of Veterinary Drugs in Foods
ChoRE	Carbohydrate response element
ChREBP	Carbohydrate-responsive element binding protein
CIPK	Calcineurin B-like-interacting protein kinase
CNS	Central nervous system
CoQ10	Coenzyme Q10
CP	Cold plasma
CPT1A	Carnitine palmitoyltransferase 1a
CRISPR	Clustered regularly interspaced short palindromic repeats
CRP	C-reactive protein
CVD	Cardiovascular diseases
CYP1A1	Cytochrome p450 superfamily
CYPs	Cytochrome P450-dependent mixed-function oxidases
d	Day
DAG	Diacyl glycerol
DALYs	Disability-adjusted life years
DHA	Docosahexaenoic acid
DHPS	Dihydrodipicolinate synthase
DM	Diabetes mellitus
DMTs	Dinucleotide methylase transferases
DPP	Dipeptidyl peptidase
DREB	Dehydration responsive element binding
DW	Dry weight
EAA	Essential amino acids
EAHB	East African highland banana
EGCG	Epigallocatechin-3-gallate
eIF2	Eukaryotic initiation factor 2
EMMPRIN	Extracellular matrix metalloproteinase inducer
EPA	Eicosapentaenoic acid
eQTL	Expression quantitative trait loci
ERK	Extracellular signal-regulated kinases
EVOO	Extra virgin olive oil
FAO	Food and Agriculture Organization
FASN	Fatty acid synthase
FBDs	Food-borne diseases
FCS	Food control system
FDA	Food and Drug Administration
FER	Ferritin
FGF21	Fibroblast growth factor 21
FODMAP	Fermentable oligo-saccharides, disaccharides, monosaccharides and polyols

FOS	Fructo-oligosaccharides
FSSAI	Food Safety and Standards Authority of India
FW	Fresh weight
FXR	Farnesoid x receptor
GABA	Gamma-aminobutyric acid
GALP	Galanin-like peptide
GAP	Good Agricultural Practice
GHP	Good Hygiene Practice
GI	Glycaemic index
GIP	Glucose-dependent insulinotropic polypeptide
GIT	Gastrointestinal tract
GK	Glucokinase
GLP1	Glucagon-like peptide-1
GLUT	Glucose transporters
GM	Genetically modified
GMOs	Genetically modified organisms
GMP	Good Manufacturing Practice
GST	Glutathione S transferase
GWAS	Genome-wide association studies
HAART	Highly active antiretroviral therapy
HACCP	Hazard analysis and critical control points
hALR	Human aldose reductase
HCA	Hydroxy citric acid
HCl	Hydrochloric acid
HCRT	Hypocretin neuropeptide precursor
HDACs	Histone deacetylases
HDL	High-density lipoprotein
HHP	High hydrostatic pressure
HL	High light
HMA	Heavy metal-associated transporters
HNF-4	Hepatocyte nuclear factor 4
HPS	High-pressure sodium
HTST	High-temperature short-time
I3C	Indole-3-carbinol
IBD	Inflammatory bowel disease
IBS	Irritable bowel syndrome
ICN2	Second International Conference on Nutrition
INFOODS	International Network of Food Data Systems
IM	QTL interval mapping
IPCC	International Plant Protection Convention
IPP	Isopentenyl diphosphate
IPPC	International Plant Protection Convention
IRT	Iron-regulated transporters

ISAAA	International Service for the Acquisition of Agri-biotech Applications
IVPD	*In vitro* protein digestibility
JECFA	Joint FAO/WHO Expert Committee on Food Additives
JEMNU	Joint FAO/WHO Expert Meeting on Nutrition
JEMRA	Joint FAO/WHO Expert Meeting on Microbiological Risk Assessment
JMPR	Joint Meeting on Pesticide Residues
KEAP-1	Kelch-like ECH-associated protein-1
kGy	kiloGrays
LCT	Low-affinity cation transporters
LDL	Low-density lipoprotein
LED	Light emitting diode
LEP	Leptin
LXR	Liver x receptor
MAOIs	Monoamine oxidase inhibitors
MARS	Marker-assisted recurrent selection
MAS	Marker-assisted selection
MCH	Melanin concentrating hormone
MCTs	Medium chain triglycerides
miRNA	microRNA
ML	Maximum level
MMP	Matrix metallopeptidase
mTORC1	Mammalian target of rapamycin complex 1
MTPs	Metal tolerance proteins
MUFA	Monounsaturated fatty acids
NAD	Nicotinamide adenine dinucleotide
NAS	Nicotianamine synthase
NB	Nitrogen balance
NBC	Niacin bound chromium iii
NCDs	Non-communicable diseases
ncRNAs	Non-coding ribonucleic acids
NFCS	National Food Control System
NGS	Next generation sequencing
NLC	Nano-structured lipid carriers
NPR	Net protein ratio
NPU	Net protein utilization
NRAMP	Natural resistance-associated macrophage protein
Nrf2	Nuclear factor erythroid 2–related factor 2
NTT	Non-thermal treatments
OIE	World Organization for Animal Health
PBMA	Plant-based milk alternatives
PCK1	Phosphoenolpyruvate carboxykinase 1

PDCAAS	Protein Digestibility Corrected Amino Acid Score
PEF	Pulsed electric fields
PER	Protein efficiency ratio
PERK	Protein kinase r-like endoplasmic reticulum kinase
PGC-1 alpha	Peroxisome proliferator-activated receptor-gamma coactivator 1 alpha
PI3K	Phosphatidylinositol-3-kinase
PL	Pulsed light
PLIN	Perilipin
POMC	Proopiomelanocortin
PON1	Paraoxonase
PPARs	Peroxisome proliferator-activated receptors
PPO	Polyphenol oxidase
PPRE	PPAR responsive element
PS	Phytosiderophores
PUFA	Polyunsaturated fatty acids
QTL	Quantitative trait locus
RA	Risk assessment
RBCs	Red blood cells
RC	Risk communication
RCP	Recommended Code of Practice
RDS	Rapidly digestible starch
RM	Risk management
RNAi	RNA interference
RNA-Seq	RNA sequencing
RS	Resistant starch
RT-PCR	Reverse-transcription polymerase chain reaction
RXR	Retinoic acid receptor
SAA	Sulphur containing amino acids
SAGE	Serial Analysis of Gene Expression
SAM	s-adenosyl methionine
SBPase	Sedoheptulose-1,7-bisphosphatase
SCD1	Stearoyl-coenzyme A desaturase 1
SCFAs	Short chain fatty acids
SDG	Sustainable Development Goals
SDS	Slowly digestible starch
SIRT	Sirtuin 1
SLN	Solid lipid nanoparticles
SLSS	Space life support systems
SPS Agreement	Agreement on sanitary and phytosanitary measures
SREBF1	Sterol regulatory element binding transcription factor 1
TAA	Total ascorbic acid
TAC	Total antioxidant capacity
TALENs	Transcription activator-like effector nuclease

TF	Task force
TFAM	Task force on antimicrobial resistance
TGs	Triglycerides
TILLING	Targeting induced local lesions in genomes
TLR	Toll-like receptor
TNF-α	Tumour necrosis factor-alpha
TPC	Two-pore channel
TPD	True protein digestibility
TR	Thyroid hormone receptor
TSG	Tumour suppressor gene
TZDs	Thiazolidinediones
UHPH	Ultra high-pressure homogenization
US	Ultrasound
USD	United States dollars
UV	Ultra-violet
VAD	Vitamin A deficiency
VEGF	Vascular endothelial growth factor
VIT	Vacuolar iron transporter
VLDL	Very low-density lipoprotein
WAT	White adipose tissue
WHO	World Health Organization
WTO	World Trade Organization
YSL	Yellow Stripe Like
ZFN	Zinc-finger nucleases
ZIP	Zn and Fe permease family

Chapter 1
Biodiversity for Nutritive Gains: Values, Benefits, and Threats

Sundaravel Pandian Kalaipandian, Ramesh S. V., Fernanda Caro Beveridge, Zhihua Mu, and Steve Adkins

Abstract Intensive agriculture and reliance on few cultivated crops, to feed the ever-growing population, have led to narrow genetic diversity and constricted nutritional repertoire of plants. Despite having a huge biodiversity of around 50,000 edible plants, only 15 species (majorly rice, maize, and wheat) contribute to almost 90% of food requirement of the population worldwide. It has led to the prevalence of hidden hunger or mineral malnutrition and other diet-related disorders among the masses worldwide. On the other hand, diverse plant species with nutritive bioactive potential lay neglected or, where the nutritional information is known, remain underutilized. This chapter discusses the nutritional importance of plant biodiversity, its benefits and threats posed, conservation and sustainable use of biodiversity for food and nutritional security, and glimpses of breeding strategies required or being followed for enhancing the nutritional content of plants.

Keywords Biodiversity · Neglected and underutilized crops · Nutritional benefits · Orphan crops · Malnutrition

1.1 Introduction

Despite the mammoth and rapid steps forward in managing world hunger through the green revolution, undertaken with a sole aim of enhancing food production, these intensive crop production systems have now encountered new issues such as those to do with food quality and human health and the impact of such production systems on the environment. According to the FAO (2018), more than 800 million people worldwide remain chronically undernourished in the past 10 years. Problems of

---

S. P. Kalaipandian (✉) · F. C. Beveridge · Z. Mu · S. Adkins
School of Agriculture and Food Sciences, The University of Queensland, Gatton, Australia
e-mail: s.kalaipandian@uq.edu.au

R. S. V.
Physiology, Biochemistry and Post-Harvest Technology Division, ICAR-Central Plantation Crops Research Institute, Kasaragod, Kerala, India

R. S. V., S. Praveen (eds.), *Conceptualizing Plant-Based Nutrition*,
https://doi.org/10.1007/978-981-19-4590-8_1

malnutrition, protein–energy imbalances, and mineral nutrition deficiencies, such as iron, have been estimated to affect around 30% of world population including 151 million children under the age of 5 who have stunted growth (WHO. Available at: http://www.who.int/nutrition/topics/ida/en/). In addition, the current global food production systems have become affected by climate change, environmental degradation, and biodiversity loss (Vermeulen et al. 2012). All these problems have come about due to the pursuit of attaining homogeneity in the global food supply by profoundly relying on narrow range of cereal and pulse crops and neglecting food crop biodiversity (Jarvis et al. 2016). The world's crop diversity has witnessed a narrowing of the range planted over past 5 decades, and hence, the food and dietary composition of the world's foods has become uniform. Even though around 7000 plant species have been identified as a potential source of food, only six species (wheat (*Triticum aestivum* L.), soybean (*Glycine max* L.), maize (*Zea mays* L.), rice (*Oryza sativa* L.), barley (*Hordeum vulgare* L.), and rapeseed (*Brassica napus* L.) occupy more than half of the cultivated land area in the world. Regionally important and diverse food crop species have become abandoned. Following a mega-study conducted over 150 countries, some scientists believe that this constitutes a new and severe threat to food security and human nutrition (Khoury et al. 2014). The over-reliance on the rice–wheat cropping systems in Southern Asia, to meet their food requirements, has caused a resurgence of malnutrition especially for deficiency of micronutrients (Kataki 2014). In some regions in Asia, South America, and Africa, through biofortification, crop varieties of maize, beans, cowpea, other legumes, pearl millet, rice, and wheat have been bred to supply pro-vitamin A, mineral nutrients (Fe and Zn) (Saltzman et al. 2014), as well as cereals in Europe and the American continents are enriched in phenylpropanoids. However, in all cases, this has led to an overall reduction in crop biodiversity. Hence, there is an urgent need for re-establishing food diversity by restoring old and incorporating new diverse crop species into our food basket. The plethora of underutilized crops, often only grown in their centers of origin, are not finding a place in other regions due to agronomic, cultural, and/or economic reasons (Padulosi et al. 2002).

1.2 Nutritional Value of Biodiversity

Currently, cereal and cereal-based foods (comprising both true and pseudo-cereals), besides contributing to roughly two-thirds of the world's food calories, serve as an epitome of human culture through the annals of time. In the last four millennia, major grain cereals have been domesticated and are now being genetically modified to improve human nutrition (Das 2016; Doebley et al. 2006). Nevertheless, until recently many underutilized crops (alternatively called orphan or neglected crops) have received little genetic modification or improvement (Dansi et al. 2012). Changing human nutritional and health priorities have unearthed many new cereal species that can produce gluten-free foods. Some of these gluten-free, underexplored cereal species of nutritional importance include quinoa (*Chenopodium quinoa* Willd.), teff (*Eragrostis tef* (Zucc.) Trotter), and amaranth (*Amaranthus* spp.) (Massawe et al.

2016; Jarvis et al. 2017). Similarly, to meet dietary protein requirements, a diverse range of new tropical legume crops, such as winged bean (*Psophocarpus tetragonolobus* (L.) DC.), lentil (*Lens culinaris* Medik.), lima bean (*Phaseolus lunatus* L.), lablab (*Lablab purpureus* L.), and Bambara groundnut (*Vigna subterranean* [L.] Verdc.), are now being considered as promising new dietary protein sources (Messina 1999; Henchion et al. 2017). These underutilized legumes are not only agronomically hardy but are endowed with flavorsome nutritional profiles especially with a high content of essential amino acids (EAA), of a type that is deficient in cereal-based diets (USDA Food Composition Database; Yao et al. 2015) (Table 1.1). The major concern with new crops such as winged bean is the presence of antinutritional factors, such as relatively high tannin content in the seed coat (Singh et al. 2017). The diverse species of plants with nutritional potential are presented in Fig. 1.1. (Hunter et al. 2019).

Furthermore, the nutritional composition among varieties of the same species may differ drastically. For instance, the orange-fleshed sweet potato (*Ipomoea batatas* L.) varieties are known to have more than 200 times the content of β-carotene than found in the white-fleshed varieties. Thus, the orange-fleshed variety has a greater scope for the alleviation of vitamin A deficiency in sub-Saharan Africa where consumption of the white-fleshed sweet potato variety is prevalent (Low et al. 2013). The role of the native, yellow-fleshed banana (*Musa* spp.) cultivar *karat* in alleviating the pro-vitamin A deficiency in Federated States of Micronesia of Pacific region is now well documented (Engelberger et al. 2013). In the same way, the nutritional supremacy of the green leaf vegetable aibika (*Abelmoschus manihot* L.) from Papua New Guinea is now well demonstrated (Rubiang-Yalambing et al. 2014). Similarly, the African leafy vegetables (e.g., spider plant (*Gynandropsis gynandra* L. (Briq.)), roselle (*Hibiscus sabdariffa* L.) and hair lettuce, moringa (*Moringa oleifera* Lam.), African nightshade (*Solanum scabrum* Mill.), and jute mallow (*Corchorus olitorius* L.) are a rich source of the micronutrient iron and are abound with other nutraceutical compounds such as allyl sulfides, flavonoids, isothiocyanates, lycopene, and various phenolic acids (Ojiewo et al. 2013). These nutritional interventions attain more significance when compared to the single nutrient-focused biofortification and cost-intensive approaches to alleviate nutritional imbalances of masses around the world. The nutritional benefits from several other underutilized crop species [viz. African cabbage *Cleome gynandra* L.; Schönfeldt and Pretorius 2011; rice bean (*Vigna umbellate* [Thunb.] Ohwiand Ohashi; Katoch 2012), various roots and tubers (Olango et al. 2013) are now beginning to be recognized (Chapman et al. 2015).

1.3 Benefits of Biodiversity

The use of biologically diverse crop species is invaluable for the agroecosystem functions and services (FAO 2020). Biodiversity at the ecosystem and the species level and then at genetic diversity within species level contributes to modern

Table 1.1 Diverse plant species, which are underutilized or neglected nevertheless possess immense nutritional benefits, are presented herein

S. No.	Plant species	Center of origin or center of diversity or geographic region of importance	Nutritional feature(s)	References
1	Proso millet (*Panicum miliaceum* L.)	Native to North China	Abundant in EAA (methionine, isoleucine, leucine), higher EAA index (51%) than wheat, and high protein content (12.5%)	Habiyaremye et al. (2017)
2	Teff [*Eragrostis tef* (Zucc.) Trotter]	Ethiopia	Gluten-free, high EAA content, rich in minerals, low glycemic index (GI), and abundant crude fiber	Ayele et al. (1996)
3	Quinoa (*Chenopodium quinoa* Krock)	Peru and Bolivia	Protein (14.12%); Phytoecdysteroid content 138–570 μg/g; Good-quality phytosterol profile [β-sitosterol 63.7 mg 100 g^{-1}), campesterol (15.6 mg 100 g^{-1}), and stigmasterol (3.2 mg 100 g^{-1})]	Navruz-Varli and Sanlier (2016)
4	*Fagopyrum* spp. (*F. Esculentum* Moench, *F. tataricum* (L.) Gaertn. *and F. Cymosum* (Trevir.) Meisn)	Southwestern China	Nutritional superiority over rice, wheat, maize in terms of amino acids profile and mineral nutrients and bioactive flavonoids of pharmaceutical importance	Joshi et al. (2019)
5	Minor millets, finger millet (*Eleusine coracana* (L.), kodo millet (*Paspalum scrobiculatum* L.), foxtail millet (*Setaria italica* (L)), little millet (*Panicum sumatrense*), proso millet (*Panicum miliaceum* L.) and barnyard millet (*Echinochloa crusgalli* (L.) Beauv and *E. colona* (L.)Link)	India	Rich in co-enzymes, sulfur-containing amino acids, non-starchy polysaccharides, and dietary fiber	Bergamini et al. (2013)
6	Winged bean (*Psophocarpus tetragonolobus* L. (DC.)	Papua New Guinea (center of genetic diversity)	Seed protein content equivalent to soybean, balanced amino acids including lysine (generally deficient in cereals), oil derived from seed is high in unsaturated fatty acids and vitamin E and rich in thiamin, riboflavin, and niacin	National Research Council (1975)

7	Bambara groundnut (*Vigna subterranea* (L.) Verdc.)	Africa	Leaves are rich in K and N, inexpensive source of protein and has potential to reduce oxidative stress	
8	Amaranth (*Amaranthus* spp.)	Americas and Africa, Asia, and Europe	Protein (14%), 8% of dietary fiber, high essential amino acids	Pedersen et al. (1987)
9	Leafy vegetables spider plant (*Gynandropsis gynandra* L. (Briq.)), moringa (*Moringa oleifera* lam.), African nightshade (*Solanum scabrum* mill.) and jute mallow (*Corchorus olitorius* L.)	Africa	Good source of iron, precursor to vitamin A, and valuable metabolites including allylic sulfides, flavonoids, isothiocyanates, lycopene, and phenolic acids	Ojiewo et al. (2013)
10	Edible aroids include *Colocasia esculenta* (L.) (taro), *Xanthosoma sagittifolium* (L.) (cocoyam), *Cyrtosperma merkusii* (giant swamp taro) and *Alocasia macrorrhiza* (L.) (giant taro)	Humid tropics	Rich in energy, minerals and vitamins and β-Carotene concentrations of giant swamp taro vary from 50 to 4486 μg/100 g	Englberger et al. (2003)
11	*Moringa oleifera* Lam	India	Multipurpose tree used as food, feed, and dietary supplement and health effects for treating type-2 diabetes	Grosshagauer et al. (2021)
12	*Solanum aethiopicum* L.	Africa	Rich alkaloids, flavonoids, phytosterols, saponins, and vitamin C. Dietary supplements of *S. aethiopicum* and *S. macrocarpon* could help in fighting obesity	Han et al. (2021)
13	Orange-fleshed sweet potato [*Ipomoea batatas* (L.) Lam.]	Africa	A 100 g of boiled sweet potato provides daily recommended intake of vitamin A in children	Low et al. (2013)
14	Karat or yellow-fleshed banana cultivars, giant swamp taro [*Cyrtosperma merkusii* (Hassk.) Schott], breadfruit [*Artocarpus altilis* (Parkinson) Fosberg] and pandanus	Federated States of Micronesia	Rich in β-carotene, dietary fiber	Engelberger et al. (2013)
14	Jussara (*Euterpe edulis* Mart.)	Brazil fruits	High antioxidant and high anti-inflammatory properties	Schulz et al. (2015, 2017)

(continued)

Table 1.1 (continued)

S. No.	Plant species	Center of origin or center of diversity or geographic region of importance	Nutritional feature(s)	References
15	*Campomanesia courbaril, Eugenia uniflora* L., *Eugenia dysenterica* DC., *Plinia cauliflora* (Mart.) Kausel, *Psidium cattleianum* Sabine, *Hymenaea courbaril* L., *Hancornia speciosa* Gomes, *Caryocar brasiliense* Cambess., *Genipa Americana* L.	Brazil fruit diversity	Diverse compounds with antioxidant potential, viz. 51 phenolics, 23 carotenoids, 8 iridoids, and a couple of anthocyanins	Biazotto et al. (2019), Junior et al. (2019)
16	*Adansonia digitata* L.	Africa	Vitamin C126–509 mg/100 g	Dulloo et al. (2014)
17	*Grewia tenax* (Forssk.) Fiori	Africa	Iron (7.4–20.8 mg/100 g); calcium (610 mg/100 g)	Dulloo et al. (2014)
18	*Sclerocarya birrea* (A. Rich.) Hochst	Africa	Vitamin C (85–319 mg/100 g)	Dulloo et al. (2014)
19	*Tamarindus indica* L.	Africa	Iron (3.1 mg/100 g)	Dulloo et al. (2014)
20	*Ziziphus mauritiana* Lam	Africa	Iron (0.8 mg/100 g)	Dulloo et al. (2014)

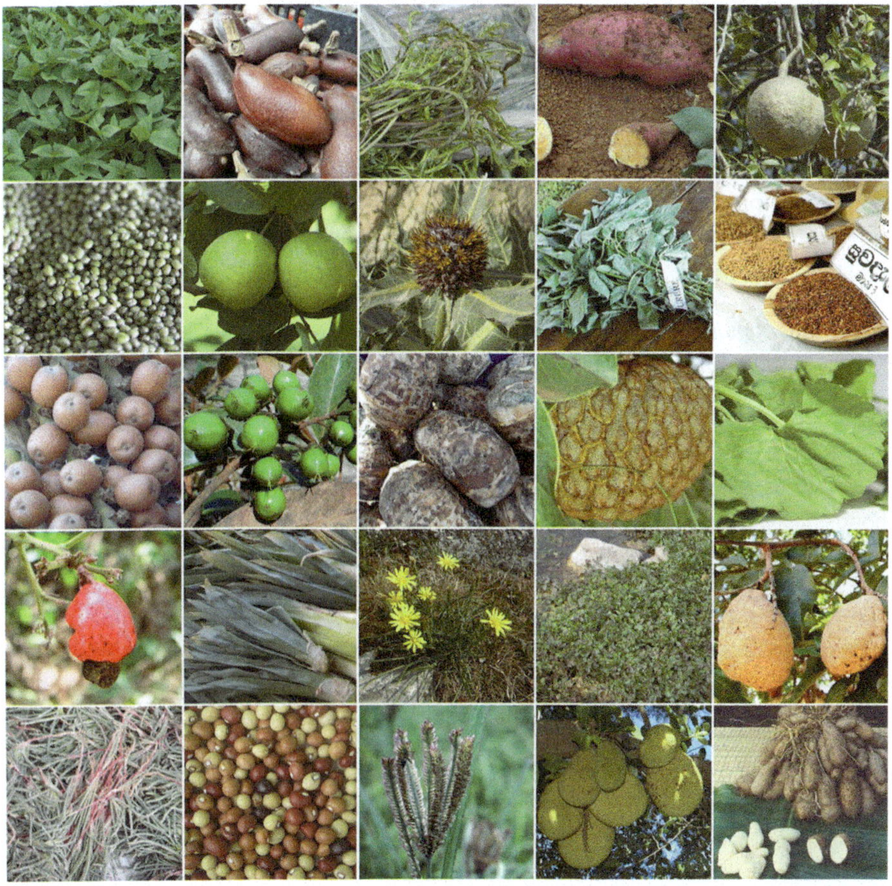

Fig. 1.1 Diverse species of food crops used under Biodiversity for Food and Nutrition (BFN) Project are presented. Source (Hunter et al. 2019) https://doi.org/10.1007/s00425-019-03169-4

agriculture in numerous ways and supports the livelihoods of many millions of farmers (Sunderland 2011). Most of the currently cultivated crops are domesticated from their wild relatives, and it is clear that crop biodiversity contributes to the food security for a growing world population (Sunderland 2011). Therefore, biodiversity conservation is a most important facet to ensure long-term food security. It has been estimated that around 80% of the population in developing countries depends upon plant biodiversity present in their local ecosystems for their primary health care (Herndon and Butler 2010), suggesting the importance of biodiversity to human health. Forests often supply natural foods such as herbs, vegetables, and fruits. These kinds of foods are rich in not only macronutrients but also act as an excellent source of micronutrients (Sunderland et al. 2013). To date, more than 7000 natural plant species have been domesticated for food, 13 of these that have become major crops have also been improved with various traits by using genes obtained from about

60 wild relatives, and more than 70,000 plant species are being used as traditional or modern medicines. As most of the human population still relies on these sources for nutrition and medicines, the further loss in biodiversity would cause serious and deleterious impacts on the human population. Nutritional diversity within species or their varieties offers a diverse range of options for food combinations that can provide a balanced human diet. van Niekerk et al. (2016) analyzed the nutritional profile of potato (*Solanum* spp.) varieties that are cultivated in sub-Saharan Africa. They found that there were intraspecific and varietal differences in potato diversity, and this had a significant effect on the macronutrient and micronutrient contents available to the consumers and played a major role in local community health.

The various organisms present in agricultural soil are essential for the maintenance of soil ecosystem health and functioning. These soil microorganisms play an essential role in symbiotic nitrogen fixation and the mobilization of phosphorus for the uptake by plant roots (El Mujtar et al. 2019). Microbial biodiversity contributes considerably to agricultural production, food security, and farmers livelihoods, especially in the context of climate change (Pilling et al. 2020). Other important biodiverse populations, such as those of insects and birds, affect the pollination of plants, and several studies have shown that a reduction in the size and biodiversity has a detrimental effect on plant populations. For example, insect-mediated pollination, found to be essential for maintaining the sustainable production in the agroecosystems to ensure the food security, can affect pollination (Koul et al. 2018).

The presence of a wide range of genetic diversity within a species or population will aid the adaptation of those species or populations to a changing climate, or deal with any adverse environmental stresses, such as those caused by prolonged heat, drought, or cold climates, and support the movement to different elevations, to habitats with different soils, or deal with more dramatic seasonal change (Meisner et al. 2018). The presence of diverse range of organisms in biological communities is indispensable for the sustainable production of food, and the production of diverse foods within these ecosystems will not only efficiently use the resources available but also increase the recycling of materials naturally and increase the complementarities and synergies of the ecosystem (Montoyo et al. 2020; Pilling et al. 2020). Biodiversity can be considered a form of security; if any abiotic or biotic event threatens crop production, then high biodiversity can help reduce that deleterious impact upon production loss. Certain natural foods are often found to complement dietary requirements when such damage occurs to the cultivated crops. Hence, it is important to conserve both the domesticated and wild relatives to maintain population diversity which can help to manage challenges, such as those brought about by climate change. In summary, food and agricultural production largely depends on the availability of a wide range of biodiversity, firstly at the genetic level, then at the species level, and finally at the ecosystem level. Biodiversity contributes invaluable benefits toward the health of the people around the world.

1.4 Threats to Biodiversity

Although biodiversity provides numerous benefits to humankind, serious threats to biodiversity are inevitable due to the inappropriate usage of biological resources. Changes in land and water use, increased pollution, and greenhouse gas emissions all provide a significant threat to plant biodiversity. Recent evidence has indicated a declining trend in plant community biodiversity. This biodiversity loss has been impacting various essential services to food and agriculture production, including those from forest and wetland ecosystems (Pilling et al. 2020). The conversion of forested land area into agricultural fields is one of the most serious threats to biodiversity. When a large, forested area is converted into intensive agriculture, especially to monocropping, it will significantly reduce biodiversity which in turn initiates a huge reduction in the supply of ecosystem goods and services in the longer term (Sunderland et al. 2013). Intensive monocropping of rice in Asia, during the last 40 years, has dramatically increased the production and farmer income through the use of elite varieties, hybrids, agrochemicals, and new irrigation technologies. However, it has seriously negatively affected the biodiversity of the land and soil, mainly because of the wide use of agrochemicals, the loss of well-adapted local rice varieties, and the homogenization of the landscape (Fischer et al. 2017). In addition, people now consume a large number of rice-based foods and this lacks dietary diversity which in turn lacks balanced nutrition in their diets (Fischer et al. 2017). Likewise, focusing on only a small number of crop species for food around the world is likely to affect the biodiversity of the global food system (Khoury et al. 2014). Several studies have shown intensive agriculture to pose a major threat to biodiversity, and it is not only affecting the species diversity in cropping area but also in the adjacent habitats (Zabel et al. 2019).

Climate change is another major threat to biodiversity. It affects plant populations as well as soil biota, both in a spatial and temporal manner. For example, both plant roots and litter provide input into the soil, which in turn interacts with soil organisms such as decomposers and symbionts. These interactions are often species-specific and are greatly influenced by environmental factors (viz. temperature, moisture, and other factors; Pugnaire et al. 2019). Climate change drought events can directly affect the composition of soil microbes including fungi and bacteria due to their impact on root growth and leaf litter production. Climate change-induced higher temperatures can affect certain physiological processes in plants, and the effects include increased evaporation and transpiration. Plant litter and rhizodeposition provide a huge amount of organic matter to the soil, and the changes in the climate will influence this soil organic matter level. Further, the elevated atmospheric CO_2 concentration, constantly increasing in the environment, affects all flora and fauna, and the interactions among these climate change factors may even cause greater deleterious effects to biodiversity (Pugnaire et al. 2019). Further, reactive nitrogen and gaseous ammonia are other factors that can reduce biodiversity by directly damaging the vegetation (Dise et al. 2011). Many ecosystems evolved in nitrogen-limiting environments, when nitrogen is applied excessively; it causes the long-term nitrogen deposition in the ecosystem by eutrophication and acidification. Several studies have reported that long-term nitrogen deposition in the ecosystem reduced the plant biodiversity. For example, a decline of biodiversity in Europe is directly correlated with nitrogen deposition, and the reports warn that several plant species will be extinct in Europe by 2050 if the nitrogen deposition will continue to increase (Dise et al. 2011).

In addition to the above-listed factors, human travel and human trade are increasing around the world and that increase the introduction of invasive organisms, such as insect pests, pathogens, and weeds, between countries which then pose threats to local population biodiversity (Freer-Smith and Webber 2017). To stop this invasive threat to new environments, it is important to better understand the pathways of trade, rather than focusing on individual pest agents. Overall, it is clear that the community biodiversity around the world is declining and immediate action needs to take place to reduce this threat.

1.5 Conservation and Sustainable Use of Biodiversity for Food and Nutrition Security

The global human population is expected to reach nine billion by the year 2050, and food production will need to be increased, but this will need to be done with further limited resources of cultivable land and water. Intensive agriculture via deforestation may be a short-term solution; however, such practices will cause more deleterious effects on the food production chain and will affect livelihoods in the longer term. Crop improvement programs will need diverse genetic resources; hence, the conservation of a wide range of genetic diversity within a species is a very important consideration (Khoury et al. 2014). Biodiversity conservation is one of the paramount factors to achieving food security for the world's growing population. It has always been a trade-off between food production and biodiversity conservation. Promoting agrobiodiversity could be an approach to securing food production and to provide a balanced nutritive diet for the rural population across developing nations (Ruiz et al. 2014). Diversification of food is the most likely way to achieve food and nutrition security rather than depending solely on a few, dominant major agricultural crops. Maintenance of diversity in all three levels including at the genetic, the species, and the ecosystem level will create more resilient crops and can increase their adaptation to climate change (Scherer et al. 2020). For example, the availability of a diverse range of crops or varieties, which possess various levels of tolerance to environmental stresses, could help avoid crop failure in certain seasons (FAO 2015). Changes in crop management practices, such as varietal selection or irrigation technologies to be used, could increase the adaptation of farming systems to climate change (FAO 2015). Maintenance of a risk register to identify plant health threats and the development of strict quarantine/biosecurity policies could help avoid the spread of new biotic threats (Freer-Smith and Webber 2017).

It has been estimated that the price of many agricultural commodities will dramatically increase in the future (Zabel et al. 2019). Hence, intensive agricultural production is expected to generate greater income and provide economic growth. It will be extremely difficult to maintain biodiversity and sustainability while increasing production. In addition, new policies must focus on both agricultural production and biodiversity conservation, and the local authority and international organizations will be required to insist on the implementation of sustainable agricultural production strategies (Beltrame et al. 2019; Zabel et al. 2019).

As food security and conservation of biodiversity are interrelated challenges, it is important to consider both to achieve reasonable outcomes. Fischer et al. (2017) proposed a socioecological model to integrate both food security and biodiversity conservation to achieve the best outcome. Smallholders traditionally produce diverse crops within small land areas for the local consumption and sometimes to provide to international markets. Such smallholder-based agroecological systems use some inputs which have also been found to be resilient to climate change and market fluctuations. The only risk is the uncertainty of supply to larger population (Fischer et al. 2017). By employing an integrative approach to agricultural production, it may be possible to meet production demands while maintaining the ecosystem like implementing the best management practices locally or coordinating the sustainable goals internationally which will complement biodiversity conservation and agricultural production (Zabel et al. 2019). Also, it is important to identify the possible future conflicts that may arise between biodiversity and agriculture while implementing sustainability policies and conservation projects (Zabel et al. 2019).

Awareness among rural population must be created on the deforestation for conversion of forest to agricultural land which may produce short-term income only, and it will affect the ecosystems and livelihoods in the long term (Sunderland et al. 2013). The loss of invaluable goods and services from the forest will affect the food security in the world (Arnold et al. 2011). Identification of conflicts and synergies between food security and conservation of biodiversity is imperative. Including local biodiversity aspects in the global policies of food and nutrition security-related schemes and promoting healthy, diversified, and sustainable diets from biodiversity will increase the awareness among people to conserve the biodiversity.

1.6 Breeding Strategies for Enhancing Nutritionally Superior Plants

As stated above, modern breeding strategies have focused on parameters such as economic yield, host plant resistance, and reduction of drudgery in cultivation rather than nutritional composition of the crops or identification or exploitation of functional biomolecules with potential impact on human nutrition. In addition, the greatest bottleneck in exploring the plant systems for functional metabolites is our inadequate understanding of plant metabolism and numerous biochemical pathways that are contributing to it and the influence of environmental factors in these processes. Moreover, the perception that a crop bred, through modern breeding, for improved nutritional quality may lead to a significant yield penalty is not true always. Instances of improved micronutrients contents (e.g., iron, zinc, and vitamin A) in cereal crops have not witnessed any yield decline (Dwivedi et al. 2012). The impending threat of climate change and its influence on agriculture in diverse geographic regions such as Africa, Mesoamerica, the Andes, and South and Central Asia poses a greater responsibility than ever for plant breeding approaches. In this context, the concept of "evolutionary breeding" is suggested to improve the genetic diversity in farmers' field not only to enhance the crops' resilience toward climate change but also to harvest the potential nutritional gains. As the strategy involves cultivating diverse genotypes of a crop in a field, the final harvested produce every year differs in terms of genetic architecture and nutritional content owing to increased natural pollination (Ceccarelli 2016). The strategy has been followed for crops like rice, durum and bread wheat, maize, barley, common bean, *Cucurbita pepo,* and tomato among others (Ceccarelli 2016). Besides the yield stability and robustness, the quality and aroma profile of the crops have witnessed an improvement suggesting the potential of this technique for nutritional security of masses wherever possible (Rahmanian et al. 2014). Breeding for enrichment of micronutrients is a sustainable, economical, and successful approach. Successful instances are maize enriched with pro-vitamin A-, Fe-, and Zn-rich legume seeds, bean, lentil and cowpea and cereals pearl millet, rice, and wheat. Further, prospecting for crop genotypes with high bioavailability for micronutrients is another complementary strategy to defeat the prevalence of malnutrition (Thomas 2007). The application of modern molecular breeding tools including genetic manipulation has been a proven tactic to improve the nutritional status of crops including enhancement of grain protein and developing quality protein maize (QPM) (Prasanna et al. 2001; Kumar et al. 2011; Tabbita et al. 2013; Vishwakarma et al. 2014). Adoption of QPM over common maize has significantly improved the nutritional status of human health especially in infants in terms of improved weight and height growth rate and enhanced feed efficiency (Gupta et al. 2013; Tessema et al. 2016). Beneficial effects of consumption of plant phenolics through diet have led to the development of cultivars in diverse crops such as rice, maize, barley, sorghum, soybean, and wheat that are rich in phenylpropanoids for cultivation in America and Europe (Dwivedi et al. 2016). Exploration of nutritive potential of nontraditional food crops such as plantation crops (coconut etc.) for greater nutraceutical application is a feasible strategy (Ramesh et al. 2021; Hebbar et al. 2022). Crop germplasm characterization approaches need to emphasize the development of database for nutritional composition of the genotypes besides the morphological and genetic marker traits. In this regard, the FAO International Network of Food Data Systems (FAO/INFOODS) (https://www.fao.org/infoods/infoods/en/), a food composition database for biodiversity, which aims to achieve and advocate an international harmonization and support for food composition activities is worth mentioning (Charrondière et al. 2013).

Inclusion of forest tree species in breeding strategies or agroforestry system is a feasible plan to improve the dietary richness of the marginalized section. Studies have proven the linkage between tree cover and dietary diversity of children in 21 African Countries (Black et al. 2013; Johnson et al. 2013; Ickowitz et al. 2014; Ickowitz et al. 2016). Also, the traditional and culturally important foods around the world in general are either wild or underutilized. Hence, it is mandatory to conserve and preserve these "cultural keystone species" for their cultivation in home gardens, etc. Biochemical characterization of traditional landraces has helped in unraveling their potential in improving the nutritional quality of some of the widely cultivated varieties and to counter the issues of climate change-induced abiotic stresses (Massaretto et al. 2018).

1.7 Concluding Remarks

Research evidence has unequivocally proved the correlation between plant biodiversity and enhanced human nutrition. Biodiversity has supplied humans with food, feed, drinks, and minerals and played a greater role in the reduction of malnutrition. Further, the direct correlation between farm-level species diversity and improvement in dietary quality warrants micro-level approaches to enhance the nutritional security of masses. This in situ preservation of agrodiversity would go long way in ensuring food and nutritional security and in providing benefits for ecosystem processes and the environment. In the context of climate-change induced food security issues, and the unexplored pool of resistance conferring genes of underutilized cereals and their resilience towards biotic and abiotic stresses, exploitation of these new crop models for the development of "future-ready" and nutritionally superior plants is imperative. Considering the importance of protein–energy malnutrition promoting the cultivation of underutilized legumes would help in enhancing the consumption of plant-based protein diets and assist in achieving Sustainable Development Goals. In the research front, efforts should be prioritized to breed for palatable and high-yielding cultivars of neglected and underutilized species (as in the case of winged bean and others). Also, an institutional mechanism to share the genotypes among the research organizations across the world is mandatory to accelerate the breeding efforts and to harvest the nutritional benefits for diverse populations.

References

Arnold JEM, Powell B, Shanley P, Sunderland TCH (2011) Forests, biodiversity and food security. Int For Rev 13(3):online

Ayele M, Doleže J, Van Duren M, Brunner H, Zapata-Arias FJ (1996) Flow cytometric analysis of nuclear genome of the Ethiopian cereal Tef [*Eragrostis tef* (Zucc.) Trotter]. Genetica 98(2): 211–215

Beltrame D, Gee E, Güner BO, Laurıdsen N, Samarasınghe WW, Wasıke V, Hunter D, Borellı T (2019) Mainstreaming biodiversity for food and nutrition into policies and practices: methodologies and lessons learned from four countries. Anadolu Ege Tarımsal Araştırma Enstitüsü Dergisi 29(1):25–38

Bergamini N, Padulosi S, Ravi SB, Yenagi N (2013) Minor millets in India: a neglected crop goes mainstream. Routledge, London, pp 313–325

Biazotto KR, de Souza Mesquita LM, Neves BV, Braga AR, Tangerina MM, Vilegas W, Mercadante AZ, De Rosso VV (2019) Brazilian biodiversity fruits: discovering bioactive compounds from underexplored sources. J Agric Food Chem 67(7):1860–1876

Black RE, Victora CG, Walker SP, Bhutta ZA, Christian P, De Onis M, Ezzati M, Grantham-McGregor S, Katz J, Martorell R, Uauy R (2013) Maternal and child undernutrition and overweight in low-income and middle-income countries. Lancet 382(9890):427–451

Ceccarelli S (2016) Increasing plant breeding efficiency through evolutionary-participatory programs. In: Pilu R, Gavazzi G (eds) More food: road to survival. Bentham Science Publishers, pp 17–40

Chapman MA (2015) Transcriptome sequencing and marker development for four underutilized legumes. Appl Plant Sci 3(2):1400111. https://doi.org/10.3732/apps.1400111

Charrondière UR, Stadlmayr B, Rittenschober D, Mouille B, Nilsson E, Medhammar E, Olango T, Eisenwagen S, Persijn D, Ebanks K, Nowak V (2013) FAO/INFOODS food composition database for biodiversity. Food Chem 140(3):408–412

Dansi A, Vodouhè R, Azokpota P, Yedomonhan H, Assogba P, Adjatin A, Loko YL, Dossou-Aminon I, Akpagana KJ (2012) Diversity of the neglected and underutilized crop species of importance in Benin. ScientificWorldJournal 2012:932947. https://doi.org/10.1100/2012/932947

Das S (2016) Amaranthus: a promising crop of future. Springer Nature, Singapore, p IX, 208. https://doi.org/10.1007/978-981-10-1469-7

Dise NB, Ashmore MR, Belyazid S et al (2011) Nitrogen as a threat to European terrestrial biodiversity. In: The European nitrogen assessment: sources, effects and policy perspectives. Cambridge University Press, Cambridge

Doebley JF, Gaut BS, Smith BD (2006) The molecular genetics of crop domestication. Cell 127(7):1309–1321

Dulloo ME, Hunter D, Leaman D (2014) Plant diversity in addressing food, nutrition and medicinal needs. In: Gurib-Fakim A (ed) Novel plant bioresources: applications in food, medicine and cosmetics. Wiley-Blackwell, Chichester. https://doi.org/10.1002/9781118460566.ch1

Dwivedi SL, Sahrawat KL, Rai KN, Blair MW, Andersson MS, Pfeiffer W (2012) Nutritionally enhanced staple food crops. Plant Breed Rev 36:169–291

Dwivedi SL, Upadhyaya HD, Chung IM, De Vita P, Garcia-Lara S, Guajardo-Flores D, Gutierrez-Uribe JA, Serna-Saldivar SO, Rajakumar G, Sahrawat KL, Kumar J (2016) Exploiting phenylpropanoid derivatives to enhance the nutraceutical values of cereals and legumes. Front Plant Sci 7:763. https://doi.org/10.3389/fpls.2016.00763

Engelberger L, Johnson E, Fanzo J, Hunter D, Borelli T (2013) Traditional foods of the Pacific: go local, a case study in Pohnpei, Federated States of Micronesia. In: Fanzo J, Hunter D, Borelli T, Mattei F (eds) Diversifying food and diets: using agricultural biodiversity to improve nutrition and health. Earthscan, London

Englberger L, Aalbersberg W, Ravi P, Bonnin E, Marks GC, Fitzgerald MH, Elymore J (2003) Further analysis on Micronesia banana, taro, breadfruit and other foods for provitamin A carotenoids and minerals. J Food Compos Anal 16:216–236

FAO (2015) Regional overview of food insecurity: African food insecurity prospects brighter than ever. FAO, Accra

FAO (2018) FAO, IFAD, UNICEF, WFP and WHO. 2018. The state of food security and nutrition in the world 2018. Building climate resilience for food security and nutrition. FAO, Rome

FAO (2020) How the world's food security depends on biodiversity. http://www.fao.org/3/cb0416en/CB0416EN.pdf

Fischer J, Abson DJ, Bergsten A, FrenchCollier N, Dorresteijn I et al (2017) Reframing the food-biodiversity challenge. Trends Ecol Evol 32(5):335–345

Freer-Smith PH, Webber JF (2017) Tree pests and diseases: the threat to biodiversity and the delivery of ecosystem services. Biodivers Conserv 26:3167–3181

Grosshagauer S, Pirkwieser P, Kraemer K, Somoza V (2021) The future of Moringa foods: a food chemistry perspective. Front Nutr 8:751076. https://doi.org/10.3389/fnut.2021.751076

Gupta HS, Raman B, Agrawal PK, Mahajan V, Hossain F, Thirunavukkarasu N (2013) Accelerated development of quality protein maize hybrid through marker-assisted introgression of opaque-2 allele. Plant Breed 132:77–82

Habiyaremye C, Matanguihan JB, D'Alpoim Guedes J, Ganjyal GM, Whiteman MR, Kidwell KK, Murphy KM (2017) Proso millet (*Panicum miliaceum* L.) and its potential for cultivation in the Pacific Northwest, US: a review. Front Plant Sci 7:1961. https://doi.org/10.3389/fpls.2016.01961

Han M, Opoku KN, Bissah NA, Su T (2021) *Solanum aethiopicum*: the nutrient-rich vegetable crop with great economic, genetic biodiversity and pharmaceutical potential. Horticulturae 7(6):126. https://doi.org/10.3390/horticulturae7060126

Hebbar KB, Ramesh SV, Ghosh DK, Beegum PP, Pandiselvam R, Manikantan MR, Mathew AC (2022) Coconut sugar- a potential storehouse of nutritive metabolites, novel bio-products and prospects. Sugar Tech 24:841–856. https://doi.org/10.1007/s12355-021-01101-3

Henchion M, Hayes M, Mullen AM, Fenelon M, Tiwari B (2017) Future protein supply and demand: strategies and factors influencing a sustainable equilibrium. Foods 6(7):53. https://doi.org/10.3390/foods6070053

Herndon CN, Butler RA (2010) Significance of biodiversity to human health. Biotropica 42:558–560

Hunter D, Borelli T, Beltrame DM, Oliveira CN, Coradin L, Wasike VW, Wasilwa L, Mwai J, Manjella A, Samarasinghe GW, Madhujith T (2019) The potential of neglected and underutilized species for improving diets and nutrition. Planta 250(3):709–729

Ickowitz A, Powell B, Salim MA, Sunderland T (2014) Dietary quality and tree cover in Africa. Glob Environ Chang 24:287–294

Ickowitz A, Rowland D, Powell B, Salim MA, Sunderland T (2016) Forests, trees, and micronutrient-rich food consumption in Indonesia. PLoS One 11(5):e0154139. https://doi.org/10.1371/journal.pone.0154139

Jarvis A, Rieseberg LH, Struik PC (2016) Increasing homogeneity in global food supplies and the implications for food security. Proc Natl Acad Sci U S A 111(11):4001–4006. https://doi.org/10.1073/pnas.1313490111

Jarvis DE, Ho YS, Lightfoot DJ, Schmöckel SM, Li B, Borm TJ, Ohyanagi H, Mineta K, Michell CT, Saber N, Kharbatia NM (2017) The genome of *Chenopodium quinoa*. Nature 542:307–312

Johnson KB, Jacob A, Brown ME (2013) Forest cover associated with improved child health and nutrition: evidence from the Malawi demographic and health survey and satellite data. Glob Health Sci Pract 1(2):237–248. https://doi.org/10.9745/ghsp-d-13-00055

Joshi DC, Chaudhari GV, Sood S, Kant L, Pattanayak A, Zhang K, Fan Y, Janovská D, Meglič V, Zhou M (2019) Revisiting the versatile buckwheat: reinvigorating genetic gains through integrated breeding and genomics approach. Planta 250:783–801. https://doi.org/10.1007/s00425-018-03080-4

Junior AG, de Souza P, dos Reis Livero FA (2019) *Plinia cauliflora* (Mart.) Kausel: a comprehensive ethnopharmacological review of a genuinely Brazilian species. J Ethnopharmacol 245:112169. https://doi.org/10.1016/j.jep.2019.112169

Kataki PK (2014) Shifts in cropping system and its effect on human nutrition: case study from India. J Crop Prod 6:119–144

Katoch R (2012) Nutritional potential of rice bean (*Vigna umbellata*): an underutilized legume. J Food Sci 78(1):C8–C16

Khoury CK, Bjorkman AD, Dempewolf H, Ramirez-Villegas J, Guarino L, Jarvis A, Rieseberg LH, Struik PC (2014) Increasing homogeneity in global food supplies and the implications for food security. Proc Natl Acad Sci U S A 111:4001–4006

Koul M, Thakur P, Bhatnagar AK (2018) Pollination limitation: a threat to biodiversity and food security. J Food Agric Environ 16(2):76–80
Kumar J, Jaiswal V, Kumar A, Kumar N, Mir RR, Kumar S, Dhariwal R, Tyagi S, Khandelwal M, Prabhu KV, Prasad R (2011) Introgression of a major gene for high grain protein content in some Indian bread wheat cultivars. Field Crops Res 123:226–233
La Frano MR, de Moura FF, Boy E, Lönnerdal B, Burri BJ (2014) Bioavailability of iron, zinc, and provitamin A carotenoids in biofortified staple crops. Nutr Rev 72:289–307
Low J, Arimond M, Labarta R, Andrade M, Namanda S (2013) The introduction of orange fleshed sweet potato in Mozambican diets: a marginal change to make a major difference. In: Fanzo J, Hunter D, Borelli T, Mattei F (eds) Diversifying food and diets: using agricultural biodiversity to improve nutrition and health. Earthscan, London
Massaretto IL, Albaladejo I, Purgatto E, Flores FB, Plasencia F, Egea-Fernández JM, Bolarin MC, Egea I (2018) Recovering tomato landraces to simultaneously improve fruit yield and nutritional quality against salt stress. Front Plant Sci 9:1778. https://doi.org/10.3389/fpls.2018.01778
Massawe F, Mayes S, Cheng A (2016) Crop diversity: an unexploited treasure trove for food security. Trends Plant Sci 21:365–368
Meisner A, Jacquiod S, Snoek BL, ten Hooven FC, van der Putten WH (2018) Drought legacy effects on the composition of soil fungal and prokaryote communities. Front Microbiol 9:294
Messina MJ (1999) Legumes and soybeans: overview of their nutritional profiles and health effects. Am J Clin Nutr 70(3):439–450
Montoya D, Gaba S, de Mazancourt C, Bretagnolle V, Loreau M (2020) Reconciling biodiversity conservation, food production and farmers' demand in agricultural landscapes. Ecol Model 416: 108889–108909
El Mujtar V, Muñoz N, McCormick BP, Pulleman M, Tittonell P (2019) Role and management of soil biodiversity for food security and nutrition; where do we stand? Glob Food Sec 20:132–144
National Research Council (US) (1975) The winged bean: a high-protein crop for the tropics (second edition). National Academies, Washington, D.C
Navruz-Varli S, Sanlier N (2016) Nutritional and health benefits of quinoa (*Chenopodium quinoa* Willd.). J Cereal Sci 69:371–376
Ojiewo CO, Mwai GN, Abukutsa-Onyango MO, Agong SG, Nono-Womdim R (2013) Exploiting the genetic diversity of vegetable African nightshades. Bioremediat Biodivers Bioavailab 7(1): 6–13. http://oar.icrisat.org/id/eprint/6365
Olango TM, Stadlmayr B, Charrondiere UR (2013) Literature about nutrition and underutilized foods: diversity in nutrient composition of underutilised root and tuber crops. Acta Hortic 979: 147–155
Padulosi S, Hodgkin T, Williams JT, Haq N (2002) Underutilised crops: trends, challenges and opportunities in the twenty-first century. In: Engels J, Rao VR, Jackson M (eds) Managing plant genetic diversity. CAB International, pp 323–338
Pedersen B, Kalinowski LS, Eggum BO (1987) The nutritive value of amaranth grain (*Amaranthus caudatus*). Plant Foods Hum Nutr 36(4):309–324
Pilling D, Bélanger J, Hoffmann I (2020) Declining biodiversity for food and agriculture needs urgent global action. Nat Food 1:144–147
Prasanna BM, Vasal SK, Kassahun B, Singh NN (2001) Quality protein maize. Curr Sci 81:1308–1319, 106
Pugnaire FI, Morillo JA, Peñuelas J, Reich PB, Bardgett RD, Gaxiola A, Wardle DA, van der Putten WH (2019) Climate change effects on plant-soil feedbacks and consequences for biodiversity and functioning of terrestrial ecosystems. Sci Adv 5:eaaz1834
Rahmanian M, Salimi M, Razavi K, Haghparast R, Ceccarelli S (2014) Evolutionary populations: living gene banks in farmers' fields. Farming Matters 13–15. https://hdl.handle.net/20.500.11766/7306
Ramesh SV, Krishnan V, Praveen S, Hebbar KB (2021) Dietary prospects of coconut oil for the prevention and treatment of Alzheimer's disease (AD): a review of recent evidences. Trends Food Sci Technol 112:201–211

Rubiang-Yalambing L, Arcot J, Greenfield H, Holford P (2014) Aibika (*Abelmoschus manihot* L.): genetic variation, morphology and relationships to micronutrient composition. Food Chem 193: 62–68

Ruiz KB, Biondi S, Oses R, Acuña-Rodríguez IS, Antognoni F, Martinez-Mosqueira EA et al (2014) Quinoa biodiversity and sustainability for food security under climate change. A review. Agron Sustain Dev 34:349–359

Saltzman A, Birol E, Bouis HE, Boy E, De Moura FF, Islam Y, Pfeiffer WH (2014) Biofortification: progress toward a more nourishing future. In: Bread and brain, education and poverty. Pontifical Academy of Sciences, Vatican City. Scripta varia 125. www.pas.va/content/dam/accademia/pdf/sv125/sv125-bouis.pdf

Scherer L, Svenning JC, Huang J, Seymour CL, Sandel B, Mueller N et al (2020) Global priorities of environmental issues to combat food insecurity and biodiversity loss. Sci Total Environ 730: 139096

Schönfeldt HC, Pretorius B (2011) The nutrient content of five traditional south African dark green leafy vegetables—a preliminary study. J Food Compos Anal 24(8):1141–1146

Schulz M, Borges GD, Gonzaga LV, Seraglio SK, Olivo IS, Azevedo MS, Nehring P, de Gois JS, de Almeida TS, Vitali L, Spudeit DA (2015) Chemical composition, bioactive compounds and antioxidant capacity of Juçara fruit (*Euterpeedulis* Martius) during ripening. Food Res Int 77: 125–131

Schulz M, Biluca FC, Gonzaga LV, Borges GD, Vitali L, Micke GA, de Gois JS, de Almeida TS, Borges DL, Miller PR, Costa AC (2017) Bioaccessibility of bioactive compounds and antioxidant potential of Juçara fruits (*Euterpe Edulis* Martius) subjected to *in vitro* gastrointestinal digestion. Food Chem 228:447–454

Singh V, Goel R, Pande V, Asif MH, Mohanty CS (2017) De novo sequencing and comparative analysis of leaf transcriptomes of diverse condensed tannin-containing lines of underutilized *Psophocarpus tetragonolobus* (L.) DC. Sci Rep. https://doi.org/10.1038/srep44733

Sunderland TCH (2011) Food security: why is biodiversity important? Int For Rev 13(3):online

Sunderland T, Powell B, Ickowitz A, Foli S, Pinedo-Vasquez M, Nasi R et al (2013) Food security and nutrition: the role of forests. *Discussion paper.* CIFOR, Bogor

Tabbita F, Lewis S, Vouilloz JP, Ortega MA, Kade M, Abbate PE, Barneix AJ (2013) Effect of the Gpc-B1 locus on high grain protein content introgressed into Argentinean wheat germ-plasm. Plant Breed 132:48–52

Tessema M, Gunaratna NS, Donato K, Cohen JL, McConnell M, Belayneh D, Brouwer ID, Belachew T, De Groote H (2016) Translating the impact of quality protein maize into improved nutritional status for Ethiopian children: study protocol for a randomized controlled trial. BMC Nutr 2:54. https://doi.org/10.1186/s40795-016-0089-z

Thomas D (2007) The mineral depletion of foods available to US as nation (1940–2002) – a review of the 6th edition of McCance and Widdowson. Nutr Health 19:21–55

van Niekerk C, Schönfeldt H, Hall N, Pretorius B (2016) The role of biodiversity in food security and nutrition: a potato cultivar case study. Food Nutr Sci 7:371–382

Vermeulen SJ, Campbell BM, Ingram JS (2012) Climate change and food systems. Annu Rev Environ Resour 37(1):195. https://doi.org/10.1146/annurev-environ-020411-130608

Vishwakarma MK, Mishra VK, Gupta PK, Yadav PS, Kumar H, Joshi AK (2014) Introgression of the high protein gene Gpc-B1 in an elite wheat variety of Indo-Gangetic plains through marker-assisted backcross breeding. Curr Plant Biol 1:60–67

Yao DN, Kouassi KN, Erba D, Scazzina F, Pellegrini N, Casiraghi MC (2015) Nutritive evaluation of the Bambara groundnut Ci12 landrace [*Vigna subterranea* (L.) Verdc. (Fabaceae)] produced in Côte d'Ivoire. Int J Mol Sci 16(9):21428–21441

Zabel F, Delzeit R, Schneider J et al (2019) Global impacts of future cropland expansion and intensification on agricultural markets and biodiversity. Nat Commun 10:2844

Chapter 2
Biofortification of Crops: Novel Insights and Approaches for Enhanced Nutrient Accumulation

Eloy Navarro-León, Francisco Javier López-Moreno, Ali Ahmad, Juan Manuel Ruiz, and Begoña Blasco

Abstract Hidden hunger is a worldwide problem that is characterized by insufficient intake of micronutrients, which are necessary for optimal human health. Biofortification of food crops is an effective and efficient strategy to alleviate human nutrient deficiencies. It has the ability to increase the nutrient content in the edible parts of the plants. This potent agronomic tool is employed to increase the accumulation of nutrients such as mineral elements, amino acids, and vitamins among others. The main factors that determine the success of biofortification are plant-/crop-dependent, such as the genotypes' nutrient accumulation mechanisms, and others, namely environmental conditions, and consumer or public acceptance. In general, two complementary approaches of plant biofortification, the agronomic and the biotechnological tools, are adopted. In the agronomic approach, the nutrients accumulation is enhanced through the application of fertilizers and biostimulants or the management of cultivation conditions. Alternatively, in the latter, crops with higher nutrient concentration or bioavailability are developed using breeding (including molecular) or genetic engineering techniques. Indeed, novel gene or genome editing tools are gaining prominence in the generation of biofortified crops. Application of these strategies has enabled enhancement of biosynthetic pathway of organic nutrients or decreased the concentration of antinutrients or increased nutrient transport to the edible parts. Thus, plant transporters are crucial targets for attaining optimal nutrient movement to and within the plant. Also, it is pertinent to continue to deepen our knowledge about the mechanisms of nutrients accumulation in the plant and their bioavailability for humans and animals and identifying ways and means to modify them to obtain plants with higher nutritional quality.

E. Navarro-León (✉) · A. Ahmad · J. M. Ruiz · B. Blasco
Department of Plant Physiology, Faculty of Sciences, University of Granada, Granada, Spain
e-mail: enleon@ugr.es

F. J. López-Moreno
IFAPA, Institute of Research and Training in Agriculture and Fisheries, Granada, Spain

R. S. V., S. Praveen (eds.), *Conceptualizing Plant-Based Nutrition*,
https://doi.org/10.1007/978-981-19-4590-8_2

Keywords Agronomic biofortification · Antinutrients · Biotechnology · Fertilizers · Nutrient transporters

2.1 Introduction

In the worldwide scenario, besides calorie hunger, there is an important problem of hidden hunger that is characterized by the insufficient intake of micronutrients that are necessary for optimal human health. Therefore, it is not only necessary to produce food in an adequate quantum but also it is essential to produce nutrient-rich foods (Sharma and Verma 2019). Humans require at least 20 essential minerals that can be obtained through the ingestion of a balanced diet; however, nutrient deficiencies are serious human health concerns worldwide (White and Broadley 2009). Some of the major nutritional disorders and the main diseases caused are as follows: iron (Fe) deficiency that causes anemia, calcium (Ca) deficiency that causes osteoporosis, vitamin A deficiency that causes night blindness, vitamin C that causes scurvy, zinc (Zn) deficiency that causes hypogonadism and dwarfism, and selenium (Se) deficiency that causes weak joints (Prasad and Shivay 2020).

Biofortification of food crops is an effective and efficient strategy to alleviate the problem of nutrient deficiencies due to its ability to increase the specific nutrient content in the edible parts of the plants (White and Brown 2010). Biofortification has been successfully employed to increase the accumulation of nutrients such as mineral elements, amino acids, and vitamins. Biofortification aims to increase the accumulation of nutrients in a cost-efficient and sustainable manner (Sharma and Verma 2019). Biofortification may be achieved in two complementary ways by following agronomic practices such as fertilization and through genetic approaches (breeding or genetic engineering) with aid of biotechnological tools generating varieties with enhanced nutrient accumulation or bioavailability (Table 2.1) (Sharma and Verma 2019).

Biofortification is especially valuable in regions where people have limited access to a varied diet and food supplements. Although biofortification field has attracted the researchers worldwide, the upscaling or application of the knowledge thus gained to improve the diets of common people is still in an early stage. The target crops are generally the ones that are widely consumed by population that exhibit more risk for malnutrition. Examples of target crops are wheat, rice, potato, legumes, sorghum, and millet (Sharma and Verma 2019). A successful case study of biofortification was demonstrated in children fed with an iron biofortified pearl millet, thereby reducing the anemia cases (Finkelstein et al. 2015). Other fruitful examples include the development of several zinc-biofortified rice and high-quality maize varieties through breeding processes (Bouis and Saltzman 2017; Tandzi et al. 2017). Likewise, biofortification of sweet potato and cassava with provitamin A was achieved and the vitamin was found to be effective even after cooking and storage (De Moura et al. 2015). More successful instances of biofortified crops are presented in Table 2.2.

Table 2.1 Different biofortification approaches and their descriptions

Approaches		Description
Agronomic	Element fertilization	Foliar or soil supplementation of the targeted element or with others that improve the nutritional quality
	Microorganisms	Application of living microorganisms that increase nutrient bioavailability or increase the root uptake surface
	Biostimulants and other compounds	Application of diverse compounds that stimulate natural processes in plants to enhance the nutrient accumulation regardless of their nutrient content
	Environmental management	Modification of environmental conditions such as CO_2 concentrations, temperature, or water supply to increase nutrient accumulation
Genetic	Breeding	Genotypes with useful characteristics for biofortification are crossed with commercial genotypes to obtain new biofortified varieties
	Modification of biosynthetic pathways	Modification of gene expression to increase the nutrient biosynthesis rate or decrease its degradation rate
	Inhibition of antinutrients	Modification of gene expression to decrease the presence of compounds that hinder nutrient assimilation by animals and humans
	Modification of transporters	Modification of gene expression to enhancement the activity of nutrient transport proteins

2.2 Factors Affecting the Success of Biofortification

The main factors associated with the success of biofortification are summarized in Fig. 2.1.

2.2.1 Plant-Related Factors

Nutritional requirements vary among the plant species, and hence, similar approaches of biofortification cannot be applied to genetically distant species. Thus, the efficiency of an agronomic biofortification is very specific to a particular nutrient–crop combination (Dixit et al. 2018). The biofortification performed utilizing biotechnology approaches is limited to species with a relatively good quality genomic resources (Sharma and Verma 2019). Once the crop species has been identified, it is recommended to know the mechanisms of nutrient accumulation, the tissues where nutrients are accumulated, and the appropriate ligand compounds, etc. (Cominelli et al. 2020a). Likewise, it is vital that the nutrients accumulate in the edible portion of the crop because some nutrients are more easily transported to the leaves than to the seeds or fruits and some nutrients remain in the root to a greater extent (Connorton et al. 2017).

In the biotechnological approach, it is fundamental to take into account the potentially deleterious off-target effects of an altered gene expression. For example,

Table 2.2 Successful examples of biofortification in crops and the approaches followed

Nutrient	Species	Approach	Reference
Ca	Baby leaf vegetables	Agronomic	D'Imperio et al. (2016)
Ca	Carrot	Genetic engineering	Morris et al. (2008)
Fe	Pearl millet	Breeding	Finkelstein et al. (2015)
Fe	Bean	Breeding	Haas et al. (2016)
Fe and Zn	Rice	Genetic engineering	Trijatmiko et al. (2016)
Zn	Wheat	Breeding	Rosado et al. (2009)
Zn	Rice	Breeding	Bouis and Saltzman (2017)
Se	Wheat	Agronomic	Idrees et al. (2018)
I	Cabbage	Agronomic	Ojok et al. (2019)
Tryptophan and lysine	Maize	Breeding	Tandzi et al. (2017)
Lysine	Maize	Genetic engineering	Tang et al. (2013)
Provitamin A	Sweet potato and cassava	Breeding	De Moura et al. (2015)
Provitamin A	Rice	Genetic engineering	Paine et al. (2005)
Provitamin A	Maize	Breeding	Gannon et al. (2014)
B6 vitamin	Cassava	Genetic engineering	Li et al. (2015)
Folate (B9 vitamin)	Rice	Genetic engineering	Blancquaert et al. (2015)

reducing the phytate content of a crop significantly affects various other physiological functions (Cominelli et al. 2020a), and the enhancement of carotenoid levels is fraught with negative effects of reduced chlorophyll and tocopherol contents (Simkin 2019). On the other hand, in the agronomic approach, it is important to consider the antagonisms between nutrients. Thus, despite providing large quantum of nutrients, accumulation of minerals in plant system is not sufficient due to antagonisms in the culture medium or the effect of antagonism on the nutrient uptake mechanism of plants (Lyons and Cakmak 2012). However, in some cases, the elemental antagonisms are species-specific. For instance, sulfur (S) and sulfates inhibit selenium (Se) accumulation because of the similarity between both elements, but the appropriate combination of S and phosphorus (P) enhances Se accumulation in rapeseed (Izydorczyk et al. 2021). Another undesirable effect of biofortification is the induction of heavy metal accumulation. For instance, certain Zn and Fe transporters can also transport cadmium (Cd) and other heavy metals. If these transporters are overexpressed, it can lead to a overaccumulation of these heavy metals in the edible parts and be toxic to animal and human consumption (Narayanan et al. 2019). Therefore, it is very crucial to perform a detailed compositional analysis of the biofortified crop before making the product available for public consumption (Dixit et al. 2018).

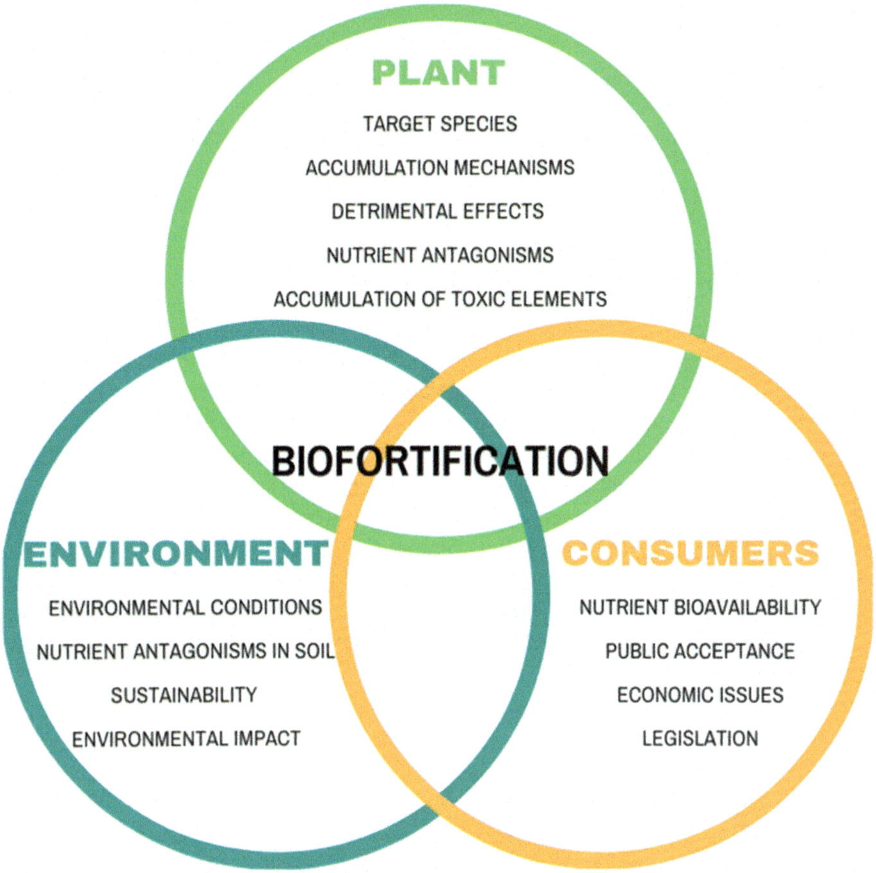

Fig. 2.1 Factors contributing to the success of biofortification process

2.2.2 Environmental Factors

The environmental conditions (soil, climate, localization) are crucial for successful biofortification. For example, the soil pH may limit the availability of nutrients for the plant. In addition, the rainfall frequency, the temperature, and the soil chemistry may severely constrain the application of agronomic biofortification techniques (Dixit et al. 2018). Moreover, a low impact on the environment and sustainability over time are two crucial factors for the success of biofortification. In biofortification approaches based on application of fertilizers, it is important to have knowledge regarding the soil composition and its structure so as to avoid application of excess quantum of fertilizers. In consequence, agronomic biofortification is not considered a sustainable approach in soils having appreciably good crop growth conditions (Menguer et al. 2018). In contrast, genetic biofortification is a more sustainable approach because it reduces the application of fertilizers in the environment (Sharma and Verma 2019).

2.2.3 Factor Related to the Consumers

Once the biofortified plant has been developed, it is crucial to evaluate the amount of the nutrient that is assimilated by animals and humans (D'Imperio et al. 2016). The proportion of assimilated nutrients depends on the amount of antinutrients and promoter substances in the food. Indeed, for biofortification purposes, it is key to minimize the presence of antinutrients such as phytates, phenols, and oxalate and maximize the promoter substances such as vitamins, choline, and cysteine (Sharma et al. 2017). Furthermore, the food processing techniques followed are also crucial since some of the processing operations, namely cutting and boiling, cause severe nutrients loss. Hence, it is important to know the effects of different processing ways to estimate the quantity of nutrients that are assimilated by animals or humans (Sharma and Verma 2019).

The acceptance of a biofortified crop by potential consumers is a critical component in assessing the success of a biofortification program. Despite the great efficiency of accumulation of nutrients, the efforts can go vain if the product is not accepted by the public (Dixit et al. 2018). An example of this case is golden rice (Ye et al. 2000). Therefore, it is pertinent to carry out market studies and to consider the opinion of approved panels that perform organoleptic changes such as appearance, flavor, and texture that determine the ultimate public acceptance (Park et al. 2009). Besides, biofortification will not be viable if at the end of the process the economic cost exceeds the benefits obtained. Regardless of the approach, biofortification is more cost-effective than food supplementation (Sharma and Verma 2019; Simkin 2019). However, in the short term, the agronomic approach can be a viable option, but in the long term, the genetic approach is more profitable. Indeed, the advantages of genetic biofortification are that is a one-time investment and the germplasm can be distributed at international levels (Sharma and Verma 2019). Nevertheless, a major disadvantage could be the regulatory barriers for the approval of genetically modified organisms (GMOs) in some countries (Bhambhani et al. 2021).

2.3 Agronomic Biofortification

In agronomic fertilization, the aim is to increase the accumulation of nutrients through the application of fertilizers and biostimulants or the management of cultivation conditions. The main advantages of this approach are its simplicity and the low technical requirements, and it does not warrant any legislative barriers akin to GMOs (Vlčko and Ohnoutková 2019).

2.3.1 Element Fertilization

In this approach, certain elemental nutrition is provided to plants to increase their nutritional quality. Typically, plants are supplied with fertilizers enriched with the target nutrients that are necessary to accumulate in the edible parts. The most successful examples of agronomic biofortification have been achieved for elements Zn and Se (Wakeel et al. 2018), iodine (Izydorczyk et al. 2021), and in baby leafy vegetables biofortified with Ca (D'Imperio et al. 2016). Biofortification with other elements such as Fe is more cumbersome due to limitations in its bioavailability for the plant. Thus, this is one of the main factors that limit agronomic biofortification together with the soil conditions and the retranslocation to edible parts (Wakeel et al. 2018). Fertilizers for plants are generally supplied through soil medium; however, biofortification through the foliar application or the foliar and soil combination are more effective and ensure the accurate localization of nutrients, especially for cereals and leafy vegetables (Sharma and Verma 2019; Pradhan et al. 2020; Izydorczyk et al. 2021). Furthermore, nutrient absorption can be enhanced by surfactants or applying nutrients in the form of microparticles or nanoparticles such as Zn nanoparticles (Vlčko and Ohnoutková 2019; Ponce-García et al. 2019). In addition, the coating of seeds with nutrients is another possibility (Sharma and Verma 2019).

In some cases, fertilization is used with elements that are not the target of biofortification but that induce a greater nutrient quality in plants. For instance, biofortification with elements such as Fe, Zn, and Se enhances the concentration of amino acids, glucosinolates, phenolic compounds, and flavonoids and increases antioxidant properties (Bachiega et al. 2016; Barrameda-Medina et al. 2017; Li et al. 2018). Alternatively, silicon (Si) is not considered an essential element; however, it is widely applied to improve the nutritional quality of crops (Dixit et al. 2018; Sharma and Verma 2019). Furthermore, appropriate N fertilization, besides determining the yield and the protein content, is a key factor in the accumulation of elements such as Fe and Zn (Ricachenevsky et al. 2019). Hence, the most suitable fertilization composition should be chosen considering the state of the soil, the target nutrient for biofortification, the interactions between nutrients, and taking into account sustainability (Prasad and Shivay 2020).

Nanofertilizers are recent potent addition to maximize the sustainability of element fertilization. The application of elements as nanofertilizers ensures the gradual release of nutrients easing nutrient availability to the plant. Nanofertilizers have a large specific surface area, thereby improving the effective nutrient uptake by the plant. It avoids the excessive application of fertilizers, thereby preventing eutrophication and pollution. Numerous nanofertilizers have been approved worldwide and proved their efficacy for nutrient biofortification (Basavegowda and Baek 2021). For instance, Se nanoparticles have better stability, plants absorb them faster, and they are less toxic compared to the conventional ionic forms (García Márquez et al. 2020). Zn nanoparticles are more efficient for common bean fertilization than conventional Zn fertilizers (Ponce-García et al. 2019). Furthermore, several P nanofertilizers are being developed given the lower efficiency of traditional P fertilizers that causes a significantly low P bioavailability for the plant (Basavegowda and Baek 2021).

2.3.2 *Biostimulants and Other Compounds*

Biostimulants are compounds applied externally to stimulate and enhance nutrient accumulation, crop quality, or tolerance to stresses, regardless of their nutrient content. The objective is that a biostimulant increases the biomass or the nutritional quality of a crop without a great supply of fertilizers (Ricci et al. 2019). The use of biostimulants with or without biological activity could be useful in biofortification by directly influencing nutrient accumulation or increasing the root development which in turn can increase nutrient uptake and enhance ion transport to the shoot. Important ingredients of biostimulants are amino acids, silica, salicylic acid, and humic acids. Thus, these compounds enhance nutrient uptake and the accumulation of antioxidant compounds such as phenols (Vega et al. 2019; Vlčko and Ohnoutková 2019; Izydorczyk et al. 2021). Also, the use of extracts from leaves of hyperaccumulator species was proven to be an effective strategy for the biofortification of certain elements such as Se (Izydorczyk et al. 2021).

Biostimulants also encompass the use of beneficial microorganisms for biofortification. Improving the interaction between soil microorganisms and root systems is a way to enhance nutrient accumulation. Microorganisms contribute to atmospheric N-fixation, the solubilization of nutrients, and the synthesis of phytohormones (Khan et al. 2019). The siderophores secreted by microorganisms chelate Fe and increase the uptake by the plant (Srivastava et al. 2013). Furthermore, microorganisms reduce soil pH and enhance root growth increasing the root absorptive area. The use of biofertilizers (bacteria and fungi) instead of synthetic compounds is an environment-friendly approach. These biofertilizers reduce the loss of nutrients and increase the bioavailability of the naturally present nutrients (Khan et al. 2019). A flourishing biofertilizer-based fortification was documented in Se and Zn biofortification. Bacteria such as *Bacillus* and other plant growth-promoting rhizobacteria increase the solubilization of Se and Zn in the soil which enhances the accumulation of these elements in the plant (Izydorczyk et al. 2021). Besides, the inoculation of plant seeds with arbuscular mycorrhiza such as fungus *Rhizopagus irregularis* improved plant biomass and its accumulation of organic acids, and vitamin B1 and its analogs (Vlčko and Ohnoutková 2019).

2.3.3 Environmental Factors

Another possibility for biofortification is the modification of environmental conditions such as CO_2 concentrations, temperature, or water supply. Thus, Se accumulation was improved under heat stress in lettuce (Hawrylak-Nowak et al. 2018) and drought stress in maize and wheat (Mathers et al. 2017; Bocchini et al. 2018). Alternatively, growth of plants such as carrot and sour orange, under high CO_2 conditions, showed an enhanced ascorbate accumulation; however, this effect is species-specific (Simkin 2019). Usually, crops grown under elevated CO_2 concentrations showed lower protein and micronutrient contents. The increment in crop yields often leads to a dilution effect and reduces the nutrient concentration in edible parts, so it is mandatory to develop crops that maintain or enhance the nutritional quality (Wakeel et al. 2018). Therefore, it is anticipated that the current global change scenario may negatively influence the nutritional quality of crops (Simkin 2019).

2.4 Genetic Biofortification

Genetic biofortification is the development of crops with enhanced nutrient concentration using breeding or genetic engineering techniques (Garg et al. 2018). Developments in the field of genetic approach are crucial to alleviate nutrient hunger given the multiple limitations of the agronomic methods. Furthermore, besides being more efficient, genetic biofortification is more sustainable and environment-friendly than the agronomic approach because it avoids the excessive fertilizer application that pollutes soil and water (Garg et al. 2018; Gupta et al. 2021). Breeding techniques allow the selection of varieties/genotypes with useful characteristics for biofortification purposes. Breeding is supported by numerous DNA sequencing and genetic screening techniques within the marker-assisted selection (MAS) and genome selection approaches (Gupta et al. 2021). Complementarily, genetic engineering techniques provide us the capacity to modify certain target gene sequences. Some examples of these tools are heterologous gene expression, RNA interference (RNAi), Targeting Induced Local Lesions in Genomes (TILLING), and Clustered Regularly Interspaced Short Palindromic Repeats (CRISPR)/Cas-based gene or genome editing (Till et al. 2018; Bhambhani et al. 2021). Application of these techniques enables enhancement of the biosynthetic pathway, improves nutrient transport to the edible parts resulting in nutrient density, or decreases the presence of antinutrients (Fig. 2.2).

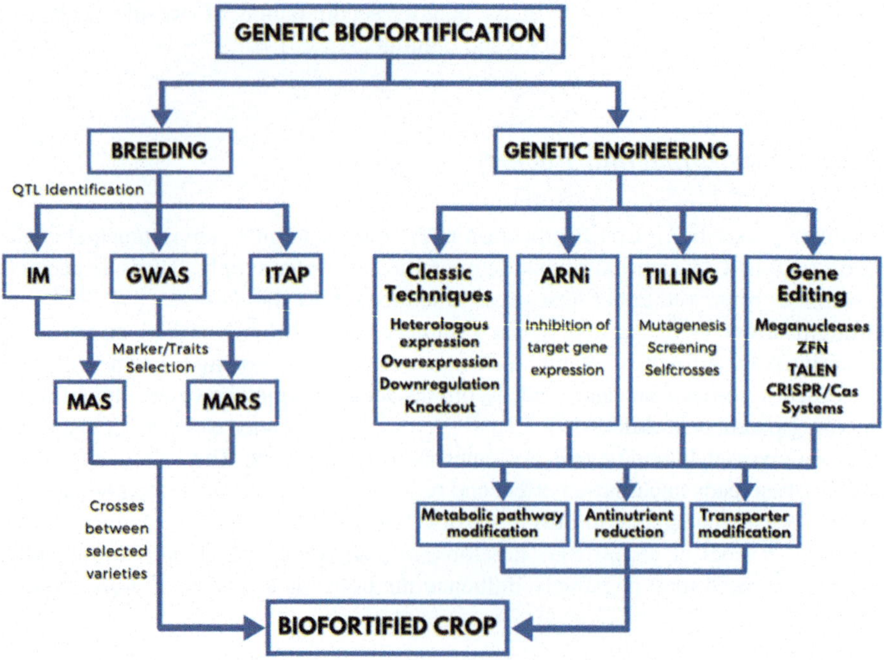

Fig. 2.2 Overview of the main genetic techniques and approaches for the generation of biofortified crops

2.4.1 *Biofortification Using Breeding Techniques*

In traditional breeding, genotypes with useful characteristics for biofortification are hybridized with commercial genotypes to obtain new biofortified varieties. The genotypic variations for differential nutrient accumulation exist within the same species. Indeed, the first step in breeding is the identification and characterization of genetic variability for nutrient uptake, transport, or accumulation in the target organ (White and Broadley 2009). Numerous genotype selection and breeding techniques have been developed to investigate and characterize the genetic variation in crops by taking advantages in the field of quantitative trait locus (QTL) linked to higher accumulation of nutrients followed by identification of molecular markers associated with it. Currently, two main approaches are used to identify QTLs in crops: QTL interval mapping (IM) and genome-wide association studies (GWAS). Once QTLs are identified, they are used for marker-assisted selection (MAS) or marker-assisted recurrent selection (MARS) to select the desired genotypes for breeding. In addition, intron-targeted amplified polymorphism (ITAP) is a new approach to identify makers with the aid of bioinformatic tools (Gupta et al. 2020). Using these techniques, numerous QTL/traits associations have been identified, for example, those that determine a greater accumulation of Zn and Fe in gramineous species (Vlčko and Ohnoutková 2019; Pradhan et al. 2020). Diverse examples of crop biofortification using breeding approaches are presented in Table 2.2.

2.4.2 Genetic Engineering Techniques

Genetic engineering has proven its huge potential of increasing nutrient accumulation in specific target plant organs and in a simple and rapid manner compared to conventional or molecular breeding approaches. The classic techniques such as gene overexpression or heterologous expression increase the transcription rate or the gene copy number to achieve higher quantities of the final gene products causing an increased nutrient accumulation. In addition, it is possible to introduce a downregulated or knockout version of a gene to reduce the antinutrient synthesis or to modify a metabolic pathway (Dutt et al. 2019). Alternatively, RNAi technique also has also been successful in silencing a gene expression (Vlčko and Ohnoutková 2019).

A different approach, within the ambit of genetic engineering, directly seeks the modification of a target gene sequence. For instance, in the TILLING technique, different genotypes are generated through mutagenesis and are subsequently screened to identify mutations in a target gene. Then, backcrosses are performed to produce homozygotes for the selected mutation, and finally, the mutation is correlated with its phenotype (Till et al. 2018). The TILLING process is long; however, faster gene editing techniques have been developed in recent years. Thus, these tools make possible effective targeted mutagenesis and site-specific genome modifications (Jiang et al. 2021). The gene editing tools initially developed were those based on nucleases such as meganucleases, zinc-finger nucleases (ZFN), and transcription activator-like effector nuclease (TALEN). However, these techniques are outperformed by the more versatile CRISPR/Cas systems which utilize an endonuclease (Cas) and a guide RNA to effect appropriate genetic modification in the target DNA sequence. The most used endonuclease is Cas9, of which multiple variants have been developed, but other such as Cas12, Cas13, and Cas14 introduce novel enhancements to the CRISPR/Cas system (Bhambhani et al. 2021).

Using the genetic engineering techniques described above following three different approaches, it is possible to generate the biofortified plants. One of them is the modification of specific genes for a specific metabolic pathway (Bhambhani et al. 2021). Hence, improved comprehension of different metabolic steps that are involved in the production or degradation of target nutrient is vital. Another possibility, although more complex, is to create a whole new biosynthetic pathway aimed at inducing the accumulation of a specific compound inside the plant system. It is necessary to know the gene sequences, their regulation, the enzyme biochemistry, and the potential off-target consequences, for plant phenotype (Vlčko and Ohnoutková 2019). Researchers have developed numerous plant biofortified genotypes using this approach. For instance, by overexpressing the phytoene synthase enzyme among others, Ye et al. (2000) generated golden rice, which accumulates provitamin A. Sikdar et al. (2016) using RNAi technology have developed barley plants that accumulate relatively high essential amino acids. Furthermore, Minhas et al. (2018) generated rice plants with higher thiamine accumulations through the overexpression of *thi4* and *thiC* genes.

Another approach, the genetic engineering techniques resort to, is to reduce the presence of compounds that act as antinutrients in animals and humans. The most important antinutrients in crops are phytic acid and certain polyphenolic compounds (Cominelli et al. 2020a). Low phytic acid plants can be generated by creating genetic mutations in transporters (that move phytic acid into vacuoles) or in key genes involved in phytic acid biosynthesis such as *SULTR* and *MRP*. Some of these mutants exhibit pleiotropic effects. However, genotypes without these off-target or pleiotropic effects were obtained in common bean by modifying *MRP1* gene and in rice and barley with mutations in *SLTR3* gene (Cominelli et al. 2020b). The low phytic acid mutants should be combined with other modifications to produce plants with a greater accumulation of nutrients while increasing their bioavailability (Cominelli et al. 2020a). Finally, the third approach is to modify genes coding for nutrient plant transporters to increase its accumulation in a target organ of the plant.

2.5 Biofortification Through Modification of Nutrient Transporters

Plant transporters are crucial to the circulation of nutrients to and within plant tissues. Transporters carry the ions inside the roots from the soils, and then, specific transporters take the ions from the root to the xylem vessels. Other transporters transport the nutrients from xylem to other distal parts, leaves, fruits, and seeds of plants (Fig. 2.3). In cells, important transporter such as the cation exchangers (CAX) transport ions inside the vacuoles for its storage (Pittman and Hirschi 2016). Based on several scientific studies, it was proposed that the modification of any of these types of transporters could be useful to improve nutrient accumulation in plants (Table 2.3).

2.5.1 CAX Transporters and Ca Biofortification

There is a strong correlation between CAX1 expression and Ca accumulation (Conn et al. 2011; Rios et al. 2012). Indeed, several experiments have shown the potential of the *CAX1* gene manipulation to increase Ca content in the edible part and therefore its potential in biofortification programs (Table 2.3). Thus, experiments were conducted in tomato and potato plants to constitutively overexpress a version of CAX1. However, it resulted in damage in the fruits because of cytosolic Ca deficiency (Gao et al. 2019; Zorrilla et al. 2019). On the other hand, there are similar

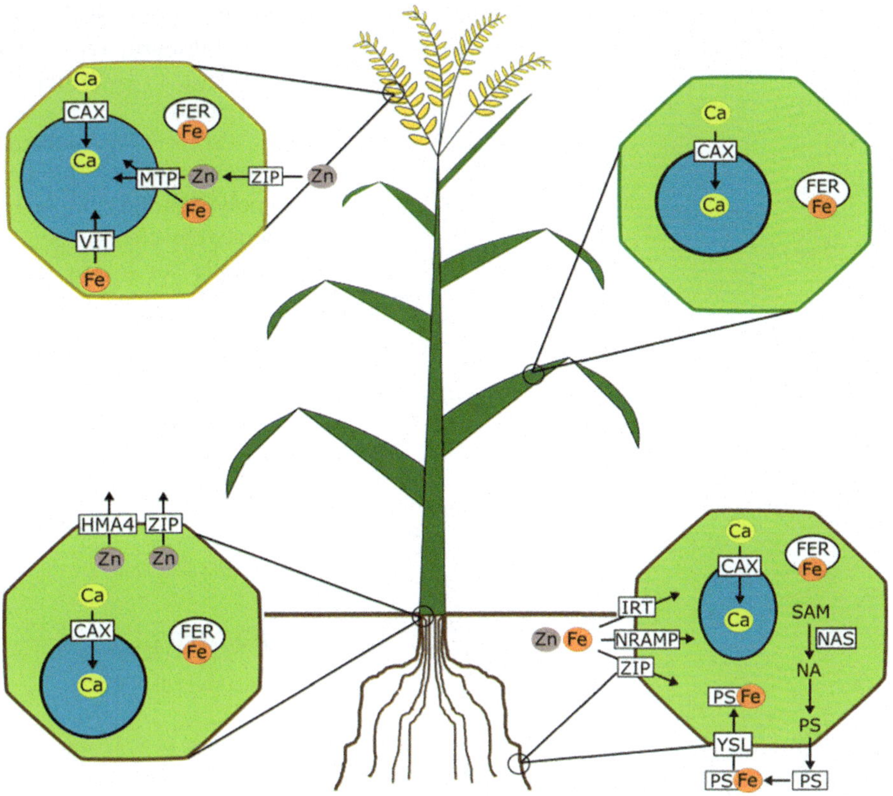

Fig. 2.3 Main transporters and other proteins modified in biotechnological biofortification and their localization in the plant

experiments with no negative (or off-target) effects in potato (Park et al. 2005), in lettuce (Park et al. 2009), in carrot (Morris et al. 2008), and in rice (Yi et al. 2012). Notably, a mutant with a single amino acid modification in CAX1 transporter was obtained using TILLING approach in *B. rapa* (Graham et al. 2014). This mutant did not exhibit any negative effects on plant growth, however, enhanced the accumulation of Ca, Mg, and Fe (Navarro-León et al. 2018).

2.5.2 *Other Ca Transporters and Ca-Related Proteins*

Another possibility for Ca biofortification is the modification of other Ca transporters such as two-pore channel (TPC), Ca channel proteins in plasma membrane or low-affinity cation transporters (LCT), and other Ca-related proteins such as calcineurin B-like interacting protein kinase (CIPK) and calmodulin (CAM). Ca accumulation is correlated with the expression of TPC1, CAX3, and Ca sensor

Table 2.3 Modulation of plant transporters' expression to enhance nutrient accumulation in crops

Transporter	Elements	Species	Technique	References
CAX1	Ca, Mg, Fe	*Brassica rapa*	TILLING	Navarro-León et al. (2018)
CAX1	Ca	Potato, carrot, lettuce, rice	Heterologous expression	Park et al. (2005), Morris et al. (2008), Park et al. (2009), Yi et al. (2012)
CAX2 and CAX4	Ca	Tomato	Heterologous expression	Chung et al. (2010), Park et al. (2005)
HMA4	Zn, Fe	*Brassica rapa*	TILLING	Blasco et al. (2019)
HMA4	Zn	Tobacco	Heterologous expression	Siemianowski et al. (2011), Barabasz et al. (2012)
IRT1	Fe and Zn	Rice	Heterologous expression	Tan et al. (2015)
IRT1 + FER1	Fe, Zn	Cassava	Heterologous expression	Narayanan et al. (2019)
NAS1 + NAS1	Fe and Zn	Rice	Heterologous expression	Banakar et al. (2017)
NAS2	Fe	Rice and chickpea	Gene overexpression	Trijatmiko et al. (2016), Tan et al. (2018)
YSL	Fe	Rice	Gene overexpression	Lee et al. (2012)
NRAMP1	Fe, Zn	Rice and tobacco	Heterologous expression	Wang et al. (2019)
VIT2	Fe	Wheat and barley	Gene overexpression	Connorton et al. (2017)
MTP1	Zn	Barley	Gene overexpression	Menguer et al. (2018)
ZIP5	Fe and Zn	Maize	Gene overexpression	Li et al. (2019)
NRAMP3 + NAS1 + FER	Fe and Zn	Rice	Heterologous expression	Wu et al. (2019)
IRT1 + NAS1 + FER	Fe	Rice	Heterologous expression	Boonyaves et al. (2017)

proteins such as CIPKs and CAM in finger millet plants (Kumar et al. 2014). Furthermore, the expression of *LCT1* gene with a CAMV35S promoter was effective in increasing Ca accumulation in wheat (Antosiewicz and Hennig 2004). Likewise, the expression of other Ca-binding proteins such as calreticulin could be effective to increase Ca accumulation (Sharma et al. 2017).

2.5.3 *HMA4 Transporter and Zn Biofortification*

The heavy metal-associated transporters (HMA) are a family of heavy metal transporters that are essential for Zn homeostasis. For instance, HMA2 and HMA4 are involved in the discharge of Zn into the xylem and thus in the transport from roots to leaves (see Fig. 2.3) (Wong and Cobbett 2008). Several experiments have proven that the increase in xylem loading through HMA4 modification increases Zn transport to the shoot which seems a viable approach for Zn biofortification (Humayan Kabir et al. 2014). Thus, Siemianowski et al. (2011) observed that the overexpression of the *AtHMA4* gene produces an increase in the concentration of Zn in the roots and leaves of tobacco plants. Confirming these findings, Barabasz et al. (2012) also showed that the expression of the *HMA4* gene from the hyperaccumulator *Arabidopsis halleri* (AhHMA4) results in an increase in Zn accumulation in the leaves of tomato plants. Furthermore, a higher activity of HMA4 transporter affected Fe accumulation and its root to shoot distribution in tomato plants (Kendziorek et al. 2014). Likewise, a mutant characterized by a single modification in HMA4 transporter of *B. rapa* derived from TILLING approach showed higher Zn, Cu, Mg, and Fe concentrations (Blasco et al. 2019).

2.5.4 *Fe and Zn Biofortification Through Transporter Modifications*

To increase the concentration of Fe and Zn in plants, researchers have generated plants with enhanced activity of root transporters, higher presence of Fe accumulating proteins, or increased capacity for vacuole accumulation (Connorton et al. 2017).

2.5.4.1 IRT Transporters

Iron-regulated transporters (IRT) belong to the Zn and Fe permease family (ZIP) and are the main transporters that carry Fe^{2+} and Zn^{2+} from the rhizosphere to the roots (Pradhan et al. 2020). IRT1 and IRT3 are located in the plasma membrane and transport Fe^{2+} to the cytosol and are upregulated under Fe deficiency conditions (Narayanan et al. 2019). On the other hand, IRT2 is located in intracellular vesicles, thereby functioning in Fe storage to prevent Fe toxicity. In *Arabidopsis*, overexpression of *AtIRT3* enhanced Fe accumulation in roots and Zn in shoots (Li et al. 2019). In addition, Tan et al. (2015) described that exogenous expression of *MxIRT* in rice increased Zn and Fe accumulations.

2.5.4.2 Phytosiderophores

Plant-derived phytosiderophores (PS) that bind to Fe^{3+} are explored as an alternate strategy for Fe uptake. The plants synthesized nicotianamine, in a reaction catalyzed by nicotianamine synthase (NAS), forms a base for biosynthesis of PS (Tan et al. 2018). Then, PS is secreted to the rhizosphere where it binds Fe^{3+} to form PS-Fe^{3+} complex, which is taken up inside the root through yellow stripe-like (YSL) transporters. NA and mugineic acids also chelate Zn, and these complexes are transported into the plant through YSL transporters (Wu et al. 2019). Experiments that achieved higher NAS activity showed high Fe and Zn accumulations in rice (Trijatmiko et al. 2016; Banakar et al. 2017) and higher Fe concentration in chickpea (Tan et al. 2018). Similarly, activation of *YSL* gene in rice also resulted in a high Fe accumulation (Lee et al. 2012). Furthermore, endosperm-specific promoters are quite useful to ensure the accumulation of nutrients in that part of the seed. Thus, the expression of *OsNAS1* and *HvNAS1* genes in rice increased Fe and Zn contents in the endosperm (Banakar et al. 2017).

2.5.4.3 NRAMP Transporters

Natural resistance-associated macrophage protein (NRAMP) also transports Fe but has a diverse cellular localization. Some NRAMP (AtNRAMP3 and AtNRAMP4) are responsible for the efflux of Fe from the vacuole to cytosol, but others (AtNRAMP1) are located in plasma membranes and transport Fe^{2+} from the rhizosphere (Wu et al. 2019). Some NRAMP transporters also transport Mn and Zn, but it varies depending on the species (Wang et al. 2019). An example of NRAMP1 modification was provided by Wang et al. (2019) wherein expression of *AhNRAMP1* in rice and tobacco increased their yields and Fe and Zn concentrations.

2.5.4.4 Other Fe and Zn Transporters

The vacuolar iron transporter 1 (VIT1) transports Fe into vacuoles (Wu et al. 2019). Two VIT (VIT1 and VIT2) were characterized in rice and wheat (Zhang et al. 2012). Higher activity of these transporters improved Fe accumulation in seeds. VIT2 is of much interest in the field of biofortification because it is expressed in the endosperm. Indeed, *TaVIT2* overexpression in wheat and barley increased twice the Fe content in flour (Connorton et al. 2017). Furthermore, metal tolerance proteins (MTPs) transport Zn, Fe, and other metals out of the cytosol to the extracellular part or into intracellular vesicles to prevent toxicities (Dixit et al. 2018). It highlights the functional role of MTP1 that is located in tonoplast and transports Zn in barley. Thus, Zn accumulation was enhanced through the expression of *HvMTP*1 transporter in barley endosperm (Menguer et al. 2018). Besides, ZIP transporters are key to transport divalent cations into the cell to maintain ion homeostasis. For instance, maize ZmZIP5 is situated in the plasma membrane and the endoplasmic reticulum. The overexpression of *ZmZIP5* increases Fe and Zn in the endosperm without detrimental effects (Li et al. 2019).

2.5.4.5 Multigene Approaches

Several experiments have shown that modification of more than one gene related to Fe or Zn accumulation is more effective in increasing their concentrations in the plant system. Ferritin (FER) is a ubiquitous protein that serves as a Fe storage in cells (Wu et al. 2019). Studies have modified the expression of previously characterized transporters and ferritin (FER). Transgenic rice expressing nicotianamine synthase (*OsNAS2*) and soybean ferritin (*SferH-1*) genes showed a sixfold greater Fe in rice endosperm without any detrimental effects (Trijatmiko et al. 2016). In another study, a cassette of *AtIRT1*, *AtNAS1*, and *PvFER* genes was expressed in rice to document increased Fe accumulation under Fe deficiency conditions (Boonyaves et al. 2017). Likewise, the overexpression of the iron assimilatory protein (FEA1) and VIT1 from *Arabidopsis* increased Fe and Zn accumulation in cassava plants. These transgenic plants provide food with greater ions contents after being cooked. Hence, these plants could fulfill a remarkable percentage of the dietary Fe necessities in food (Narayanan et al. 2019).

2.6 Food Fortification

Food fortification is a cost-effective, efficient alternative strategy to improve the micronutrient and vitamin contents of the food, thereby alleviating the ill effects of mineral deficiencies (micronutrient malnutrition) in middle- and low-income countries. One of the widely employed fortification strategy is to mix up the synthetic micronutrients to the commonly consumed foods such as cereals (rice, wheat, maize flour), lipids (oils and fats), and others such as milk, sugar, and salt. However, the success of food fortification and its effect on population's health depends on multiple factors including the actual bioavailability of fortificants, quantum of fortified food consumed, and the level of fortification (Verma 2015). Instances of classical food fortification include rice meal flour fortified with iron (ferric pyrophosphate), wheat flour and maize meal with iron (NaFeEDTA), soy sauce with iron, porridge cereals with zinc, cereals flour with zinc (100 mg Zn/Kg), wheat flour bun fortified with vitamin A, and staple condiments with multiple micronutrients (iron, folic acid, zinc, vitamin A, iodine, vitamin D, and calcium) (Chadare et al. 2019). The challenges encountered in classical food fortification have resulted in devising a novel food-to-food fortification programs wherein locally available, and accessible food resource is used to fortify another food. For example, tapioca (cassava tuber) is fortified with soybean flour for carbohydrates and fiber; a maize-based fermented cereal dough is fortified with baobab fruit powder (the latter is rich in vitamins A, C, E, and F;

proteins; fiber; carbohydrates; iron; zinc; calcium; and potassium) (Adejuyitan et al. 2012). Thus, food fortification is an essential strategy for achieving nutritional security of masses and preventing many diseases associated with malnutrition in both the developing and under-developed countries. However, the success of food fortification program depends on multiple factors such as cultural aspects of food, poverty reduction programs in vogue, and other socio-cultural dimensions.

2.7 Concluding Remarks

Biofortification offers a great potential to alleviate the problems of nutritional deficiencies around the world, especially in regions experiencing difficulties in accessing varied diet. Research and application of biofortification should consider all the factors that determine the success of this approach. Thus, it is crucial to know the mechanisms of accumulation of nutrients in the plant, and the potential consequences of the various approaches of biofortification and acceptance of biofortified food crop by consumers. It is also necessary to take advantage of the different approaches to biofortification (agronomic and genetic) according to the context and the objectives to be achieved. Genetic engineering techniques offer a multitude of possibilities for modifying transporters and other proteins in the plant that may be involved in biofortification. We must continue to deepen our knowledge about the mechanisms of nutrients accumulation in the plant and their bioavailability for humans and animals and how to modify them to obtain plants with higher nutritional quality.

References

Adejuyitan JA, Abioye AO, Otunola ET, Oyewole YN (2012) An evaluation of some properties of baobab fruit powder and ogi mixes. Trans J Sci Technol 2(7):99–102

Antosiewicz DM, Hennig J (2004) Overexpression of LCT1 in tobacco enhances the protective action of calcium against cadmium toxicity. Environ Pollut 129:237–245. https://doi.org/10.1016/J.ENVPOL.2003.10.025

Bachiega P, Salgado JM, de Carvalho JE et al (2016) Antioxidant and antiproliferative activities in different maturation stages of broccoli (*Brassica oleracea* Italica) biofortified with selenium. Food Chem 190:771–776. https://doi.org/10.1016/J.FOODCHEM.2015.06.024

Banakar R, Alvarez Fernandez A, Díaz-Benito P et al (2017) Phytosiderophores determine thresholds for iron and zinc accumulation in biofortified rice endosperm while inhibiting the accumulation of cadmium. J Exp Bot 68:4983–4995. https://doi.org/10.1093/jxb/erx304

Barabasz A, Wilkowska A, Ruszczyńska A et al (2012) Metal response of transgenic tomato plants expressing P1B-ATPase. Physiol Plant 145:315–331. https://doi.org/10.1111/j.1399-3054.2012.01584.x

Barrameda-Medina Y, Blasco B, Lentini M et al (2017) Zinc biofortification improves phytochemicals and amino-acidic profile in *Brassica oleracea* cv. Bronco. Plant Sci 258:45–51. https://doi.org/10.1016/j.plantsci.2017.02.004

Basavegowda N, Baek K-H (2021) Current and future perspectives on the use of nanofertilizers for sustainable agriculture: the case of phosphorus nanofertilizer. 3 Biotech 11:357. https://doi.org/10.1007/s13205-021-02907-4

Bhambhani S, Kondhare KR, Giri AP (2021) Advanced genome editing strategies for manipulation of plant specialized metabolites pertaining to biofortification. Phytochem Rev 81–99. https://doi.org/10.1007/s11101-021-09749-1

Blancquaert D, Van Daele J, Strobbe S et al (2015) Improving folate (vitamin B9) stability in biofortified rice through metabolic engineering. Nat Biotechnol 33:1076–1078. https://doi.org/10.1038/nbt.3358

Blasco B, Navarro-León E, Ruiz JM (2019) Study of Zn accumulation and tolerance of HMA4 TILLING mutants of *Brassica rapa* grown under Zn deficiency and Zn toxicity. Plant Sci 287: 110201. https://doi.org/10.1016/J.PLANTSCI.2019.110201

Bocchini M, D'Amato R, Ciancaleoni S et al (2018) Soil selenium (Se) biofortification changes the physiological, biochemical and epigenetic responses to water stress in *Zea mays* L. by inducing a higher drought tolerance. Front Plant Sci 9:389. https://doi.org/10.3389/fpls.2018.00389

Boonyaves K, Wu T-Y, Gruissem W, Bhullar NK (2017) Enhanced grain iron levels in rice expressing an IRON-REGULATED METAL TRANSPORTER, NICOTIANAMINE SYNTHASE, and FERRITIN gene cassette. Front Plant Sci 8:130. https://doi.org/10.3389/fpls.2017.00130

Bouis HE, Saltzman A (2017) Improving nutrition through biofortification: a review of evidence from HarvestPlus, 2003 through 2016. Glob Food Sec 12:49–58. https://doi.org/10.1016/J.GFS.2017.01.009

Chadare FJ, Idohou R, Nago E, Affonfere M, Agossadou J, Fassinou TK, Kénou C, Honfo S, Azokpota P, Linnemann AR, Hounhouigan DJ (2019) Conventional and food-to-food fortification: An appraisal of past practices and lessons learned. Food Sci Nutr 7(9):2781–2795

Chung MY, Han JS, Giovannoni J et al (2010) Modest calcium increase in tomatoes expressing a variant of *Arabidopsis* cation/H^+ antiporter. Plant Biotechnol Rep 4:15–21. https://doi.org/10.1007/s11816-009-0112-9

Cominelli E, Pilu R, Sparvoli F (2020a) Phytic acid and mineral biofortification strategies: from plant science to breeding and biotechnological approaches. Plan Theory 9:553. https://doi.org/10.3390/plants9050553

Cominelli E, Pilu R, Sparvoli F (2020b) Phytic acid and transporters: what can we learn from low phytic acid mutants? Plan Theory 9:69. https://doi.org/10.3390/plants9010069

Conn SJ, Gilliham M, Athman A et al (2011) Cell-specific vacuolar calcium storage mediated by CAX1 regulates apoplastic calcium concentration, gas exchange, and plant productivity in *Arabidopsis*. Plant Cell 23:240–257. https://doi.org/10.1105/tpc.109.072769

Connorton JM, Jones ER, Rodríguez-Ramiro I et al (2017) Wheat vacuolar iron transporter TaVIT2 transports Fe and Mn and is effective for biofortification. Plant Physiol 174:2434–2444. https://doi.org/10.1104/pp.17.00672

D'Imperio M, Renna M, Cardinali A et al (2016) Calcium biofortification and bioaccessibility in soilless "baby leaf" vegetable production. Food Chem 213:149–156. https://doi.org/10.1016/J.FOODCHEM.2016.06.071

De Moura FF, Miloff A, Boy E (2015) Retention of provitamin a carotenoids in staple crops targeted for biofortification in Africa: cassava, maize and sweet potato. Crit Rev Food Sci Nutr 55:1246–1269. https://doi.org/10.1080/10408398.2012.724477

Dixit S, Shukla R, Sharma YK (2018) Biofortification of plant nutrients: present scenario. In: Plant nutrients and abiotic stress tolerance. Springer Singapore, Singapore, pp 119–136

Dutt S, Manjul AS, Chauhan M et al (2019) Biotechnology for nutritional and associated processing quality improvement in potato. Springer, Cham, pp 429–483

Finkelstein JL, Mehta S, Udipi SA et al (2015) A randomized trial of iron-biofortified pearl millet in school children in India. J Nutr 145:1576–1581. https://doi.org/10.3945/jn.114.208009

Gannon B, Kaliwile C, Arscott SA et al (2014) Biofortified orange maize is as efficacious as a vitamin A supplement in Zambian children even in the presence of high liver reserves of vitamin A: a community-based, randomized placebo-controlled trial. Am J Clin Nutr 100:1541–1550. https://doi.org/10.3945/ajcn.114.087379

Gao H, Wu X, Zorrilla C et al (2019) Fractionating of calcium in tuber and leaf tissues explains the calcium deficiency symptoms in potato plant overexpressing CAX1. Front Plant Sci 10:1793. https://doi.org/10.3389/FPLS.2019.01793

García Márquez V, Morelos Moreno Á, Benavides Mendoza A, Medrano Macías J (2020) Ionic selenium and nanoselenium as biofortifiers and stimulators of plant metabolism. Agronomy 10: 1399. https://doi.org/10.3390/agronomy10091399

Garg M, Sharma N, Sharma S et al (2018) Biofortified crops generated by breeding, agronomy, and transgenic approaches are improving lives of millions of people around the world. Front Nutr 5: 12. https://doi.org/10.3389/fnut.2018.00012

Graham NS, Hammond JP, Lysenko A et al (2014) Genetical and comparative genomics of Brassica under altered Ca supply identifies *Arabidopsis* Ca-transporter orthologs. Plant Cell 26:1–14. https://doi.org/10.1105/tpc.114.128603

Gupta PK, Balyan HS, Sharma S, Kumar R (2020) Genetics of yield, abiotic stress tolerance and biofortification in wheat (*Triticum aestivum* L.). Theor Appl Genet 133:1569–1602. https://doi.org/10.1007/s00122-020-03583-3

Gupta PK, Balyan HS, Sharma S, Kumar R (2021) Biofortification and bioavailability of Zn, Fe and Se in wheat: present status and future prospects. Theor Appl Genet 134:1–35. https://doi.org/10.1007/s00122-020-03709-7

Haas JD, Luna SV, Lung'aho MG et al (2016) Consuming iron biofortified beans increases iron status in Rwandan women after 128 days in a randomized controlled feeding trial. J Nutr 146: 1586–1592. https://doi.org/10.3945/jn.115.224741

Hawrylak-Nowak B, Dresler S, Rubinowska K et al (2018) Selenium biofortification enhances the growth and alters the physiological response of lamb's lettuce grown under high temperature stress. Plant Physiol Biochem 127:446–456. https://doi.org/10.1016/J.PLAPHY.2018.04.018

Humayan Kabir A, Swaraz AM, Stangoulis J (2014) Zinc-deficiency resistance and biofortification in plants. J Plant Nutr Soil Sci 177:311–319. https://doi.org/10.1002/jpln.201300326

Idrees M, Cheema SA, Farooq M, Wakeel A (2018) Selenium nutrition for yield enhancement and grain biofortification of wheat through different application methods. Int J Agric Biol 20:1701–1709. https://doi.org/10.17957/IJAB/15.0649

Izydorczyk G, Ligas B, Mikula K et al (2021) Biofortification of edible plants with selenium and iodine – a systematic literature review. Sci Total Environ 754:141983. https://doi.org/10.1016/J.SCITOTENV.2020.141983

Jiang L, Strobbe S, Van Der Straeten D, Zhang C (2021) Regulation of plant vitamin metabolism: backbone of biofortification for the alleviation of hidden hunger. Mol Plant 14:40–60. https://doi.org/10.1016/J.MOLP.2020.11.019

Kendziorek M, Barabasz A, Rudzka J et al (2014) Approach to engineer tomato by expression of AtHMA4 to enhance Zn in the aerial parts. J Plant Physiol 171:1413–1422. https://doi.org/10.1016/J.JPLPH.2014.04.017

Khan A, Singh J, Upadhayay VK et al (2019) Microbial biofortification: a green technology through plant growth promoting microorganisms. In: Sustainable green technologies for environmental management. Springer Singapore, Singapore, pp 255–269

Kumar A, Mirza N, Charan T et al (2014) Isolation, characterization and immunolocalization of a seed dominant CaM from finger millet (*Eleusine coracana* L. Gartn.) for studying its functional role in differential accumulation of calcium in developing grains. Appl Biochem Biotechnol 172:2955–2973. https://doi.org/10.1007/s12010-013-0714-0

Lee S, Ryoo N, Jeon J-S et al (2012) Activation of rice yellow Stripe1-like 16 (OsYSL16) enhances iron efficiency. Mol Cells 33:117–126. https://doi.org/10.1007/s10059-012-2165-9

Li K-T, Moulin M, Mangel N et al (2015) Increased bioavailable vitamin B6 in field-grown transgenic cassava for dietary sufficiency. Nat Biotechnol 33:1029–1032. https://doi.org/10.1038/nbt.3318

Li K, Hu G, Yu S et al (2018) Effect of the iron biofortification on enzymes activities and antioxidant properties in germinated brown rice. J Food Meas Charact 12:789–799. https://doi.org/10.1007/s11694-017-9693-0

Li S, Liu X, Zhou X et al (2019) Improving zinc and iron accumulation in maize grains using the zinc and iron transporter ZmZIP5. Plant Cell Physiol 60:2077–2085. https://doi.org/10.1093/pcp/pcz104

Lyons G, Cakmak I-F (2012) Agronomic biofortification of food crops with micronutrients. In: Fertilizing crops to improve human health: a scientific review, pp 97–122

Mathers AW, Young SD, McGrath SP et al (2017) Determining the fate of selenium in wheat biofortification: an isotopically labelled field trial study. Plant Soil 420:61–77. https://doi.org/10.1007/s11104-017-3374-y

Menguer PK, Vincent T, Miller AJ et al (2018) Improving zinc accumulation in cereal endosperm using HvMTP1, a transition metal transporter. Plant Biotechnol J 16:63–71. https://doi.org/10.1111/pbi.12749

Minhas AP, Tuli R, Puri S (2018) Pathway editing targets for thiamine biofortification in rice grains. Front Plant Sci 9:975. https://doi.org/10.3389/fpls.2018.00975

Morris J, Hawthorne KM, Hotze T et al (2008) Nutritional impact of elevated calcium transport activity in carrots. Proc Natl Acad Sci U S A 105:1431–1435. https://doi.org/10.1073/pnas.0709005105

Narayanan N, Beyene G, Chauhan RD et al (2019) Biofortification of field-grown cassava by engineering expression of an iron transporter and ferritin. Nat Biotechnol 37:144–151. https://doi.org/10.1038/s41587-018-0002-1

Navarro-León E, Ruiz JM, Graham N, Blasco B (2018) Physiological profile of CAX1a TILLING mutants of *Brassica rapa* exposed to different calcium doses. Plant Sci 272:164–172. https://doi.org/10.1016/J.PLANTSCI.2018.04.019

Ojok J, Omara P, Opolot E et al (2019) Iodine agronomic biofortification of cabbage (*Brassica oleracea* var. capitata) and cowpea (*Vigna unguiculata* L.) is effective under farmer field conditions. Agronomy 9:797. https://doi.org/10.3390/agronomy9120797

Paine JA, Shipton CA, Chaggar S et al (2005) Improving the nutritional value of Golden Rice through increased pro-vitamin A content. Nat Biotechnol 23:482–487. https://doi.org/10.1038/nbt1082

Park S, Kang TS, Kim CK et al (2005) Genetic manipulation for enhancing calcium content in potato tuber. J Agric Food Chem 53:5598–5603. https://doi.org/10.1021/jf050531c

Park S, Elless MP, Park J et al (2009) Sensory analysis of calcium-biofortified lettuce. Plant Biotechnol J 7:106–117. https://doi.org/10.1111/j.1467-7652.2008.00379.x

Pittman JK, Hirschi KD (2016) CAX-ing a wide net: Cation/H^+ transporters in metal remediation and abiotic stress signaling. Plant Biol 18:741–749. https://doi.org/10.1111/plb.12460

Ponce-García C, Soto-Parra J, Sánchez E et al (2019) Efficiency of nanoparticle, sulfate, and zinc-chelate use on biomass, yield, and nitrogen assimilation in green beans. Agronomy 9:128. https://doi.org/10.3390/agronomy9030128

Pradhan SK, Pandit E, Pawar S et al (2020) Genetic regulation of homeostasis, uptake, bio-fortification and efficiency enhancement of iron in rice. Environ Exp Bot 177:104066. https://doi.org/10.1016/J.ENVEXPBOT.2020.104066

Prasad R, Shivay YS (2020) Agronomic biofortification of plant foods with minerals, vitamins and metabolites with chemical fertilizers and liming. J Plant Nutr 43:1534–1554. https://doi.org/10.1080/01904167.2020.1738464

Ricachenevsky FK, Vasconcelos MW, Shou H et al (2019) Editorial: improving the nutritional content and quality of crops: promises, achievements, and future challenges. Front Plant Sci 10:738. https://doi.org/10.3389/fpls.2019.00738

Ricci M, Tilbury L, Daridon B, Sukalac K (2019) General principles to justify plant biostimulant claims. Front Plant Sci 10:494. https://doi.org/10.3389/fpls.2019.00494

Rios JJ, Lochlainn SO, Devonshire J et al (2012) Distribution of calcium (Ca) and magnesium (Mg) in the leaves of *Brassica rapa* under varying exogenous Ca and Mg supply. Ann Bot 109: 1081–1089. https://doi.org/10.1093/aob/mcs029

Rosado JL, Hambidge KM, Miller LV et al (2009) The quantity of zinc absorbed from wheat in adult women is enhanced by biofortification. J Nutr 139:1920–1925. https://doi.org/10.3945/jn.109.107755

Sharma A, Verma RK (2019) Biofortification: a promising approach toward eradication of hidden hunger. In: Microbial interventions in agriculture and environment. Springer Singapore, Singapore, pp 313–327

Sharma D, Jamra G, Singh UM et al (2017) Calcium biofortification: three pronged molecular approaches for dissecting complex trait of calcium nutrition in finger millet (*Eleusine coracana*) for devising strategies of enrichment of food crops. Front Plant Sci 7:2028. https://doi.org/10.3389/fpls.2016.02028

Siemianowski O, Mills RF, Williams LE, Antosiewicz DM (2011) Expression of the P1B-type ATPase AtHMA4 in tobacco modifies Zn and Cd root to shoot partitioning and metal tolerance. Plant Biotechnol J 9:64–74. https://doi.org/10.1111/j.1467-7652.2010.00531.x

Sikdar MSI, Bowra S, Schmidt D et al (2016) Targeted modification of storage protein content resulting in improved amino acid composition of barley grain. Transgenic Res 25:19–31. https://doi.org/10.1007/s11248-015-9911-7

Simkin AJ (2019) Genetic engineering for global food security: photosynthesis and biofortification. Plan Theory 8:586. https://doi.org/10.3390/plants8120586

Srivastava MP, Tiwari R, Sharma N (2013) Effect of different cultural variables on siderophores produced by *Trichoderma* spp. Int J Adv Res 1:1–6

Tan S, Han R, Li P et al (2015) Over-expression of the MxIRT1 gene increases iron and zinc content in rice seeds. Transgenic Res 24:109–122. https://doi.org/10.1007/s11248-014-9822-z

Tan GZH, Das Bhowmik SS, Hoang TML et al (2018) Investigation of baseline iron levels in Australian chickpea and evaluation of a transgenic biofortification approach. Front Plant Sci 9: 788. https://doi.org/10.3389/fpls.2018.00788

Tandzi LN, Mutengwa CS, Ngonkeu ELM et al (2017) Breeding for quality protein maize (QPM) varieties: a review. Agronomy 7:80. https://doi.org/10.3390/agronomy7040080

Tang M, He X, Luo Y et al (2013) Nutritional assessment of transgenic lysine-rich maize compared with conventional quality protein maize. J Sci Food Agric 93:1049–1054. https://doi.org/10.1002/jsfa.5845

Till BJ, Datta S, Jankowicz-Cieslak J (2018) TILLING: the next generation. Springer, Cham, pp 139–160

Trijatmiko KR, Dueñas C, Tsakirpaloglou N et al (2016) Biofortified indica rice attains iron and zinc nutrition dietary targets in the field. Sci Rep 6:19792. https://doi.org/10.1038/srep19792

Vega I, Nikolic M, Pontigo S et al (2019) Silicon improves the production of high antioxidant or structural phenolic compounds in barley cultivars under aluminum stress. Agronomy 9:388. https://doi.org/10.3390/agronomy9070388

Verma A (2015) Food fortification: a complementary strategy for improving micronutrient malnutrition (MNM) status. Food Sci Res J 6:381–389. https://doi.org/10.15740/HAS/FSRJ/6.2/381-389

Vlčko T, Ohnoutková L (2019) Recent advances and perspectives in crop biofortification. Biol Plant 63:586–593. https://doi.org/10.32615/bp.2019.056

Wakeel A, Farooq M, Bashir K, Ozturk L (2018) Micronutrient malnutrition and biofortification: recent advances and future perspectives. In: Plant micronutrient use efficiency. Academic Press, pp 225–243

Wang N, Qiu W, Dai J et al (2019) AhNRAMP1 enhances manganese and zinc uptake in plants. Front Plant Sci 10:415. https://doi.org/10.3389/fpls.2019.00415

White PJ, Broadley MR (2009) Biofortification of crops with seven mineral elements often lacking in human diets – iron, zinc, copper, calcium, magnesium, selenium and iodine. New Phytol 182: 49–84. https://doi.org/10.1111/j.1469-8137.2008.02738.x

White PJ, Brown PH (2010) Plant nutrition for sustainable development and global health. Ann Bot 105:1073–1080. https://doi.org/10.1093/aob/mcq085

Wong CKE, Cobbett CS (2008) HMA P-type ATPases are the major mechanism for root-to-shoot Cd translocation in *Arabidopsis thaliana*. New Phytol 181:71–78. https://doi.org/10.1111/j.1469-8137.2008.02638.x

Wu T-Y, Gruissem W, Bhullar NK (2019) Targeting intracellular transport combined with efficient uptake and storage significantly increases grain iron and zinc levels in rice. Plant Biotechnol J 17:9–20. https://doi.org/10.1111/pbi.12943

Ye X, Al-Babili S, Klöti A et al (2000) Engineering the provitamin A (beta-carotene) biosynthetic pathway into (carotenoid-free) rice endosperm. Science 287:303–305. https://doi.org/10.1126/science.287.5451.303

Yi GH, Lee HS, Sohn JK, Kim KM (2012) Physico-chemical properties of *Arabidopsis* Ca^{2+}/H^{+} antiporter transgenic rice grain. Biosci Res 9:8–16

Zhang Y, Xu Y-H, Yi H-Y, Gong J-M (2012) Vacuolar membrane transporters OsVIT1 and OsVIT2 modulate iron translocation between flag leaves and seeds in rice. Plant J 72:400–410. https://doi.org/10.1111/j.1365-313X.2012.05088.x

Zorrilla C, Schabow JE, Chernov V, Palta JP (2019) CAX1 vacuolar antiporter overexpression in potato results in calcium deficiency in leaves and tubers by sequestering calcium as calcium oxalate. Crop Sci 59:176–189. https://doi.org/10.2135/cropsci2018.06.0355

Chapter 3
Food Matrix: Implications for Nutritional Quality

Veda Krishnan, Maharishi Tomar, Lovemore N. Malunga, and Sijo Joseph Thandapilly

Abstract Evidence supporting diet–disease relationships has emphasized the development of functional foods, i.e., foods which confer health benefits far beyond hunger satisfaction and survival. Targeted nutrient-based characterization approaches conducted since the genesis of nutritional sciences exposed that nutrient behave functionally different in isolation compared to their behavior within their inherent matrices. Hence, such studies were incapable of understanding the dynamics of nutrients as well as their bioaccessibility/bioavailability. Thus, the concept of "*food matrix*" evolved to describe the integrated physicochemical domain that contains and/or interacts with nutrients providing unique functionalities and behaviors from those exhibited in isolation. The food matrix governs nutrient bioaccessibility (fraction of released luminal nutrients from matrix after digestion in the gastrointestinal tract) and bioavailability (fraction of nutrients absorbed by the body through circulatory system), which act as the ultimate indicators of nutritional quality. The state and type of nutrient being important, a few macronutrients like carbohydrates, proteins, and lipids have been extensively studied to date, while other bioactives and micronutrients have largely been ignored. Various in vitro and in vivo studies have deciphered that other than nutrient dynamics, intrinsic properties like pH, moisture, enzyme activity, particle size, processing type, food preparation, and absorption and so on also have a significant role in nutrient bioavailability. In this chapter, we briefly introduce the concept of food matrix and its relevance in fine-tuning the nutritional spectrum of crops. We comprehensively elaborate and conceptually explain the different approaches, which have unraveled the role of food matrices as complex real food systems or as fundamental approaches to define the underlying phenomenon. The implications of the food matrix with respect to food processing, flavor perception, satiety, and gut microbiota are also discussed. The

V. Krishnan · M. Tomar
Division of Biochemistry, ICAR-Indian Agricultural Research Institute, New Delhi, India

L. N. Malunga · S. J. Thandapilly (✉)
Agriculture and Agri-Food Canada, Department of Food and Human Nutritional Sciences, University of Manitoba, Winnipeg, MB, Canada
e-mail: lovemore.malunga@agr.gc.ca; Sijo.joseph@agr.gc.ca

R. S. V., S. Praveen (eds.), *Conceptualizing Plant-Based Nutrition*,
https://doi.org/10.1007/978-981-19-4590-8_3

relevance of the food matrix in designing novel food prototypes with customized nutrition addressing food allergies and intolerances is also discussed.

Keywords Bioavailability · Food matrix · Food processing · Food prototypes

3.1 Introduction

Dietary transition is leaving a notorious footprint on health and well-being, which led to an unprecedented increase in lifestyle disorders. Effect of nutrients from diet purely depends on its bioavailability, which in turn depends on its bioaccessibility. The nutrients present in the food get digested, released, and further get bioavailable (Fig. 3.1). During in vivo digestion process, nutrient gets liberated from the matrix, known as bioaccessibility depending on the action of digestive enzymes as well as the complexity of the matrix (in terms of other components as well as interactions among them). Further, the released and solubilized nutrient gets transported to the intestine, where binding and uptake occur at the intestinal mucosa and get transferred

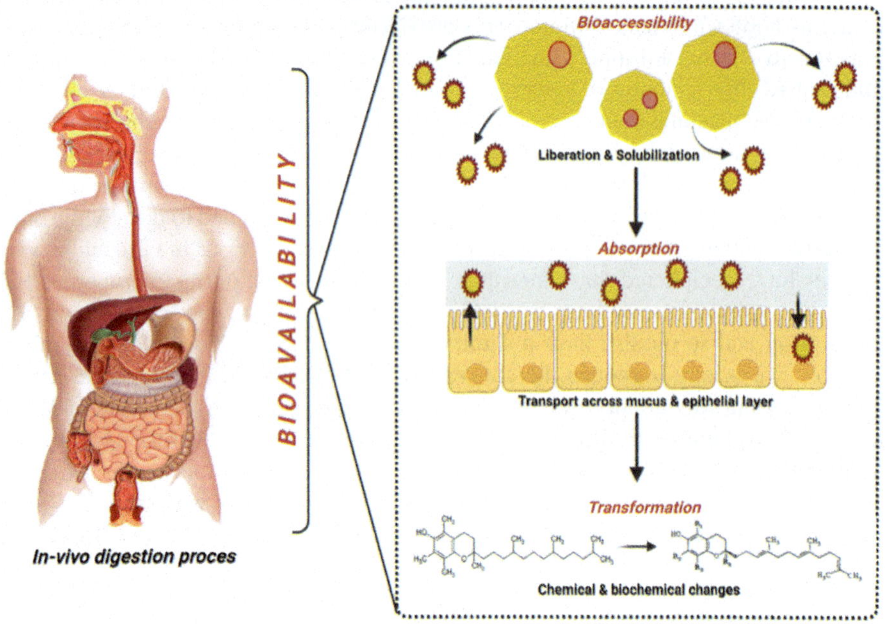

Fig. 3.1 In vivo digestion process depicting nutrient bioavailability. Illustration representing mechanism of in vivo digestion and nutrient bioavailability. After consuming food, it is digested by oral, gastric, and intestinal digestion process involving salivary and pancreatic α-amylases, brush border enzymes, i.e., glucogenic maltase–glucoamylase (MGAM) and sucrase–isomaltase (SI), proteases and lipases. Finally, the released (bioaccessible) nutrient gets solubilized and get absorbed in the small intestine into the bloodstream. The bioavailable form of nutrient either gets transformed or in intact form reaches the target tissue of action

across the gut wall to the blood or lymphatic circulation. Even though the role of nutrients highlighted their importance in food matrix as well as in pure forms toward nutritional benefits, recent studies throw insights on the importance of food matrix studies.

3.2 Role of Food Matrix Toward Understanding Nutritional Quality

The concept of food has evolved over the decades from a source of nutrition to an intricate multicomponent system, where the macro- and microconstituents coexist in an embedded physical state, known as the food matrix. As the macro- and microconstituents along with accessory moieties of flavor, color, and functional nature interact within the matrix, understanding their dynamics at the molecular level is critical for assessing the ultimate indicators of nutritional quality. The "matrix" is a three-dimensional physical space where macro- and micronutrients are packaged to deliver the complex functionality. As the unique packaging pattern affects the functionality in terms of digestibility, it is vital to determine the stability, diffusivity, strength, and scaffolding pattern of the matrix.

With respect to nutrition and food science, foods are nutrient delivery medium and that medium could be uniform or complex. Traditional matrices like dairy are uniform, while nutrient blends for fortification like multigrain flours are complex matrices. Complex matrices can either be naturally (millets) or artificially (nutriblends) prepared (Mondal et al. 2022; Tomar et al. 2022). Not being a mature dimension in nutritional sciences, food matrix is often confused with food microstructure; while former is organization and association of components in multiple spatial length scales, latter is simply the structural organization (Capuano et al. 2018a, b). But the food matrix is a part of food microstructure that typically corresponds to a spatial and physical domain that includes, interacts directly, and/or imparts a specific functionality to a matrix component (nutrient) or food element. Thus, the uniqueness of the food matrix depends on its components as different structural elements in the same food which may interact differently in different matrices. The complexity of specific foods at spatial scale due to their inherent composition (carbohydrates, lipids, protein, and minerals) or added processing constituents like colorants or flavoring molecules could be tagged using visual markers for matrix characterization. Studies have identified that the stability and complexity of food matrix depend on different types of molecular interactions among the components (macro and micro) which includes hydrogen bonding, coordination forces, electrostatic interactions, π–π stacking, and hydrophobic reactions. As the functional attributes like stability and solubility depend on such interactions, it can cause either desirable or undesirable effects to the ultimate quality of food. The impact of food matrix interaction was even highlighted over the molecular assembly (at different length scales) by Ai et al. (2015) endorsing the fact that food matrix alters the ultimate nutritional, functional, and textural aspects of food.

3.3 Different Types of Food Matrices and Their Interactions

Food matrices can be classified as liquid, emulsion, gel, cellular, fibrous, viscoelastic, dense, and artificial (Fig. 3.2). Milk and beverages have been characterized to understand their matrix dynamics in relation to their proximate composition. Another complex liquid matrix well studied is wine, which has been characterized for its components [polyphenolic compounds, polymeric pigments (tannins), minor quantities of proteins, and carbohydrates] as well as their interactions toward color, taste, and aroma. Interaction among flavoring agents, sugar, and phytochemicals such as vitamin C, carotenoids, and flavonoids in fruit juices revealed various dynamics like masking and synergistic effects (Caswell 2009). Retention of aromatic compounds has been studied in emulsion matrices, and their type and composition have been found to influence binding and adsorption ability. Nanoemulsions, multilayer emulsions, solid lipid particles, and filled hydrogel particles comprising varied types of emulsion matrices composed of lipids and bioactives have been initially used as good delivery systems. Later, such emulsion matrix carrier has also

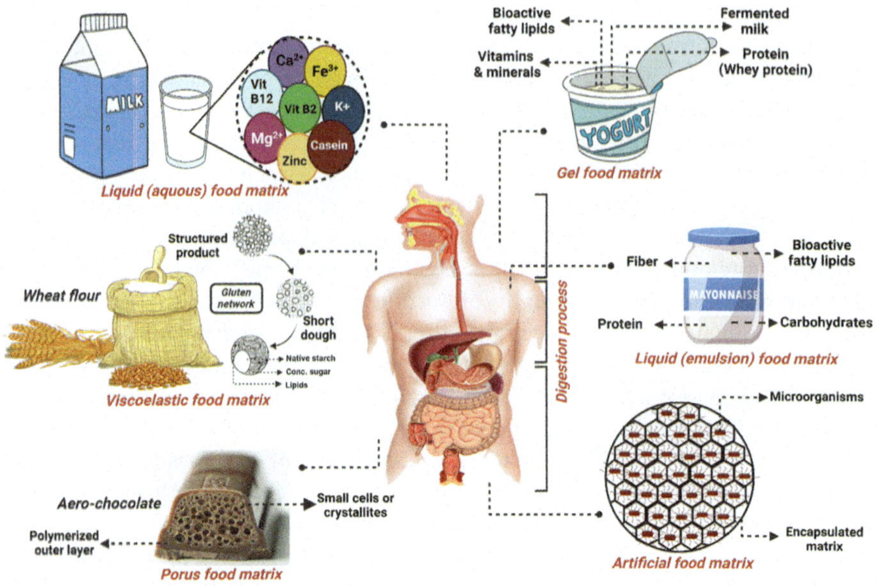

Fig. 3.2 Types of food matrices. Cartoon depicts the different types of food matrices like liquid, gel-based, viscoelastic, emulsion, porous, and artificial

explored to delay digestion (e.g., starch), increase bioavailability (lipids/phenolics), and induce satiety by activating gut–brain axis, targeting lipophilic bioactive components in the gut and so on (McClements and Li 2010; Lim et al. 2021). Other than emulsion matrices, dense matrices which are glassy, semi-crystalline or crystalline, and of moist nature have been frequently used in pharmacology to contain drugs (Baghel et al. 2016). Gel matrices using polymers like gelatin or agar are the major texture providers in desserts and confectionery. Alginate-based gel matrices have been used as suitable carrier systems for bioaccessibility and bioavailability studies. Cellular matrices are another class of most studied food matrices, where fruits and vegetables have been extensively studied for their inherent microstructure as well as composition. It is a hydrated heterogeneous network of supramolecular structures consisting of glucuronoxylans, xyloglucans, pectins, and some structural proteins, reinforced with cellulose as well as hemicellulosic microfibrils (Cosgrove 2005; Flutto 2003). Fibrous extracellular matrices composed of collagen or elastin which primarily provides integrity and texture in food commodities like meat are another matrix to worth explore. Protein, being in diverse nature, impart texture as well as viscoelastic properties to food like in case of gluten. Formations of such viscoelastic matrix, which result from a complex gluten work, assist in gas retention during dough proofing and setting into final porous structure in baked products. Similar viscoelastic network exists in rubber-like chewing gums which results from a continuous matrix of sweeteners (sugars), glycerol, and flavorings dispersed in a discontinuous aqueous phase. Advancement in encapsulation and entrapment led to the development of artificial food matrices for inducing determinant fine-tuned release of metabolites.

Studies have reported that effect on the nutritional quality of food is not always the sum of the effect of individual components or additive, and hence, simply proximal composition analysis after extracting the components cannot deliver the clear picture. It has been found that the component interactions could be synergistic or neutralizing or even toxic against expectations. The presence of two positive nutrients like Ca^{2+} and Mg^{2+} could deliver an added effect being cofactors of many metabolically relevant enzymes and thus assist in nutrient bioavailability, while the presence of an additional component phytic acid to the same matrix could neutralize the effect and make them less bioaccessible. Similarly, if the total effect is higher than the individual effect, it could be synergistic. In contrary to synergism, antagonism happens when the total sum of the effect is found to be less than predicted. The presence of phenolics has been observed with masking effect also as its presence affects the expression of only one component in the matrix. Moreover, based on interactive components, food matrix interactions have also been investigated as binary (like starch–protein or starch–lipid), ternary (starch–protein–lipid), quaternary (starch–protein–lipids–polyphenols) (Krishnan et al. 2020, 2021a, b, c, d), and so on (Fig. 3.3).

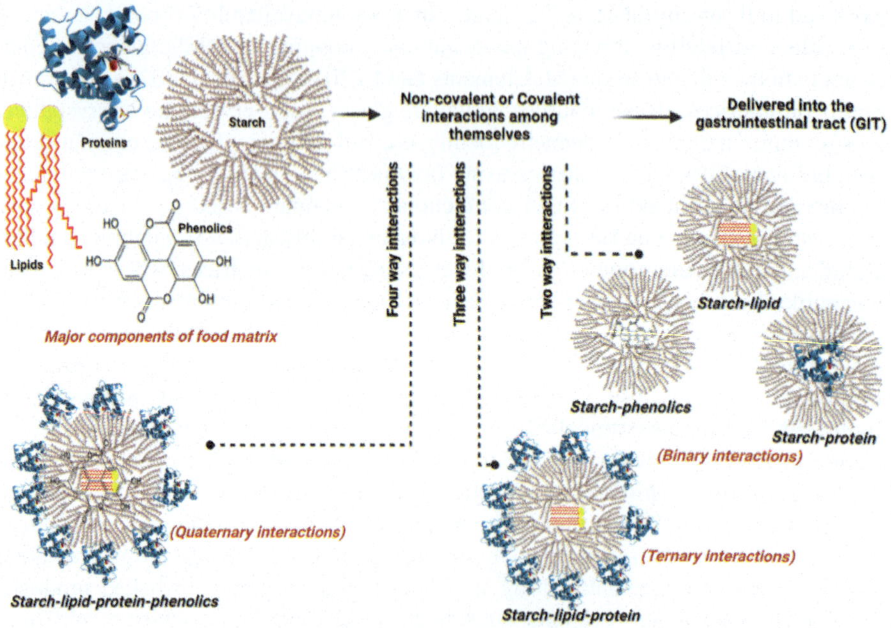

Fig. 3.3 Types of food matrix interactions. Based on the components involved in interaction, food matrix interactions are classified as binary (two-way), ternary (three-way), and quaternary (four-way)

3.4 Food Matrix Alters Nutrient Bioavailability

Nutritional quality of food has been believed to solely depend on the proximate composition. But advances in understanding food matrix clarified that food is not an ideal system with components distributed equally. It is a multicomponent, multidimensional intricate system with various macro- and microcomponents. Thus, the ultimate indicator of quality is nutrient bioavailability. It was also believed that the efficacy of the food matrix is limited to its effect on food digestion which in turn is influenced by the proximate composition. But the recent attention on the nutritional content of foods has challenged this idea with the fact that several food matrix components or nutrients do not act similarly when studied individually vs. as a part of whole foods. Foods with comparable chemical structures and composition differ significantly in the bioavailability of nutrients, physiological functions, gut microbe influence, and overall health implications. This disparity arises from the heterogeneity in interactions between nutrients, food matrix and components, and other host-related effects, underlining the fact that food matrix ultimately governs nutrient bioavailability (Krishnan et al. 2021a, b). Thus, bioaccessibility and bioavailability are influenced by the dynamics with the diverse components more than just their relative abundance in the food matrix (Parada and Aguilera 2007). Hence, nutrient bioavailability is the ultimate determinant of nutritional quality which depends on the type and complexity of the food matrix, discharge rate of components from the matrix, their chemical changes during digestion and absorption, biodistribution, and metabolism.

Decrease in nutrient bioavailability is caused by a variety of physiological events. These processes include slower release due to cell wall integrity or complex nature of special confinement in matrix or sparingly soluble nature or result in insoluble complexes in (GIT) or limited due to low permeable nature through mucous layers (Thakur et al. 2020). In vitro methods to evaluate bioavailability/bioaccessibility have helped to decipher the molecular interactions between food components and nutrients, and the influence of enzyme activity, pH, processing, and food preparation on the absorption of nutrient or biomolecules (Sandberg 2005; Santos et al. 2019). A plethora of in vitro and in vivo studies have discovered that other than the nutrient dynamics, intrinsic components like pH, moisture, enzyme activity, particle size, processing type, food preparation, and absorption also have significant roles in nutrient bioavailability (Parada and Aguilera 2007). Other than the nutrient's abundance in the matrix, the shape, size, surface-to-weight ratio, and processing also influence nutrient bioavailability as they all determine the accessibility of the nutrient from the food matrix (Parada and Aguilera 2007).

The digestibility of protein from grains is dependent on the intactness of their cell walls (Bhattarai et al. 2017). The cell wall prevents or reduces the access of digestive enzymes to cellular proteins and limits protelysis. Many more, humans also lack enzymes that hydrolyze cell wall polymers. Consequently, extracted proteins have a higher digestibility index compared to same protein in its native matrix (Bhattarai et al. 2017; Zahir et al. 2018). Exposing intact cells to gastrointestinal enzymes and buffer causes a less than 3% protein and starch being digested. Thus, mechanical or enzymatic breakdown of the cell wall is required to allow the digestive enzymes access the intracellular proteins or starch. Milling is often used for food grains to disrupt their structural matrix, and degree of milling is often reflected by their particle size distribution. The digestibility of grain protein is inversely correlated to its particle size (Tinus et al. 2012; Zahir et al. 2018). The digestibility of soy protein ranged from 2 to 55% depending on their particle (70–2000 μM) (Zahir et al. 2018). Similarly, the digestibility of cowpea ranged from 58% to 72% depending on milling condition and particle size (Tinus et al. 2012). The fragility of cell wall to mechanical breakdown is dependent on grain species. Consequently, the protein digestibility varies with grain type and cultivar (Nosworthy et al. 2018a). This interspecies variation may be associated with differences in cell wall ligands.

Disruption of the cell wall structure is achieved by mechanical breakdown (milling, grinding, homogenizing, and pureeing), thermal processing, or enzymatic treatments or their combination. Mechanical processes fracture the cell wall integrity and increase the surface area. When combination of these processes is required, the order in which these processes are applied is important to achieve a desired food matrix. Thermal process tends to open cell wall ligands, which restrict accessibility of enzymes and help to unfold the protein structure making it susceptible to enzymatic digestion. The extent of protein denaturation is dependent on primary structure of protein, heat intensity (temperature and time), and intrinsic food properties (water activity and pH) (Capuano et al. 2018a, b). However, rate of heat conduction or grain hydration is dependent on the particle size. Thus, cooking after a milling step is more likely to have a higher protein digestion rate compared to milling after milling step (Zahir et al. 2018). Heating of proteins in the presence reducing sugars may lower protein digestibility due to the Maillard reaction (Jiménez-Castaño et al. 2005; Wang and Ismail 2012). During this browning reaction, Maillard-induced glycosylation of lysine and arginine residues renders them unavailable to hydrolysis by trypsin. Also, Maillard reaction does promote formation of insoluble protein aggregates which cannot be hydrolyzed by human digestive enzymes.

On the other hand, the porosity of the food matrix plays an important role in protein digestion. Porous food matrix allows digestive enzymes access the substrate. Consequently, extruded products tend to have protein digestibility rates compared to similar product in compact format (Nosworthy et al. 2018a, b).

The presence of other macronutrients or cell wall polymers may reduce the rate of protein hydrolysis. This is thought to be a consequent of slowed diffusion or migration of enzymes and substrate in the reaction medium or due to nonspecific binding enzymes to the cell wall polymer or other macromolecules. The nature of compartmentalization of macronutrients (lipid, starch, and protein) in grain does affect their bioaccessibility as tend to affect each other's digestibility (Bhattarai et al. 2016). The discrepancies in results from in vitro digestion are partly because of the order in which digestive enzymes are introduced as well as their enzyme concentrations. For example, comparing protein digestion with pepsin without amylase enzyme resulted in low digestibility of protein compared to when both enzymes were used (Parada and Aguilera 2007).

The nonspecific binding of substrate by other grain compounds or other extrinsic food matrix such as those from condiments and spices may alter the digestibility of protein. For example, flavonoids, proanthocyanidins/anthocyanidins, phytic acid, tannins, and saponins reduce protein digestibility by binding to the substrate (Butler et al. 1984; Frazier et al. 2010; Świeca et al. 2013). The presence of polyphenols may precipitate the protein via noncovalent (ionic or hydrophobic) or covalent interactions. Phytic acid is evenly distributed in the most grain such that it is difficult to reduce it through mechanical processes. Germination or pretreatment with phytase is often used to reduce phytic acid content in grains. Hence, dense composition of food matrix alters the nutrient accessibility and bioavailability which indeed complex but a beneficial trait to explore.

3.5 Implications of Food Matrix in Reference to Food Processing

Understanding the effect of processing on the nutritional profile of the food has been a challenge for food processors and nutritionists for many years. Therefore, how processing strategies modulate food matrix and their downstream effects in functional and nutritional quality along with digestibility of foods is subjects of great interest (Parada and Aguilera 2007; Sensoy 2014). Food processing aims to either prolong shelf life or add value to the diet that has found to have both beneficial and deleterious effects. Positive impacts include microbial safety, better shelf life, improvement (Dunn et al. 2015) in taste, and texture and also found to alter the bioaccessibility and bioavailability of some nutrients (Capuano et al. 2018a, b). Various extrinsic factors including irradiation, heat, and heat–moisture treatment have found to alter not only the structure and functional properties of macronutrients but even bioactives. On the other hand, negative consequences in terms of loss of nutrients, aggregation of proteins, polymerization of oxidized lipids, and the formation of some toxic compounds have also been reported as postprocessing effects (Hoffman and Gerber 2015; Capuano et al. 2018a, b). Such consequences have been corroborated with alterations in the food matrices subjected during food processing. Physical alterations like phase or state transitions along with chemical changes due to thermal reactions have been reported to affect solubilization and further in the state of aggregation or dispersion.

Many food components are released from their original matrices in plant tissues and are converted into useful ingredients that are later combined and processed into products. For instance, cooking of grains, tubers, and legumes increases the digestibility due to the solubilization of the intercellular matrix-binding components and the hydration and subsequent gelatinization of the starch granules (Petitot et al. 2009). Cooking and associated processing strategies involving heat in dry or moist form have been shown to reduce the in vitro starch and protein digestibility in various food matrices (Petitot et al. 2009; Lehmann and Robin 2007; Delcour et al. 2010; Stamataki et al. 2017). This could be due to structural rearrangement in protein forming a continuous matrix trapping starch granules. Thus, it impedes the accessibility of starch granules to amylolytic enzymes in turn reduce digestibility. Throughout the process of food production, heat, moisture, and pressure can significantly alter the digestibility of major macronutrients in the processed foods (Mishra et al. 2012; Lovegrove et al. 2017). In case of starch, when heated in the presence of high moisture, it undergoes substantial changes such as disruption of hydrogen bonds between the starch chains and water absorption by granules, which leads to the swelling of starch granule and subsequent amylose leaching. The change in the molecular architecture of starch due to varying exposure of heat (gelatinization) or cold (retrogradation) alters the digestibility profiles. Time-dependent kinetics thus divides starch into rapid, slow, and resistant categories. It has been validated that the type and degree of alterations that occur in starch are primarily determined by the type of the starch, processing conditions, matrix components, and storage (Aguilera 2006).

Other than starch, protein (casein) and fat globules have known to become "activated" through heating, shearing, and enzymatic treatments. Such processing conditions have found to alter emulsion matrix in case of butter, foams in whipped cream, powder in dried milk, and gels in case of soft cheese or yogurt (Aguilera 2006). Other than the emulsifying, foaming, and gelling properties, egg proteins have also been studied for its potent allergenicity and found that processing practices could alter their immune responses (Jenkins et al. 2007; Benedé et al. 2015). Destruction of the intact microstructure by processing has also reported with liberation of several functional components like isothiocyanates, polyphenols, glucosinolates, carotenoids, and vitamins, improving their bioaccessibility and physiological effect (Parada and Aguilera 2007). For example, even though it is been known that isothiocyanates are anti-carcinogenic, the biological effect could only observe if the microstructure breakdown happens resulting in the release of myrosinase and glucosinolates. The release of precursor as well as the enzyme is critical to generate the bioactive hydrolyzed form (i.e., isothiocyanates). Phenolic compounds have also known to have similar effect like the release of carotenoids which directly depend on the rate of disruption of matrix. On the contrary, in certain cases, the disruption of matrix carrying decompartmentalization causing polyphenol oxidase release leads to oxidative degradation of polyphenols.

Among the processing methods, microbial fermentation and germination (or sprouting) have been found to induce favorable textures, flavors, and metabolite profiles. A decrease in absorption inhibitors like phytates and protease inhibitors has been found to improve mineral bioavailability as well as better protein digestibility (Kumari et al. 2015; Krishnan et al. 2015). Marco et al. (2017) also highlighted the beneficial health contributions of fermentative microorganisms such as probiotics, which produce bioactive metabolites and improve the bioaccessibility of nutrients. During parboiling, restricted migration of matrix components such as phenolics has been found to translocate from the pericarp to the inner grain layers, which has subsequently been found to affect the bioaccessibility of bound phenolics. The presence of inherent phenolics in the food matrix has been reported to reduce zinc uptake by the intestinal cells. The content of mineral-binding phenolics also varied due to their tendency to bind organic compounds like proteins; also, a change in these protein structures could reduce the mineral sequestering properties of phenolics (Pandey and Rizvi 2009).

Food matrix and nutrient bioavailability triangle for consideration while designing foods intended for different nutrient needs is presented in Fig. 3.4. In general, at molecular level, macronutrients in their native form are less accessible to digestive enzymes. At a cell or tissue level, less disruptive or processed foods resist penetration by gastrointestinal enzymes. If processing is necessary, it is important to realize that dense low porous food structure are slows down the rate of digestion.

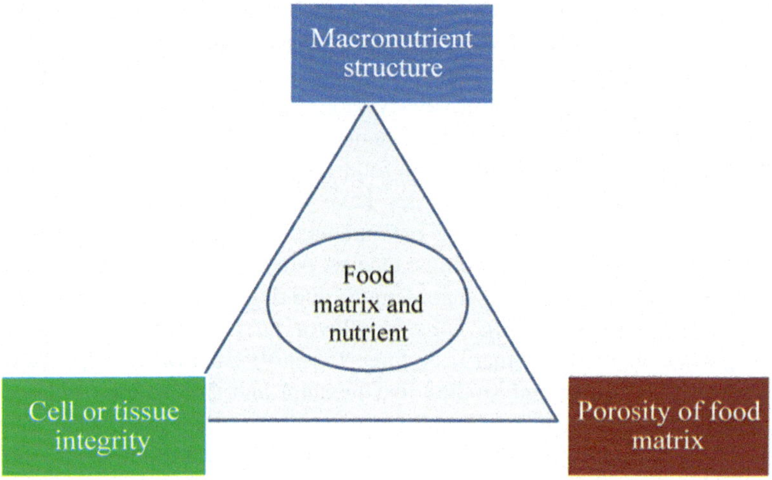

Fig. 3.4 Food matrix and nutrient bioavailability triangle, critical in developing newer prototypes. Native macronutrient structure or less disrupted cell/tissue structure or dense low porous food secondary structures result in less bioaccessible/bioavailable nutrients

3.6 Implications of Food Matrix in Reference to Flavor Perception, Satiety, and Gut Microbiota

Flavor retention and flavor perception are critical and depend on both the matrix and the component. Perception can be defined as a way of understanding how the stimuli in one sensory trait affect other stimuli. Flavor retention depends on flavor discharge, which in turn depends on the affinity of flavor component with the matrix. The most significant interaction with flavor ingredients has been observed with proteins like soy protein, zein, and free amino acids (Plug and Haring 1994; Matheis 1993a). The degrees of denaturation of protein, temperature, and pH have been mostly correlated with protein–flavor component interactions. Proteins and fats have been found to bind to flavor components (hydrocarbons, ketones, alcohols) reversibly through hydrophobic interactions where latter has been found to have better retention. The amino and carboxyl groups of free amino acids have been found to bind with a series of volatile flavoring substances like ketones or alcohols in aqueous media. Among hydrocolloids, starch and its component amylose have been shown to form complexes, but seem to be limited in applications as it changes the viscosity. The helical nature of amylose creates hydrophobic pockets where lipophilic flavors could be easily retained. Other than starch and glycogen, agar, alginates, guar gum, and cellulose have been studied toward flavor interaction and concluded that the type and amount have major role (Plug and Haring 1994; Matheis 1993a).

In case of beverages, highly esterified pectin has been used as a matrix additive to improve the mouth feel as well as viscosity. Further, cross-modal studies have found that viscosity influences both taste and aroma, even when aroma release is not majorly affected (Christensen 1980; Lethuaut et al. 2004). Three-component cross-modal interaction studies between viscosity, aroma, and sweetness in beverages have found that pectin could be used to improve mouth feel without compromising other two traits. Even though fat (majorly di and triglycerides) has been known to retain flavor components in a superior manner, their interactions are usually related to partitioning phenomena based on the relative amount in lipid and water phases. Compared to diglycerides, triglycerides have superior binding and solubilizing ability in case of lipophilic flavoring components. Similarly, compared to oils, fats have been found to have high binding capacity. Among the parameters which affect fat–flavor interactions, fatty acid chain lengths and degree of unsaturation have been found critical (Matheis 1993b). Thus far, flavor interaction studies attempted to explore majorly with two (binary) or three (ternary) components considering the complexity. Multicomponent studies like hexanal and 2-hexanone bound to soy protein and guar gum have been found to have significant binding, while protein or starch with monoglyceride as emulsifiers has been shown to bind fewer flavors in the absence of emulsifier (Matheis 1993b). Clearly, more studies are warranted to dissect such interactive systems through depletion and complementing assays in future.

Another major dimension in food product development is developing newer food prototypes with matrices involving appetite control agents like proteins or fibers having intrinsic satiating properties. Also, at an equivalent caloric value, solid food matrices have stronger satiating effects than liquid ones, which could be due to the low gastric emptying rate (Chambers et al. 2015). Compared to liquid matrices like milk, solid dairy products like cheese and yogurt induce satiety, which highlights the importance of locational digestion-induced ileal brake (Lim et al. 2021; Turgeon and Rioux 2011). A possible explanation is the increased gastric volume induced both by activating stretch receptors and by delaying gastric emptying (van Kleef et al. 2012). This could also be activating the gut–brain axis, while studies to substantiate the fact are still limiting (Fiszman and Varela 2013). In line with this, few examples have shown that satiation could be managed by providing a complex architecture to the matrix (Campbell et al. 2017). New prototypes to delay starch digestion to elicit ileal brake stimulating gut–brain axis are also a promising dimension in food matrix engineering.

Along with genetic component and evolution, the diverse food matrices we consume in our diet also play a large role in shaping microbial communities in the gut. The dietary components in the diet have proved to impact the growth, diversity, and metabolic capacity of the gut microbiome, and consequently, it has been well connected to the chronic metabolic syndromes. Diet induces a shift in the gut microbiota, and such temporary or permanent changes could cause a havoc in the metabolic landscape. Pioneering work on characterization of the obese microbiome underlined an increased Firmicutes to Bacteroidetes ratio and reduced diversity and metabolic capacity in response to high-energy diets (Ward et al. 2020). Although many factors have been shown to affect the composition of the microbiota, a recent study found that the food matrix acts as the primary factor. Semi-purified rodent diets, having cellulose as a source of dietary fiber, promotes a microbiome that degrades the mucin barrier, promotes intestinal inflammation, and thus alters the microbiome profile. There have been very few carefully controlled studies examining oxidized fats on the microbiome. The highly complicated structures of fibers like arabinoxylans as well as modified pectins have also been found to modify the gut microbiome. In a large-scale population-based study, fried food consumption was correlated with lowered α-diversity, whereas foods such as raw vegetables, eggs, fish, and raw fruit were associated with higher α-diversity (Partula et al. 2019). Rats treated with the control or deep-fried oils had distinct microbiomes as assessed by β diversity analysis, but there were no differences in α-diversity. Whether prolonged dietary changes can induce permanent alterations in the gut microbiota is unknown, mainly due to a lack of long-term human dietary interventions or long-term follow-ups of short-term dietary interventions.

3.7 Role of Food Matrix in Designing Novel Food Prototypes

Designing food matrices with customized nutrients addressing the existing challenges of food allergies, malnourishment, and intolerances is very relevant. Food allergy is "an adverse health effect arising from a specific immune response that occurs reproducibly on exposure to a given food." World Health Organization estimates that 250 million people have food allergy (Boye 2012). Incidences of food allergies are on an increase over the past two decades in Western world (Sicherer and Sampson 2014). In Canada, it is estimated that 8% of the population is allergic to certain foods (Soller et al. 2012). In USA, the prevalence of food allergies has increased by 18% from 1997 to 2013 (Keet 2014). It is estimated that 6, 9, 8, and 8.5% of the 0–2, 3–5, 11–13, and 14–18 years old, respectively, is allergic to food in the USA. About 40% of these develop severe allergic reaction upon consumption of allergens, and 30% had multiple food allergies. In general, most common food allergens are peanuts, cow's milk, eggs, soy, wheat, tree nut, fish, shellfish, sesame, and fruits among others.

Food allergies can be classified as immunoglobulin E (IgE)-mediated or cell-mediated. Both genetic and environmental factors are implicated in pathology of food allergens (Lack 2012). For an allergy to happen, an individual must be sensitized to a specific allergen during the first exposure which leads to development of allergen-specific IgE. Allergic response only occurs during the second exposure to the food. In sensitized individuals, allergen avoidance is the only existing remedy and intravenous administration of epinephrine in case of accidental exposure. Food allergens are majorly water-soluble glycoproteins with molecular size ranging from 10 to 70 kDa. Food allergens were found to share less than 35% sequence identity when compared to their human homolog (Jenkins et al. 2007). These proteins resist acidic and protease digestion of the gastrointestinal track and are possibly heat stable. It is suggested that the carbohydrate moiety of the allergens acts as a ligand of dendritic cell-specific intercellular adhesion molecule which stimulates type 2 helper T cells (Th2) response (Wills-Karp et al. 2010). Other than imparting nutrition, molecules released from food matrices during digestion have also been known to elicit adverse reactions like allergies in the body (Vissers et al. 2012). The food allergy epitopes can be sequential or conformational in nature. Specifically, IgE antibodies recognize a specific amino acid sequence in a sequential epitope, whereas in conformational epitopes, amino acids from different regions of the protein are brought together by folding of the protein. Thus, theoretically, disruption of protein structure through processing may improve tolerance where IgE antibodies recognize conformational epitopes. On the other hand, processes that increase the digestibility of protein maybe beneficial in cases where sequential epitopes elicit IgE antibody reaction.

Verhoeckx et al. (2015) reported that inherent matrices and altered profiles during food processing (mainly heating) could be responsible for allergies. The change observed in the extent of allergenicity could be due to heating-induced denaturation. The degree of allergenicity could be higher due to effect of resultant products (like in case of Maillard reaction) or lower due to extensive denaturation. However, the effect of processing induced alterations in the microstructure of matrix, which release allergens that need to be studied in detail. Protein allergenicity has not been significantly reduced by conventional food processing, while microbial fermentation and enzymatic or acid hydrolysis diminished the allergenicity but could not completely eliminate it (Verhoeckx et al. 2015).

Matrix components such as proteolytic or oxidative enzymes and fat content have also reported to elicit or impact allergenicity (Vissers et al. 2012). Thus, a closer look at the respective food matrix should be carried out in order to predict the potential allergenicity or food intolerances.

It has been also shown in multiple research studies that the level of food processing and its digestion could impact the way in which allergens are exposed to immune system (Wal 2003; Maleki 2007; Mills and Mackie 2008). Allergenic foods or proteins could react to physical, chemical, or biochemical changes differently during processing (Verhoeckx et al. 2015). For instance, certain protein denaturation treatments (e.g., thermal processing treatments) could alter three-dimensional epitope confirmation and its IgE binding capacity or it could also result in generation of new epitopes. In addition, the Maillard reaction (most important chemical modifications during thermal processing) may also impact the allergenicity of foods as shown in several studies (Taheri-Kafrani et al. 2009; Nakamura et al. 2006; Ilchmann et al. 2010).

Overall, the nature of allergen, food matrix, and degree/type of thermal processing may be of great significance when evaluating the impact of processing on food allergenicity. Nevertheless, lack of literature on the influence of various food processing approaches on different allergens and in different matrices makes it challenging to predict the allergenicity of foods and offer adequate guidance to allergic patients (Mills and Mackie 2008). In conclusion, each nutrient in food performs differently in a whole food than in its isolated form. Physiologically, the food matrix is a key factor that determines the bioaccessibility and bioavailability as well as the modulation of a healthy microbiota in the gut. As reviewed in the text, future research should focus on methodologies to the characterization of food matrices and their interactions with each component to advance our knowledge on food functionality and nutrient bioaccessibility during digestion. This will enable nutritionists to design special food matrices with improved health attributes. Furthermore, the ability to translate a specific food into the fine-tuned rheological, structural, and functional properties will be also of great interest.

3.8 Concluding Remarks

Dietary approaches addressing global macro- or micronutrient deficiencies call for a better understanding of the relationship between food matrix and nutrient delivery in the human body. In this book chapter, we have provided some evidence that the food matrix alters nutrient bioavailability and organoleptic properties of food. In general, food processing affects the food matrix apart from the inherent characteristics of a food or ingredient. However, controlled studies with a focus on food matrices are needed to provide more data on the association between food matrix and nutrient bioavailability and sensory properties of food.

References

Aguilera JM (2006) Food product engineering: building the right structures. J Sci Food Agric 86: 1147–1155

Ai W, Fang Y, Xiang S, Yao X, Nishinari K, Phillips GO (2015) Protein/polysaccharide electrostatic complexes and their applications in stabilizing oil-in-water emulsions. J Nutr Sci Vitaminol 61(Supplement):S168–S169

Baghel S, Cathcart H, O'Reilly NJ (2016) Polymeric amorphous solid dispersions: a review of amorphization, crystallization, stabilization, solid-state characterization, and aqueous solubilization of biopharmaceutical classification system class II drugs. J Pharm Sci 105(9):2527–2544

Benedé S, López-Expósito I, Molina E, López-Fandiño R (2015) Egg proteins as allergens and the effects of the food matrix and processing. Food Funct 6(3):694–713

Bhattarai RR, Dhital S, Gidley MJ (2016) Interactions among macronutrients in wheat flour determine their enzymic susceptibility. Food Hydrocoll 61:415–425

Bhattarai RR, Dhital S, Wu P, Chen XD, Gidley MJ (2017) Digestion of isolated legume cells in a stomach-duodenum model: three mechanisms limit starch and protein hydrolysis. Food Funct 8(7):2573–2582

Boye JI (2012) Food allergies in developing and emerging economies: need for comprehensive data on prevalence rates. Clin Transl Allergy 2(1):25. https://doi.org/10.1186/2045-7022-2-25

Butler LG, Riedl DJ, Lebryk DG, Blytt HJ (1984) Interaction of proteins with sorghum tannin: mechanism, specificity and significance. J Am Oil Chem Soc 61(5):916–920

Campbell CL, Wagoner TB, Foegeding EA (2017) Designing foods for satiety: the roles of food structure and oral processing in satiation and satiety. Food Struct 13:1–12

Capuano E, Oliviero T, van Boekel MA (2018a) Modeling food matrix effects on chemical reactivity: challenges and perspectives. Crit Rev Food Sci Nutr 58(16):2814–2828

Capuano E, Oliviero T, Fogliano V, Pellegrini N (2018b) Role of the food matrix and digestion on calculation of the actual energy content of food. Nutr Rev 76(4):274–289

Caswell H (2009) The role of fruit juice in the diet: an overview. Nutr Bull 34(3):273–288

Chambers L, McCrickerd K, Yeomans MR (2015) Optimising foods for satiety. Trends Food Sci Technol 41(2):149–160

Christensen CM (1980) Effects of solution viscosity on perceived saltiness and sweetness. Percept Psychophys 28(4):347–353

Cosgrove DJ (2005) Growth of the plant cell wall. Nat Rev Mol Cell Biol 6(11):850–861

Delcour JA, Bruneel C, Derde LJ, Gomand SV, Pareyt B, Putseys JA et al (2010) Fate of starch in food processing: from raw materials to final food products. Annu Rev Food Sci Technol 1:87–111

Dunn KL, Yang L, Girard A, Bean S, Awika JM (2015) Interaction of sorghum tannins with wheat proteins and effect on in vitro starch and protein digestibility in a baked product matrix. J Agric Food Chem 63(4):1234–1241

Fiszman S, Varela P (2013) The role of gums in satiety/satiation. A review. Food Hydrocoll 32: 147–154

Flutto L (2003) PECTIN - properties and determination. In: Caballero B (ed) Encyclopedia of food sciences and nutrition. Academic Press, Oxford, pp 4440–4449

Frazier RA, Deaville ER, Green RJ, Stringano E, Willoughby I, Plant J, Mueller-Harvey I (2010) Interactions of tea tannins and condensed tannins with proteins. J Pharm Biomed Anal 51(2): 490–495

Hoffman R, Gerber M (2015) Food processing and the Mediterranean diet. Nutrients 7(9): 7925–7964

Ilchmann A, Burgdorf S et al (2010) Glycation of a food allergen by the Maillard reaction enhances its T-cell immunogenicity: role of macrophage scavenger receptor class A type ĉ and Ċ. J Allergy Clin Immunol 125(1):175–83.e1-11

Jenkins JA, Breiteneder H, Mills EC (2007) Evolutionary distance from human homologs reflects allergenicity of animal food proteins. J Allergy Clin Immunol 120(6):1399–1405

Jiménez-Castaño L, López-Fandiño R, Olano A, Villamiel M (2005) Study on β-lactoglobulin glycosylation with dextran: effect on solubility and heat stability. Food Chem 93(4):689–695

Keet CA et al (2014) Temporal trends and racial/ethnic disparity in self-reported pediatric food allergy in the US. Ann Allergy Asthma Immunol 112(3):222–29.e3. https://doi.org/10.1016/j.anai.2013.12.007

Krishnan V, Jain P, Vinutha T, Hada A, Manickavasagam M, Ganapathi A, Rai RD, Sachdev A (2015) Molecular modeling and "in-silico" characterization of "Glycine max" inositol (1, 3, 4) tris 5/6 kinase-1(Gmitpk1) - a potential candidate gene for developing low phytate transgenics. Plant Omics 8(5):381–391

Krishnan V, Mondal D, Bollinedi H, Srivastava S, Ramesh SV, Madhavan L, Praveen S (2020) Cooking fat types alter the inherent glycaemic response of niche rice varieties through resistant starch (RS) formation. Int J Biol Macromol 162:1668–1681

Krishnan V, Awana M, Singh A, Goswami S, Vinutha T, Kumar RR, Praveen S (2021a) Starch molecular configuration and starch-sugar homeostasis: key determinants of sweet sensory perception and starch hydrolysis in pearl millet (Pennisetumglaucum). Int J Biol Macromol 183:1087–1095

Krishnan V, Rani R, Awana M, Pitale D, Kulshreshta A, Sharma S, Praveen S (2021b) Role of nutraceutical starch and proanthocyanidins of pigmented rice in regulating hyperglycemia: enzyme inhibition, enhanced glucose uptake and hepatic glucose homeostasis using in vitro model. Food Chem 335:127505

Krishnan V, Mondal D, Thomas B, Singh A, Praveen S (2021c) Starch-lipid interaction alters the molecular structure and ultimate starch bioavailability: a comprehensive review. Int J Biol Macromol 182:626–638

Krishnan V, Awana M, Rani AR, Bansal N, Bollinedi H, Srivastava S, Praveen S (2021d) Quality matrix reveals the potential of Chak-hao as a nutritional supplement: a comparative study of

matrix components, antioxidants and physicochemical attributes. J Food Meas Charact 15(1): 826–840
Kumari S, Krishnan V, Sachdev A (2015) Impact of soaking and germination durations on antioxidants and anti-nutrients of black and yellow soybean (Glycine max. L) varieties. J Plant Biochem Biotechnol 24(3):355–358
Lack G (2012) Update on risk factors for food allergy. J Allergy Clin Immunol 129(5):1187–1197
Lehmann U, Robin F (2007) Slowly digestible starch–its structure and health implications: a review. Trends Food Sci Technol 18(7):346–355
Lethuaut L, Weel KG, Boelrijk AE, Brossard CD (2004) Flavor perception and aroma release from model dairy desserts. J Agric Food Chem 52(11):3478–3485
Lim J, Ferruzzi MG, Hamaker BR (2021) Dietary starch is weight reducing when distally digested in the small intestine. Carbohydr Polym 273:118599
Lovegrove A, Edwards CH, De Noni I, Patel H, El SN, Grassby T et al (2017) Role of polysaccharides in food, digestion, and health. Crit Rev Food Sci Nutr 57(2):237–253
Maleki SJ (2007) Allergenicity of processed food. INFORM 18(3):195–197
Marco ML, Heeney D, Binda S, Cifelli CJ, Cotter PD, Foligné B et al (2017) Health benefits of fermented foods: microbiota and beyond. Curr Opin Biotechnol 44:94–102
Matheis G (1993a) Interactions between volatile flavoring substances and food constituents. Part I: carbohydrates, proteins and amino acids. Dragoco Rep (Flavoring Information Service) 3:98–114
Matheis G (1993b) Interactions between volatile flavours and food composition. Part 1: carbohydrates, proteins, amino acids. Part 2: lipids, inorganic salts, fruit acids, purinalcaloids, phenolic compounds, and complex systems. DRAGOCO-Bericht (Germany) 38:98–114
McClements DJ, Li Y (2010) Review of in vitro digestion models for rapid screening of emulsion-based systems. Food Funct 1(1):32–59
Mills EN, Mackie AR (2008) The impact of processing on allergenicity of food. Curr Opin Allergy Clin Immunol 8(3):249–253
Mishra S, Hardacre A, Monro J (2012) Food structure and carbohydrate digestibility. In: Carbohydrates-Comprehensive studies on glycobiology and glycotechnology. InTech, Rijeka, pp 289–316
Mondal D, Awana M, Aggarwal S, Das D, Thomas B, Singh SP et al (2022) Microstructure, matrix interactions, and molecular structure are the key determinants of inherent glycemic potential in pearl millet (*Pennisetumglaucum*). Food Hydrocoll 127:107481
Nakamura A, Sasaki F, Watanabe K et al (2006) Changes in allergenicity and digestibility of squid tropomyosin during the Maillard reaction with ribose. J Agric Food Chem 54(25):9529–9534
Nosworthy MG, Medina G, Franczyk AJ, Neufeld J, Appah P, Utioh A et al (2018a) Effect of processing on the in vitro and in vivo protein quality of beans (Phaseolus vulgaris and ViciaFaba). Nutrients 10(6):671
Nosworthy MG, Medina G, Franczyk AJ, Neufeld J, Appah P, Utioh A et al (2018b) Effect of processing on the in vitro and in vivo protein quality of red and green lentils (Lens culinaris). Food Chem 240:588–593
Pandey KB, Rizvi SI (2009) Plant polyphenols as dietary antioxidants in human health and disease. Oxidative Med Cell Longev 2(5):270–278
Parada J, Aguilera JM (2007) Food microstructure affects the bioavailability of several nutrients. J Food Sci 72:R21–R32
Partula V, Mondot S, Torres MJ, Kesse-Guyot E, Deschasau M, Assmann K et al (2019) Associations between usual diet and gut microbiota composition: results from the Milieu Intérieur cross-sectional study. Am J Clin Nutr 109(5):1472–1483
Petitot M, Abecassis J, Micard V (2009) Structuring of pasta components during processing: impact on starch and protein digestibility and allergenicity. Trends Food Sci Technol 20(11–12): 521–532
Plug H, Haring P (1994) The influence of flavour-ingredient interactions on flavour perception. Food Qual Prefer 5(1–2):95–102

Sandberg AS (2005) Methods and options for in vitro dialyzability; benefits and limitations. Int J Vitam Nutr Res 75(6):395–404

Santos DI, Saraiva JMA, Vicente AA, Moldão-Martins M (2019) Methods for determining bioavailability and bioaccessibility of bioactive compounds and nutrients. In: Innovative thermal and non-thermal processing, bioaccessibility and bioavailability of nutrients and bioactive compounds. Woodhead Publishing, Duxford, pp 23–54

Sensoy I (2014) A review on the relationship between food structure, processing, and bioavailability. Crit Rev Food Sci Nutr 54:902–909

Sicherer SH, Sampson HA (2014) Food allergy: epidemiology, pathogenesis, diagnosis, and treatment. J Allergy Clin Immunol 133(2):291–307

Soller L, Ben-Shoshan M, Harrington DW, Fragapane J, Joseph L, Pierre YS, Clarke AE (2012) Overall prevalence of self-reported food allergy in Canada. J Allergy Clin Immunol 130(4): 986–988

Stamataki NS, Yanni AE, Karathanos VT (2017) Bread making technology influences postprandial glucose response: a review of the clinical evidence. Br J Nutr 117(7):1001–1012

Świeca M, Gawlik-Dziki U, Dziki D, Baraniak B, Czyż J (2013) The influence of protein–flavonoid interactions on protein digestibility in vitro and the antioxidant quality of breads enriched with onion skin. Food Chem 141(1):451–458

Taheri-Kafrani A, Gaudin JC et al (2009) Effects of heating and glycation of beta-lactoglobulin on its recognition by IgE of sera from cow milk allergy patients. J Agric Food Chem 57(11): 4974–4982

Thakur V, Dogra S, Verma S, Vashist H (2020) Solubility enhancement techniques. World J Pharma Res 9(13):265–282

Tinus T, Damour M, Van Riel V, Sopade PA (2012) Particle size-starch–protein digestibility relationships in cowpea (Vigna unguiculata). J Food Eng 113(2):254–264

Tomar M, Bhardwaj R, Verma R, Singh SP, Krishnan V, Kansal R et al (2022) Interactome of millet-based food matrices: a review. Food Chem 385:132636

Turgeon SL, Rioux LE (2011) Food matrix impact on macronutrients nutritional properties. Food Hydrocoll 25(8):1915–1924

van Kleef E, van Trijp JCM, van den Borne JJGC, Zondervan C (2012) Successful development of satiety enhancing food products: towards a multidisciplinary agenda of research challenges. Crit Rev Food Sci Nutr 52:611–628. https://doi.org/10.1080/10408398.2010.504901

Verhoeckx KC, Vissers YM, Baumert JL, Faludi R, Feys M, Flanagan S et al (2015) Food processing and allergenicity. Food Chem Toxicol 80:223–240

Vissers YM, Wichers HJ, Savelkoul HFJ (2012) Influence of food processing, digestion and the food matrix on allergenicity & cellular measures of allergenicity. In: Multidisciplinary approaches to allergies. Springer, Berlin, pp 203–227

Wal JM (2003) Thermal processing and allergenicity of foods. Allergy 58(8):727–729

Wang Q, Ismail B (2012) Effect of Maillard-induced glycosylation on the nutritional quality, solubility, thermal stability and molecular configuration of whey protein. Int Dairy J 25(2): 112–122

Ward RE, Benninghoff AD, Hintze KJ (2020) Food matrix and the microbiome: considerations for preclinical chronic disease studies. Nutr Res 78:1–10

Wills-Karp M, Nathan A, Page K, Karp CL (2010) New insights into innate immune mechanisms underlying allergenicity. Mucosal Immunol 3(2):104–110

Zahir M, Fogliano V, Capuano E (2018) Food matrix and processing modulate in vitro protein digestibility in soybeans. Food Funct 9(12):6326–6336

Chapter 4
Plant-Based Nutraceuticals

Ramesh S. V. and Shelly Praveen

Abstract Nutraceuticals are a portmanteau of "nutrients" and "pharmaceuticals" denoting substances that are rich in nutrients that confer immense health benefits. Plants are rich source of nutraceuticals as studies have demonstrated the link between the dietary intakes of plant-derived foods with that of abundant health benefits. A wide array of phytochemicals such as glucosinolates and various polyphenols including anthocyanins, flavones, isoflavones, stilbenoids, ellagicacid, allyl sulfides, anthocyanidins, catechins, and carotenoids provide diverse health benefits, namely in the treatment of metabolic syndromes and diseases such as cancer and in improving the brain health and the general immune system. Unlike the functional foods, which are a component of regular diet that improves the overall health status besides its primary nutritional function, nutraceuticals are concentrated forms of the plant-derived compounds in an altered formulation. Nevertheless, nutraceuticals display specific physiological benefits and confer protection against acute and chronic diseases, etc. The role of plant-based nutraceuticals in the prevention and treatment of cardiovascular diseases, obesity, cancer, diabetes and antiaging and immune-boosting properties has been demonstrated. Besides the whole plants, the fruit and vegetable residues are gaining much attention owing to their potential richness in plant-based nutraceuticals. Furthermore, nutraceuticals interact with gut microbiota leading to altered bioavailability and pharmacokinetics of the phytochemicals. Different delivery vehicles, viz. liposomes, emulsion-based delivery, and nanoencapsulation, have been devised to improve the bioavailability of nutraceuticals. Also, a science-based food regulatory regimen exclusively for the plant-based nutraceuticals is warranted. This chapter discusses the concept of plant-based nutraceuticals enumerating our current understanding of biochemical features of phytochemicals and their mode of action in improving the health and

R. S. V. (✉)
Physiology, Biochemistry and Post-Harvest Technology Division, ICAR-Central Plantation Crops Research Institute, Kasaragod, Kerala, India
e-mail: ramesh.sv@icar.gov.in

S. Praveen
Division of Biochemistry, ICAR-Indian Agricultural Research Institute, New Delhi, Delhi, India

R. S. V., S. Praveen (eds.), *Conceptualizing Plant-Based Nutrition*,
https://doi.org/10.1007/978-981-19-4590-8_4

physiological well-being. Furthermore, the role of gut microbiota and its interaction with nutraceuticals and various delivery vehicles to improve the bioavailability of phytochemicals is discussed along with the need for the regulatory regime.

Keywords Nutraceuticals · Functional foods · Dietary supplements · Food residues · Antioxidants · Polyphenols · Phytotherapy

4.1 Introduction

Nutraceuticals refer to biologically active molecules present in food, and these molecules share the characteristic features of both the nutrients and medicines. Thus, nutraceuticals could be defined as naturally occurring bioactive molecule or chemical compound which besides satisfying the nutritional requirement plays a significant role in either overall health promotion or disease prevention or possess novel therapeutic effects (Fig. 4.1). Further, the constructive effects of nutraceuticals in the treatment of multiple ailments such as atherosclerosis, cardiovascular complications, diabetes, inflammation-related disorders, cancer, and neurodegenerative diseases have been well demonstrated (Sachdeva et al. 2020).

World Health Organization (WHO)-based Global Health Expenditure database reveals that United States spends 17% of its GDP and India spends 4% of its GDP on health care alone suggesting the interests on the development of various food products with potential health benefits. Further, the global nutraceutical market is expected to grow into USD 722.49 billion in the year 2027 (https://www.grandviewresearch.com/industry-analysis/nutraceuticals-market) (Accessed on 01/Sep/2021). This spurt in the growth of nutraceutical industry is due to the ever-increasing demand for functional foods and the thriving food and beverage industry. Additionally, the growth of old age population, increasing cost of health care, changes in the lifestyles, and innovations in the food sector have contributed to this demand for nutraceutical products. Asia-Pacific region alone has a market share of a little over 30% in the nutraceutical products. Indian nutraceutical demand is anticipated to touch a whopping USD 18 billion by 2025 from a modest USD 2.5 billion in the year 2015 (https://www.nuffoodsspectrum.in/news/46/5644/assocham-all-set-to-organize-5th-edition-of-nutraceuticals-symposium-.html).

DrugBank database (http://www.drugbank.ca/) enlists a collection of 537 nutraceutical products suggesting the wide range of these products in terms of applications and their characteristics features (Drug Bank database (http://www.drugbank.ca/) (Accessed on Aug 31, 2021). The plant-based nutraceuticals are obtained from different parts such as roots, bark, stem, leaves, flowers, pollen, fruits, and seeds. Plant nutraceuticals systemically interact with diverse targets in various organs to exert multiple health benefits including antioxidant, anti-inflammatory, antiproliferative, antimicrobials, and hypocholesterolemic properties (Taroncher et al. 2021). In this context, this chapter presents an overview of plant-based nutraceuticals including their biochemical nature, mode of action providing nutraceutical properties, treatment of various ailments, mode of delivery, and glimpses of regulatory regimen.

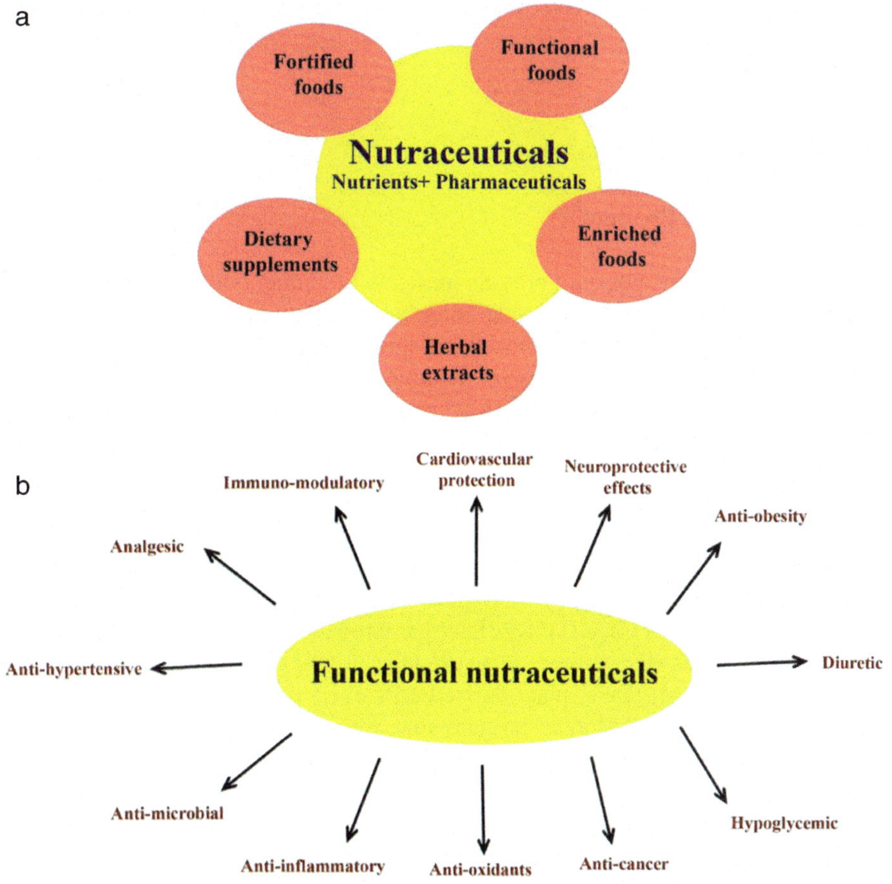

Fig. 4.1 Plant-derived nutraceuticals and its functional roles. (**a**) Nutraceuticals share the characteristic features of various dietary intakes such as fortified, functional, enriched foods, dietary supplements, and herbal extracts. (**b**) Nutraceuticals possess diverse nutritional and functional roles ranging from cardiovascular protection, neuroprotective effects, and immune-modulatory functions among others in human body

4.2 Nature of Nutraceuticals

Nutraceuticals constitute a wide array of plant metabolites that are bioactive food components providing immense health and medical benefits (Gul et al. 2016). Besides the primary metabolites, viz. carbohydrates, proteins, lipids, and vitamins which are mandatorily required for growth and maintenance of cellular functions, plant-derived secondary metabolites such as polyphenols (their derivatives), flavonoids, stilbenes, lignans, isoprenoids, alkaloids, carotenoids, amino alcohols, thiosulfinic acids, and phycobiliproteins form a major component of nutraceuticals (Gupta et al. 2019). The biochemical nature of the potential and clinically proven nutraceuticals, their sources, and biological implications is discussed below and also presented in Table 4.1.

4.2.1 Primary Metabolites

4.2.1.1 Bioactive Peptides

Food-derived proteins not only provide nutrients to human body but also modulate its physiological functions. The underlying basis for beneficial effect of food proteins could be attributed to the bioactive peptides (BP). Thus, BPs exert positive influences such as antihypertensive, antimicrobial, antioxidant, antithrombotic, immunomodulatory, and mineral binding among others on body functions (Chakrabarti et al. 2018). Despite poor understanding of structure–function relationship of BPs, evidences reveal that they are generally 2–20 amino acids of length and rich in hydrophobic amino acids among others such as arginine, lysine, and proline. A critical feature, that BPs are resistant to the activities of digestion peptidases, makes them potentially bioactive. Thus, amino acid sequence and composition of BPs significantly determine their biological potency upon release from their precursor proteins. Beneficial effects of BPs have garnered the interest of the biologists and food engineers to develop nutraceutical products utilizing protein-rich underutilized food products. For instance, plant-derived BPs exert potential health benefits. Of greater interest are seed storage proteins that are readily available and are major sources of BPs. Based on their solubility, seed storage proteins are classified into albumins (water soluble); globulins (soluble in dilute salt solutions); glutelins (soluble in dilute acid or alkali); and prolamins (soluble in water/alcohol mixtures). Seed proteins of dicots such as legumes are rich in albumins and globulins, whereas cereals or monocots predominantly have glutelins and prolamins. BPs of seed storage proteins have antiviral, antimicrobial, antitumor, antithrombotic, antihypertensive, antioxidant, and immune-modulatory characteristic features (Kumar et al. 2019).

4.2.1.2 Bioactive Lipids

Bioactive lipids (BLs) have widened the scope of dietary lipids from their conventional roles such as components of cell membrane and as a source of energy reserve to myriads of functions like cellular signaling and regulation. Thus, a critical factor that distinguishes the role BLs from normal lipids is its ability to improve human wellness besides serving as a source of energy. Various BLs, namely ceramides, diacylglycerols (DAG), eicosanoids, steroid hormones, and LPAs, are potent biochemicals that link the external stress signals to internal metabolism, having regulatory role and activating protein cascading pathways, acting as lipid-soluble signaling molecule, and intercellular signals, respectively, etc. Consumption of

Table 4.1 A repertoire of plant bioactives with potential and demonstrated nutraceutical properties

Class	Compounds	Source	Nutraceutical potential	References
Heteroglycans	Galactomannan	*Trigonella foenumgraecum*	Antidiabetic	Garg (2016)
Amino alcohol	Hydroxyisoleucine	*Trigonella foenumgraecum*	Antidiabetic, improves blood lipid spectre, renoprotective, improves insulin secretion	Garg (2016)
Thiosulfinic acid esters	Allicin, diallyl thiosulfinate, allyl methyl disulfide	*Allium sativum, Allium cepa, Allium ursinum*	Free radical scavenging, antioxidants, anti-infective agents, hypolipidemic and hypoglycemic, calcium channel inhibition, spasmolytic	Wang et al. (2017a, b) and Chan et al. (2013)
L-alanine derivatives	Alliin (methylalliin, methiin, and allylalliin)	*Allium sativum, Allium cepa, Allium ursinum*	An antioxidant, a cardioprotective agent, a neuroprotective agent, and an antimicrobial agent, calcium channel inhibition, spasmolytic	Wang et al. (2017a, b)
Allyl sulfur compounds	Allyl sulfide	*Allium sativum, Allium cepa*	Antioxidant, anticarcinogenic	Wang et al. (2017a, b)
p-benzoquinones	Thymoquinone	*Nigella sativa*	Anticancer, proapoptotic effect, antiautoimmune diseases, antiasthma, antidiabetic	Gupta et al. (2016)
Phycobiliproteins	C-phycocyanin	*Spirulina platensis/Arthrospira platensis*	Antianemia, antimicrobial, antidiabetic, chemopreventive, anticancer, and neuroprotective	Martinez et al. (2015)
Biopeptides	Amaranth Alb, amaranth glob, 11S globulin tetrapeptides	*Amaranthus hypochondriacus* L.	Antihypertensive, antioxidative, hypocholesterolemia, immunomodulatory, antitumor, hypoglycemic, and antianemia	Rastogi and Shukla (2013)
	Abrin, ricin, concanavalin A, vicilin, legumin, convicilin, α,β, γ vignin,	Legume (*Pisum sativum, Vicia faba, Vigna unguiculata, Glycine max, Phaseolus vulgaris)* seed storage proteins	Antiviral, antimicrobial, antitumor, antithrombotic, antihypertensive, antioxidant, and immunomodulatory	Kumar et al. (2019)

(continued)

Table 4.1 (continued)

Class	Compounds	Source	Nutraceutical potential	References
	Cucurbitin, cruciferin	*Cucurbita* spp., *Brassica napus*, seed storage proteins	Antiviral, antimicrobial, antitumor, antithrombotic, antihypertensive, antioxidant, and immunomodulatory	Kumar et al. (2019)
	Glutelins	Rice endosperm	Antiviral, antimicrobial, antitumor, antithrombotic, antihypertensive, antioxidant, and immunomodulatory	Kumar et al. (2019)
	Zeins, ribosome inactivating proteins, cystatins	Seed storage proteins	Antiviral	Kumar et al. (2019)
Biolipids	α-linolenic acid (ALA)	*Linum usitatissimum,* blackberry, raspberry, bitter gourd, sparkleberry, and romaine lettuce, almonds, chia seeds, walnuts, soybean green raw, green leafy vegetables, rapeseed	Inhibits synthesis of prostaglandins hence reduced inflammation, prevents chronic diseases, hypertension, thyroid cancer, decreases serum triglycerides, and reduces cardiovascular diseases	Yu et al. (2017)
	EPA (eicosapentaenoic acid)	*Chlorella minutissima, Nannochloropsis* sp.	Skin and hair growth as well as for proper visual, neural, and reproductive functions of the body	Gu et al. (2021)
	Lauric acid	*Cocos nucifera* L.	Neuroprotective functions, antiviral properties	Ramesh et al. (2020, 2021)
	DHA (docosahexaenoic acid)	*Crypthecodinium cohnii* sp., *Ceratium horridum*	–	Maltsev and Maltseva (2021)
	EPA and DHA	*Phaeodactylum tricornutum, Pavlova lutheri*	–	Maltsev and Maltseva (2021)
Isoprenoids				
Monoterpenes	Citronellal, citronellol, geraniol	Lemon grass oil, *Cymbopogon winterianus, Corymbia citriodora*	Antifungal, antibacterial, neuroprotective	Salem et al. (2018)
	α-Pinene, borneol	*Salvia lavandulifolia*	Antimicrobial, antioxidant	Cutillas et al. (2017)

	Limonene (p-mentha-1,8-diene)	Oil from citrus, orange, lemon, grapefruit, *Anethum graveolens*	Prevents DNA damage, anticancer, treatment of gastric diseases	Bacanlı et al. (2017)
	Eugenol	Clove oil	Antibacterial, antifungal, antioxidant, cardioprotective	Ranasinghe et al. (2017)
	Nocellaralactone	*Olea europaea*	Anti-inflammatory	Serrilli et al. (2013)
	Linalool	Lamiaceae (mentha), Lauraceae (laurel), Rutaceae (citrus), *Lavandula angustifolia*	Hypoglycemic	Capetti et al. (2020)
	Menthol	*Mentha piperita*	Antiseptic and anesthetic	
	Sabinene	*Myristica fragrans*		
	Carvacrol (aromatic monoterpenoids)	Thyme and oregano oil from *Origanum* sp.	Antimycotic, and antiplatelet	Bacanlı et al. (2017)
	γ-terpinene	Thyme and oregano oil	Antimycotic and antiplatelet	Bacanlı et al. (2017)
	Terpinen-4-ol	White cabbage, yellow bell pepper, red bell pepper, and nutmeg, tea tree oil (*Melaleuca alternifolia*)	Antifungal, antibacterial, antipneumonic, antilice, anti-inflammatory	Li et al. (2017)
	Terpinolene	Cabbage, carrot, hyssop, and fennel, *Melaleuca alternifolia*	Antifungal, antibacterial, antipneumonic, antilice, anti-inflammatory	Li et al. (2017)
	Safranal	Fig, saffron, tea	Anticonvulsant, free radical scavenging, agonist at GABA receptor	Hoshyar and Mollaei (2017)
8-prenylated xanthones	Mangostanin, and α-mangostin	*Garcinia mangostana*	Anti-inflammatory, antiproliferative, neuroprotective, hypoglycemic, antiobesity, and quinone reductase induction	Ovalle-Magallanes et al. (2017)
Sesquiterpenes	Elemene, curdione, turmerone, bisacurone, germacrone	*Curcuma sp.*	Anti-inflammatory	
	Farnesol, nerolidol	*Citrus x aurantium*	Anti-inflammatory	

(continued)

Table 4.1 (continued)

Class	Compounds	Source	Nutraceutical potential	References
Diterpene	Taxol	*Taxus brevifolia*	Anticancer	
	Forskolin	*Coleus forskohlii*	Anti-HIV, antihypertensive, platelet aggregation inhibitor, anti-inflammatory, anticancer	Risuleo (2016)
	Crocin, crocetin, transcrocetin	*Crocus sativus* L.	Treatment of hyperglycemia, metabolic syndrome, hypertriglyceridemia, and hypercholesterolemia, anticarcinogenic	Hoshyar and Mollaei (2017)
Triterpenes	Glycyrrhizin	*Glycyrrhiza glabra*	Antihypertensive, antiedema, potential expectorant, and gastrokinetic activities	Kim et al. (2017)
	Ginsenoside rb2, ginsenoside Rgl, ginsenoside Rbl, and ginsenoside Rd	*Panax notoginseng*	Protects against memory impairment, antipancreatitis, antiapoptotic, antiautophagy	Liu et al. (2018)
	Lupeol	Lupins, *Ficus racemosa,* rubber	Anti-inflammatory and antimicrobial	Bopage et al. (2018)
	Boswellic acids: β-boswellic acid and derivatives	*Boswellia serrata*	Anti-inflammatory, analgesic, antipyretic, and platelet inhibitory actions, antiarthritic, prostate tumor inhibitor, neuroprotective	Ameen et al. (2017)
	Ursolic acid	*Malus pumila, Ocimum basilicum*	Anti-infective, antineoplastic agents, antiarthritis, antiulcer, anticancer, antidiabetes	Bacanlı et al. (2017)
Alkaloids	Morphine	*Papaver somniferum*	Analgesic	Dang et al. (2012)
	Camptothecin	*Camptotheca acuminata*	Anticancer	Dang et al. (2012)
	Atropine	*Hyoscyamus niger*	Prevention of intestinal spams, antidote to other poisons	Dang et al. (2012)

	Vinblastine	*Catharanthus roseus*	Anticancer	Dang et al. (2012)
	Codeine	*Papaver somniferum*	Analgesic, antitussive	Dang et al. (2012)
	Caffeine	*Coffea arabica*	Stimulant, natural pesticides	Dang et al. (2012)
	Anaferine, anahygrine, withanine, somniferine, withaferin A	*Withania somnifera* L.		Dang et al. (2012)
	Berberine, thalifendine, berberrubine, and jatrorrhizine	*Berberis vulgaris, Berberis aristata,* etc.	Antidiabetic, cardiovascular and metabolic disorders, gastroenteritis, and neurodegenerative diseases	Kumar et al. (2015)
	Trigonelline	*Trigonella foenumgraecum*	Antidiabetic, renoprotective, neuroprotective, and antioxidant	Garg (2016)
Phytosteroids	Withanolides, withanol, diosgenin	*Withania somnifera* L.	Antidepressant, antifungal, antimicrobial, antimalarial, chondroprotective, cholinesterase inhibiting and promoting learning and memory in Alzheimer's, antioxidative, anti-inflammatory, antiaging, anxiolytic, and antitumor	Bharti et al. (2016)
	Diosgenin	*Trigonella foenumgraecum*	Antidiabetic, antioxidative, hepatoprotective	Garg (2016)
	β-sitosterol	*Ficus racemosa,* lemon thyme, pitanga, mixed nuts	Antimicrobial and wound healing	Bopage et al. (2018)
Phenolics				
Hydroxycinnamic acids	Caffeic acid, ferulic acid, chlorogenic acid, neochlorogenic acid, P-coumaric acid, sinapic acid, caftaric acids	Coffee, strawberry, grape, potato, lettuce, spinach, coffee beans, tea, cider, *Baccharis dracunculifolia* DC.	Antioxidant, anti-inflammatory, nutraceuticals in obesity and associated metabolic disorders, and immunomodulatory	Razzaghi-Asl et al. (2013)

(continued)

Table 4.1 (continued)

Class	Compounds	Source	Nutraceutical potential	References
Hydroxybenzoic acids	Gallic acid	Fruits and vegetables	Reduce inflammation in ulcerative colitis and Crohn's disease, and in allergic rhinitis and asthma	Choubey et al. (2018)
	Ellagic acid	*Syzygium cumini* L., raspberries, strawberries, cranberries, and pomegranates, *Terminalia chebula*	Antioxidant, antiproliferative, or anticancer	Ríos et al. (2018)
Phenolic acids	Protocatechuic acid and its derivative vanillic acid	*Olea europaea*, *Hibiscus sabdariffa* and grapes	Alleviate gingivitis, reduce inflammatory pain	Kumar and Goel (2019)
	Rosmarinic acid	*Rosmarinus officinalis, Salvia officinalis, Melissa officinalis*	Inhibits seasonal allergic rhinoconjunctivitis, application in atopic dermatitis	Kumar and Goel (2019)
	2-Hydroxy-3,4-dihydroxyacetophenone, methyl 3,4-dihydroxybenzoate, 3,4-dihydroxyphenyl acetate	*Tamarindus indica* L.	Free radical scavenging, antioxidative, and antidiabetic	Kumar and Goel (2019)
	Carthatins	*Carthamus tinctorius* L. (seed oil cake)	Acetylcholineesterase inhibitory activity	Kumar and Goel (2019)
Phenyl alcohols	Tyrosol, hydroxytyrosol	Olive oils	Prevention of cardiac arrhythmias, antioxidants	Bonechi et al. (2019)
	Carthamins	*Carthamus tinctorius* L.	Antioxidative	Lu et al. (2019)
Ferulic acid esters	Oryzanol	Wheat bran oil or rice bran oil	Antiulcer and hypolipidemic agents	Wang et al. (2017a, b)
	Cinnamic acid, cinnamyl acetate, cinnamaldehyde	*Cinnamomum zeylanicum*	Bactericidal, fungicidal, antidiabetic, antiparasitic, antioxidative, antihyperlipidemia, antihypertensive, and cardioprotective	Ranasinghe et al. (2017)
Substituted guaiacol	Eugenol	*Cinnamomum zeylanicum*	Bactericidal, fungicidal, in the treatment of gastrointestinal and respiratory complaints	Ranasinghe et al. (2017)

	Sinapic acid	*Brassica juncea*	Peroxynitrite scavenging activity	Zou et al. (2002)
Diarylheptanoids	Curcumin, mitocurcumin	*Curcuma longa*	Neuroprotective, antioxidative, anti-inflammatory, antiosteoarthritis, anticardiovascular diseases, anticancer, and wound healing	Mohanty and Sahoo (2017)
Phenolic lipids	Anacardic acids	*Anacardium occidentale*	Anti-Alzheimer's disease, antiapoptotic, antioxidative, and antibacterial	Oiram Filho et al. (2018)
Phenolic derivative	Asaricin	*Piper hispidinervum*, *P. sarmentosum*, *P. hancei*	Anticholinesterase	Xiang et al. (2017)
Benzoic acid derivatives	Salicylic acid	Lettuce, apple, plumb, Artichoke	Anticancerous	Anantharaju et al. (2017)
Anthocyanidins	Delphinidin, cyanidin, petunidin, peonidin, and malvidin, cyanidin 3-galactoside, cyanidin 3-glucoside, cyanidin 3-arabinoside, cyanidin 3-xyloside, pelargonidin	Blueberry (*Vaccinium corymbosum*), wild blueberries (*Vaccinium angustifolium* Aiton and *V. myrtilloides* Michaux), blackberries, black currant, blueberries, black grape, elderberries, strawberries, cherries, plums, cranberry, pomegranate juice, raspberry, red wine	Anticancer, antioxidative	Aqil et al. (2012)
Flavonols	Quercetin, myricetin, fisetin, kaempferol, Isorhamnetin	Apple, onion and tea, *Juniperus communis* L., celery, chives, onions, red onions, fennel, hot peppers, cherry tomatoes, spinach, sweet potato leaves, lettuce, celery, broccoli, kale, buckwheat, beans, cranberries, currants, cherries, black currant juice, *Ginkgo biloba*, red wine, cocoa powder,	Antioxidative, anti-inflammatory, immunostimulatory, and antifungal	Patel et al. (2018), Imran et al. (2019)
Flavanols	Catechins	Cocoa and tea, *Azadirachta indica*	Antibiotics	Musial et al. (2020)

(continued)

Table 4.1 (continued)

Class	Compounds	Source	Nutraceutical potential	References
	Epigallocatechin-3-gallate, epicatechin, epigallocatechin, catechin, gallocatechin	Green tea (*Camellia sinensis*), *Azadirachta indica, Sclerocarya birrea* (A. Rich.) Hochst., red wine, tea, chocolate, white wine, cocoa	Antioxidants, antimutagenic, anticarcinogenic, neuroprotective, antiobesity, antimicrobial, wound healing, antiaging, antielastase, and anticollagenase	Oda and Murakami (2017)
	Proanthocyanidin	*Vitis vinifera, Tibouchina granulose, Tamarindus indica* L.	Antioxidative, antiprotozoan agents, antiosteoarthritic	Woo et al. (2011)
Flavanones	Naringenin, eriodictyol, hesperetin	Grape, orange, and other citrus fruits, tomato, pepper mint		Testai and Calderone (2017)
Flavanone glycoside	Liquiritin, isoliquiritin, isoliquiritigenin	*Glycyrrhiza uralensis*, *Tibouchina granulose*	Anti-inflammatory and anticoronaviral agent, antitumor	Kim et al. (2017)
Flavones	Apigenin, luteolin	Persil, celery, green Pepper, *Juniperus communis* L., olives, oregano, rosemary, dry parsley, thyme	Antioxidative, anti-inflammatory, immunostimulatory, and antifungal	Bacanlı et al. (2017)
	Engeletin	*Hymenaea martiana*	Antidiabetic, anticancer	
Flavonoid-7-o-glycosides	Naringin, rutin, hesperidin	Grape fruit and other citrus fruits, tangerine juice	Antioxidative, anti-inflammatory, antimicrobial, and anticancer	Bacanlı et al. (2017)
Hydrolysable tannins	Emblicanin A, emblicanin B, punigluconin, pedunculagin	*Phyllanthus emblica*	Antioxidant, anti-inflammatory, antiarthritis	Fleck et al. (2013)
	Ellagitannins, punicafolin, phyllanemblinin	*Syzygium cumini* L., *Phyllanthus emblica* raspberries, strawberries, cranberries, and pomegranates, *Terminalia muelleri* Benth	Antioxidant, antiproliferative or anticancer, analgesic	Fleck et al. 2013
Benzopyran tannin	Chebulagic acid, chebulinic acid, chebulic acid	*Terminalia chebula*	Lipoxygenase and DNA topoisomerase inhibitors, adaptogenic, immunomodulatory	Murdock et al. (2016)

Isoflavones	Genistein, daidzein, equol	*Glycine max*, soy products (nuts, flour/bread, tofu, miso, milk, tofu yogurt, cheese/sauce), grape seed and skin	Antimicrobial, anticancer	Islam et al. (2020)
Hydroxyl isoflavan	Glabridin	*Glycyrrhiza uralensis*	Antispasmodic drug	Kim et al. (2017)
Lignans	Enterodiol	Cereals, soybean, strawberry, *Linum*	Modulate or mimic endogenous estrogens	Yu et al. (2017)
	Dihydrobenzofuran, tetrahydrofuran	*Euterpe oleracea*	Antioxidative, cytoprotective	Chin et al. (2008)
	Secoisolariciresinol, enterodiol, enterolactone, enterolignan	*Linum usitatissimum*	Antidepressant, phytoestrogen, prevents breast cancer	Yu et al. (2017)
Stilbenes	Resveratrol, piceatannol (metabolite of resveratrol), pterostilbene	*Vitis vinifera*, peanut, *Pistacia vera*, *Ramulus mori*	Antiapoptotic to pancreas cells, and antidiabetic, anti-inflammatory, treatment of Alzheimer's	Risuleo (2016)
Coumarins	Umbelliferone	Carrot	Antidiarrheal and antiulcerogenic	Cruz et al. (2020)
Carotenoids				
	Astaxanthin	*Haematococcus pluvialis*	Antioxidative	Satoh (2016)
	Phytofluene		Antioxidative	Thaipong et al. (2006)
	Lycopene	Tomatoes, pink grapefruit, apricots, red oranges, watermelon, rosehips, and guava	Antioxidative, anti-inflammatory, neuroprotective, antidementia, anticancer	Saini et al. (2020)
	β-carotene	Papaya, oranges, guava, tomatoes, pink grapefruit, apricots, red oranges, watermelon, rosehips	Antioxidative, inhibits free radical damage to DNA	Thaipong et al. (2006)
Carotenol	β-cryptoxanthin	Papaya, oranges, guava	Antioxidative	Thaipong et al. (2006)

certain BLs such as fat-soluble vitamins, carotenoids, phytosterols, monounsaturated fatty acids (MUFAs), and polyunsaturated fatty acids (PUFAs) has greater implications for health and wellness. Though MUFAs (oleic acid, palmitoleic acid, etc.) are not essential fatty acids, they have profound biological roles such as in improving cardiovascular health and in reducing blood glucose and triglycerides in diabetics. Fatty acids such as eicosapentaenoic acid (EPA, C20:5), docosahexaenoic acid (DHA, C22:6), α-linolenic acid (ALA, C18:3), stearidonic acid, and arachidonic acid tremendously reverse the health complications due to atherosclerosis, reduced blood pressure, arrhythmias, immune response disorders, weight gain, and stroke and improve the immune responses and infant visual and brain development (Decker et al. 2012). Phytosterols, namely stigmasterol, β-sitosterol, and campesterol derived from vegetable oils and algae, ameliorate the coronary heart diseases. Fat-soluble vitamins (Vitamin A, D, E, and K) and phenolic lipids not only help in fighting against coronary heart diseases but also in urinary tract diseases and cancer. Coenzyme Q10 (CoQ10) or ubiquinone is a naturally occurring quinone compound which is a component of inner mitochondrial membrane, where it acts as a cofactor of electron transport chain. CoQ10 has been found in leafy vegetables, e.g., Spinach. It is a potent antioxidant widely used in the treatment of cardiovascular disease, and it also possesses anti-inflammatory effects (Zhai et al. 2017).

4.2.1.3 Bioactive Polysaccharides

Various classes of dietary fibers such as β-glucans, pectins, and gums found in cereals such as rice, wheat, and oats accord immense health benefits such as cholesterol-lowering properties and hence reduce risk of cardiovascular diseases (CVDs) (Ho et al. 2016). Further, consumption of β-glucan derived from oats has been correlated with the decrease in blood glucose levels. US-FDA (Food and Drug Administration) also recommends the daily dietary intake of 3-g of glucan owing to its potential health benefits. Arabinoxylans are non-starch polysaccharides with antitumour and immune modulating properties (Cao et al. 2011)

4.2.2 Secondary Metabolites

4.2.2.1 Polyphenols

Polyphenols are class of secondary metabolites of plants that play pivotal role in antioxidant mechanism, UV protection, and defense against phytopathogens, etc. Whole plant foods such as cereals, whole grains, legumes, fruits and vegetables, coffee, cocoa, extra virgin olive oils, tea, and wine are rich sources of dietary polyphenols. As many as over 8000 polyphenol compounds have been identified from plant-based dietary sources and are linked to conferring multiple health benefits. Experimental evidences reveal that most of these properties of polyphenols are correlated with their intrinsic antioxidant capabilities. In general, dietary intake of polyphenols has been estimated to be around 1 g/day. Structurally, polyphenols are characterized with aromatic rings with one or more hydroxyl moieties. Polyphenols are classified into the following: (a) phenolic acids comprising derivatives of hydroxycinnamic acids (caffeic acid, chlorogenic acid, ferulic acid, neochlorogenic acid, P-coumaric acid, sinapic acid, caftaric acids sources from blueberry, cranberry, pear, cherry (sweet), apple, orange, potato, lettuce, spinach, coffee beans, tea, coffee, cider), and hydroxybenzoic acid (corilagin, ellagic acid, gallic acid) obtained from strawberry, raspberry grape juice (black/green), longan seed, and pomegranate juice. Although fruits and vegetables are rich sources of free phenolic acids, grains and seeds/nuts are sources of bound phenolic acids which require the hydrolytic action of acids, alkali, or enzymes to release their free forms; (b) flavonoids; (c) stilbenes and (d) lignans (Table 4.1).

4.2.2.2 Flavonoids

Flavonoids are large class of phenolic compounds occurring naturally in plant products. Flavonoids are further categorized into various subclasses such as flavonols, flavones, flavanols, flavanones, isoflavones, flavan-3-ols, and anthocyanidins. Chemically, flavonoids remain either free (aglycones) or as glycosides. Some of the commonly occurring plant-derived flavones, flavonols and flavanone are apigenin, luteolin, velutin, quercetin, rutin, naringenin, whereas isoflavones are genistein, daidzein, and puerarin. Apigenin is a commonly occurring flavone in wide range of plant sources, and its dietary intake has been correlated with immune-boosting properties. Its glycosidic counterparts, namely vitexin and isovitexin, contribute to anti-inflammatory effects and are of considerable nutraceutical importance (Xiao et al. 2016). Another flavone of common occurrence in edible plants such as *Punica granatum* (pomegranate), *Cynara scolymus* (artichoke), and rosemary is luteolin. Luteolin and its glycoside derivatives are known to possess anti-inflammatory effects against neurodegenerative diseases (Xiao et al. 2016). Flavones of *Euterpe oleracea*, of particular interest velutin, showed anti-inflammatory effects. Quercetin is one of the commonly known flavonols from the fruits and vegetables (*Malus x domestica*). Similarly, flavanones and flavones such as naringenin, naringin, and hesperidin derived from citrus fruits have nutraceutical properties.

Isoflavones are natural phytoestrogens which exhibit wide range of beneficial effects such as antioxidant, anticancer, antimicrobial, anti-inflammatory, antiosteoporotic, and estrogenic properties. Isoflavones such as daidzin, genistin, biochanin A, and formononetin are subclass of flavonoids found in legumes and are generally available as glycosides. Soybean is considered to be rich source of isoflavones (5–30 mg/100 g) (Thrane et al. 2017). Flavanols or flavan-3-ols are generally called catechins. Structurally, the absence of double bond between C2 and C3 and carbonyl group in ring C favors their existence as diastereoisomers. Tea and cacao beans are major sources of monomeric flavanols and their derivatives. Dimeric flavanols such as theaflavin are formed when tea flavanol is fermented. Similarly, formation of polymers by monomeric flavanols such as catechin and epicatechin is referred to as proanthocyanidins since acid hydrolysis of polymer produces anthocyanidins. The red, blue, and purple pigments of flowers, vegetables, fruits, and grains such as black rice are due to the presence of anthocyanidins. Cyanidin, delphinidin, and pelargonidin and their methylated derivatives are the vast majority of anthocyanidins of plant origin.

4.2.2.3 Stilbenes and Lignans

Structurally stilbenes are characterized with 1,2-diphenylethylene nucleus having hydroxyl groups on the phenolic rings. Stilbenes may exist as monomers or oligomers, e.g., transresveratrol.

4.2.2.4 Terpenoids

Terpenoids, alternatively called as isoprenoids, are diverse class of organic compounds derived from C5 precursor compound isopentenyl diphosphate (IPP) and its isomer dimethylallyl diphosphate. The enormous structural variations of terpenoids offer a huge functional complexity. Terpenoids are classified based on their number of isoprene units. Monoterpenes are C10 compounds, that form main constituents of both the volatile essences and essential oils of flowers (e.g., citral, geraniol, menthol, limonene etc). Similarly, the sesquiterpenes (C15) comprise 3 isoprene units (e.g., farnesol). The diterpenes (C20) are composed of four isoprene units (e.g., taxol and gibberellic acid). Noteworthy defensive compounds such as sesquiterpenoids and diterpenoids derived from flowering plants act as phytoalexins and antimicrobial compounds. Terpenoids of plant origin have antibacterial, antifungal, anti-inflammatory, antioxidant, anticancer, and antitumor activities. The tocotrienols and tocopherols induce apoptosis of human malignant cells and arrest the growth of tumor cell lines (Yu et al. 1999).

4.2.2.5 Carotenoids

Carotenoids are class of terpene compounds that have been widely investigated in fruits, vegetables, fungi, and flowers. Carotenoids are naturally occurring lipid-soluble pigments exhibiting red, orange, and blue colors. The commonly known carotenoids are lycopene found in tomato, watermelon, papaya, guava, β-carotene of carrot, mango, apricot, α-carotene from carrot, pumpkin, and corn. Chemically, carotenoids are classified into the following: (a) xanthophylls—carotenoids contain one or more oxygen atoms substituted as hydroxy, keto, epoxy, and aldehyde groups and (b) carotenes—containing hydrocarbons. Both these classes may exist as acyclic (lycopene), monocyclic (γ-carotene), or dicyclic (β-carotene and α-carotene) forms. The most striking structural feature of carotenoids is their long alternating double and single bonds forming a conjugated system, wherein electrons are delocalized providing the molecules with its biological functions. Lycopene and β-carotene have anticancerous properties (Saini et al. 2020).

4.2.2.6 Alkaloids

Alkaloids are nitrogen-containing secondary metabolites having potential pharmacological activities. Plant kingdom offers more than 12,000 alkaloids predominantly found in dicots. Owing to their structural diversity, plant alkaloids have been utilized as pharmaceuticals, narcotics, stimulants, and at times as poisons. Some of the commonly known alkaloids of plant origin are as follows: morphine—*Papaver somniferum*; camptothecin—*Camptotheca acuminate*; vinblastine—*Catharanthus roseus*; caffeine—*Coffea arabica*; nicotine—*Nicotiana tabacum,* etc., having wide repertoire of biological functions such as analgesic, anticancer, stimulant, natural pesticide, and tranquilizer.

4.2.2.7 Omega-3 and Polyunsaturated Fatty Acids

Structurally fatty acids are long straight aliphatic chain, either saturated or unsaturated, with a carboxylic group (-COOH). Omega-3 and omega-6 fatty acids are considered as essential fatty acids since human body cannot synthesize these fatty acids, and hence, dietary intake is the only source. Among the major omega-3 fatty acids, viz. α-linolenic acid (ALA; 18:3 omega-3), eicosapentaenoic acid (EPA; 20:5 omega-3), and docosahexaenoic acid (DHA; 22:6 omega-3), plants are sources of ALA, whereas EPA and DHA are obtained from marine fish oil and algal sources (Amjad Khan et al. 2017). Among the plant sources of omega-3 fatty acids, flax contains around 55% of fatty acids in the form of ALA. The other plant sources of omega-3 fatty acids are perilla, walnut, and soy foods, especially edamame-steamed and boiled young soybean and tofu, canola, pumpkin seeds, hemp seeds, pine nuts, etc.

4.3 Mode of Action of Nutraceuticals

Epidemiological studies have demonstrated that diets rich in plant-derived bioactive components have reduced the risk of chronic ailments such as CVDs, obesity, and diabetes (Gul et al. 2016). Similarly, adequate dietary intake of whole grains, fruits, and vegetables had been linked with the reduced risk of CVDs and cancers, the major health issues of the world. In vivo animal model-based findings reveal that plant-based diets rich in raw vegetables, allium, green, or crucifer vegetables provide protection against diverse cancer ailments.

4.3.1 Heart Disease

Strongest correlation was evinced between vegetable consumption and the diminution in chronic ailments, namely CVDs and age-related cataract. The high potassium content in fruits and vegetables render proper endothelial function since the improved potassium reabsorption by kidney triggers sodium urinary depletion and circumventing the problem of hypertension. The plant diet-derived vitamins, polyphenols, and glucosinolates improve the redox status of cells, by preventing the oxidation of LDL, thereby decreasing the risk of CVD-induced mortality (Alissa and Ferns 2017). Polyphenols enhance the in vivo availability of nitric oxide and reduce the endothelin-1 (a vasoconstrictor), hence averting the causes of thrombosis and stroke. Similarly, polyphenols also diminish the inflammatory markers, C-reactive protein (CRP), which are associated with the onset of CVD by modulating the DNA-binding activity of nuclear factor kappa-light-chain-enhancer. Another major component of plants, dietary fiber, provides the sense of satiety and decrease the quantum of ingested food, which ultimately causes slow postprandial glycemic peak. Further, the insoluble dietary fiber forms substrate for gut microbiota leading to the production of short-chain fatty acids which potentially inhibits β-Hydroxy β-methylglutaryl-CoA reductase activity having profound implications for cholesterol biosynthesis (Angelino et al. 2019).

4.3.2 Cancer

Plant bioactives and natural products have the ability to prevent the cancer owing to their antimutagenic and anticarcinogenic properties (Gul et al. 2016). The general mode of action of plant biochemicals are antioxidant effects, enhancing the cellular enzymatic components in the detoxification of carcinogens, inhibiting the production of N-nitrosamine, DNA repair and cellular maintenance, apoptosis of cancerous or malignant cells, upregulating noncoding RNAs that suppresses tumor, among others (Gul et al. 2016). For instance, ginger-derived [6]-gingerol modulated the proteins such as tumor necrosis factor alpha (TNF-α), extracellular signal-regulated kinases (ERK1/2), caspases-3, caspases-9, and protein 53 (tumor)-p53 that are involved in cell signaling processes to regulate the antioxidant and inflammatory processes, thereby providing antitumorigenic effects (de Lima et al. 2018). Similarly, apigenin—a naturally occurring plant-derived flavonoid—has multiple effects such as targeting cell cycle proteins (cyclins, CDKs, etc.), proteins involved in angiogenesis, metastasis, and invasion, modulating cell signaling pathways in preventing the cancer. Dietary polyphenols, glucosinolates, and carotenoids detoxify the carcinogenic compounds either by inhibiting the formation of DNA adducts or by countering their oxidant effects. The proapoptotic activities of polyphenols and glucosinolates release mitochondrial cytochrome C into cytosol ultimately activating caspase family inducing cell suicide through the p53-dependent pathway.

Biologically inactive glucosinolates are converted by intracellular myrosinase enzyme into isothiocyanates which in turn activates the enzymes involved in detoxification system. Isothiocyanates inhibit the cellular destruction of Kelch-like ECH-associated protein-1 (KEAP-1) and enhance the transcription of erythroid 2 p45-related factor 2 (Nrf2) both of which together with other proteins improve the activities of antioxidant responsive elements (Dinkova-Kostova et al. 2017).

4.3.3 Diabetes

The activities of human enzymes α-amylase and α-glucosidase which are involved in sequential breakdown of starch molecules into glucose units for energy production are considered important targets for managing the type 2 diabetes mellitus (DM). Limonoids extracted from *Azadirachta indica* and myricetin, a flavonoid, from guava leaves have shown the α-amylase inhibitory activity in vitro (Sudha et al. 2015). Betulin derived from *Ruellia tuberose* L. non-competitively inhibited the activity of α-amylase (Wulan et al. 2015), whereas diosgenin from *Dioscorea bulbifera* exhibited similar non-competitive inhibition of the enzymes, viz. α-amylase and α-glucosidase (Ghosh et al. 2014). Molecular docking studies reveal that several plant-derived compounds such as rutin, myricetin, and quercetin have comparable binding energies to that of acarbose—an antidiabetic drug. Human aldose reductase (hALR2) is another potent target enzyme to manage type 2 diabetes; hence, the organic solvent extracts of roots of *Gentiana lutea* were found to be promising in inhibiting ALR2 activities. Further, peroxisome proliferator-activated receptors-γ (PPAR-γ) agonists have been identified from plant origin so that the activities of glucose transporters are (GLUT1, GLUT4) enhanced to utilize glucose in liver and muscle cells. Catechins from green tea and sargahydroquinoic acid and sargaquinoic acid from *Sargassum yezoense* are novel PPAR γ agonists with a potential to treat diabetes (Wang et al. 2006). Investigations in type 2-induced diabetic mice models have revealed that fructooligosaccharides (FOS) obtained from *Aureobasidium pullulans* are effective inhibitors of dipeptidyl peptidase (DPP)-4 enzymes which in turn regulates the activities of incretin hormones, namely glucagon-like peptide-1 (GLP1) and glucose-dependent insulinotropic polypeptide (GIP) suggesting the importance of plant-derived FOS in the treatment of diabetes.

4.3.4 Neurological Disorders

A total of sixteen plant-derived compounds exhibit neuroprotective functions (Dey et al. 2020). Compounds such as apigenin, allicin, curcumin, capsaicin, kaempferol, piperine, epigallocatechin, resveratrol, rosmarinic acid, quercetin, eugenol, gambogic acid, carnosic acid, zingerone, and morin are some of the naturally occurring nutraceuticals with a potential to treat neurological disorders (Ahmad et al. 2015; Sun et al. 2016; Lee et al. 2018; Dey et al. 2020). In general, these compounds significantly upregulate one or more physiological and biochemical components such as p38MAPK/PKC pathway, BDNF/TrkB-dependent pathway, Keap1/Nrf2 pathway, and MAPK pathways, alternatively improve the locomotor, memory, and mitochondrial functions, or enhance the QR1 gene expression and apoptosis to exert their neuroprotective roles (Salehi et al. 2019). Conversely, these compounds downregulate certain cellular processes such as tau hyperphosphorylation, convulsions, seizures, and spatial memory impairments. Downregulation of cellular signaling molecules such as TLR2/4, NF-κB, MAPK along with reduction of ROS, GSH, NADPHd/nNOS etc. confer neuroprotective functions (Dey et al. 2020).

4.4 Mode of Delivery of Nutraceuticals

The innate biochemical nature of plant bioactives is lost when exposed to extreme conditions of temperature, oxidation, and sunlight consequently diminishing their yield levels; hence, the active ingredient of a nutraceutical warrants protection by appropriate techniques. Moreover, nutraceutical compounds, in their natural or organic form, are characterized with poor aqueous solubility, hence poor membrane permeability leading to very limited bioavailability. Further, the release features of nutraceuticals are severely affected by the characteristics of parent food matrices. Following release, nutraceuticals form insoluble complexes with the other substances in gastrointestinal tract or the process of biotransformation renders them biologically unavailable. A greater proportion of biochemicals conferring anticancer properties is lipophilic, hence warranting adjustment in pH, reduction of particle size, and use of cosurfactants or solvents which are generally toxic causing significant damage to the healthy cells. Hence, the design and fabrication of suitable delivery mechanisms to protect physicochemical, sensory, and nutritional attributes of nutraceuticals are in vogue. Exploitation of nanodelivery carriers such as liposomes, micelles and polymeric nanoparticles, solid lipid nanoparticles, and carbon nanotubes is being explored.

4.4.1 Liposomes

Liposome-based encapsulation of curcumin was suggested to avert its biotransformation during oral administration or excreted as bile secretion when administered intravenously or intraperitonealy. Liposomal curcumin was successfully shown to inhibit the growth of cancerous pancreatic cells, human prostate cancer, colorectal cancer, and human squamous cell carcinoma (Moses et al. 2019). Liposome-based delivery of resveratrol, fisetin, crocin, cyanidin-3o-glucoside, genistein, β-glucan,

(−)-epigallocatechin-3-gallate, β-cryptoxanthin and berberine has shown exemplary results in the treatment of various forms of human cancer (Moses et al. 2019)

Microencapsulation techniques are widely employed since 1980s not only to improve the stability and bioactivity but also to ameliorate the volatility and toxicity effects of plant bioactives. In general, microencapsulation technologies utilize physical and chemical processes such as spray drying, extrusion, coacervation, liposome-based delivery, and other conventional emulsions (Assadpour and Jafari 2019). However, the advent of nanotechnology and its application in food and pharmaceutical industries have opened up avenues for the utilization of nano-sized materials or nanocarriers (<1000 nM) in encapsulation processes. Nanocarriers enhance the bioavailability of food bioactives due to increased surface area-to-volume ratios, ability to penetrate target cells following improved mucoadhesiveness in the walls of human intestines, controlled release of an active ingredient, and improved solubility of hydrophobic nutraceuticals. It also protects the active ingredient from chemical and biological degradation. The classification of nanocarriers is based on the kind of nanomaterial used to produce the formulation.

4.4.2 Nanoemulsion

These are major lipid-based nanocarriers formed due to oil, water, and surfactants or biopolymers in a single (O/W or W/O) or double (O/W/O or W/O/W) nanoemulsion formats. The droplet sizes of the particles are of 200 nm and are relatively stable. Based on the hydrophobicity or hydrophilicity of active ingredient, the bioactive components can be trapped in oil or water layer, respectively. Hydrophobic phenolics and antioxidants, namely carotenoids, tannins, lignins, and bound hydroxycinnamic acids, are appropriate candidates (catechins, resveratrol, curcumin, pterostilbene, and eugenol) for O/W nanoemulsion-based delivery and rutin and anthocyanin for multiple nanoemulsions (Abbas et al. 2014).

4.4.3 Nanoliposomes

Nanoliposomes are form of lipid-based carriers formulated using oils, phospholipids, and appropriate solvents so that lipid bilayer is formed with an aqueous interior. It can cater to both the hydrophilic and hydrophobic active ingredients in its cavities and as an encapsulation, respectively (Demirci et al. 2017), e.g., curcumin, quercetin and resveratrol, epigallocatechin-3-gallate (EGCG), and tea polyphenol in nanoliposomes

4.4.4 Nanolipid Carriers

Advanced lipid-based carriers formed by crystalline or semi-crystalline materials are stabilized by surfactants. As name states, solid lipid nanoparticles (SLN) use solid lipids, whereas nanostructured lipid carriers (NLCs) use combination of solid lipids and oils. It offers advantages such as reduced leakage of entrapped nutraceuticals and improved release properties (Katouzian and Jafari 2016), e.g., resveratrol in SLN-based carriers following emulsification and evaporation, curcumin, quercetin, and silymarin in NLC carriers.

4.4.5 Natural Nanovehicles

Naturally occurring materials such as caseins-forming self-assembled micellar structure, cyclodextrins, and amylase structures are utilized as nanoencapsulating carriers, e.g., procyanidins in zein nanoparticles.

Furthermore, nanocarriers are produced employing sophisticated equipments such as electrospinning/spraying, nanospray dryer, and micro- or nanofluidics systems. Naturally occurring biopolymers such as proteins (e.g., whey protein or zein) or carbohydrates (e.g., cellulose, chitin, chitosan, gums, pectin, and starch) are used in the processes of electrospinning or electrospraying to produce nanofibers and nanoparticles for the delivery of phenolics and antioxidants of plant origin. Quercetin and ferulic acid were encapsulated in food-grade nanofibers generated from the amaranth protein in an electrospinning process (Aceituno-Medina et al. 2015).

4.4.6 Solid Lipid Nanoparticles (SLNs)

Solid lipid nanoparticles (SLNs) have attained greater attention as an alternative for carriers such as emulsions, liposomes, and polymeric nanoparticles. SLNs have been widely employed to improve the bioavailability and pharmacokinetic potential of phenolic compounds. SLNs are prepared utilizing lipid matrix, with final particle sizes ranging between 50 and 1000 nm. SLNs have improved wide array of properties of nutraceuticals such its water solubility, thermal stability, enhanced oral bioavailability, and improved protection against the digestive process.

4.4.7 Biopolymer Particles

Biopolymer particles and their production involve assembly of multiple kinds of biopolymer molecules to form colloidal structures to modify the stability, texture, and optical properties of nutraceutical bioactives. Food-grade proteins, polysaccharides, and associative complexes form excellent materials for the development of biopolymer-based encapsulation of nutraceuticals.

4.5 Regulations of Nutraceuticals

Food production system in emerging economies such as India and worldwide had witnessed a rapid change in consumption pattern, due to rapid urbanization, changes in demography, consumer awareness of nutraceuticals, dependence on processed foods, social changes, nuclear families, etc. Nutraceuticals occupy a wobble position between the regular foods and pharmaceuticals often blurring the differences warrant statutory regulations in light of safety and health claims. Countries have made their own legislative framework to assess and for safety use of nutraceuticals. In the USA, FDA differentiates the nutraceuticals from other foods and hence requires the manufacturer's to ensure that their products are safe before marketing, and warrants authoritative statement on health claims from the Academies of Sciences or appropriate bodies before the introduction of product to the market. On the other hand, European Food Safety Standards Authority (EFSA) is mandated to approve the health claim of a product before it is marketed in European Union. In Canada, nutraceuticals are treated more like a drug than as foods; in contrast, Australia and China categorize the nutraceuticals as a class of food. In India, regulation of nutraceuticals and functional foods are brought under the ambit of Food Safety Standards Authority of India (FSSAI), Food Safety and Standards Act, 2006, Rules and Regulations, 2011, Food Product Approval System (May 2013), and Food Safety and Standards Act, 2016. The section 22 of the Food Safety and Standards Act, 2006, mandates a Central Government notification for the manufacture and marketing of novel foods including nutraceuticals. Most importantly, these nutraceuticals are prohibited to contain drugs and claims of treatment to disease, or cure or mitigation of illness is strictly prohibited. Further, the advisory of FSSAI dated May 2013 warrants submission of safety or toxicity data pertaining to risk assessment for prior approval to release a product in the market. FSSAI notification dated Dec 31, 2018, prohibits the use of 14 ingredients (raspberry ketone, silica, chlorella growth factor, pine bark, tea tree oil, etc.) as nutraceuticals for the lack of scientific evidence to prove their health promotion activities. Similarly, the regulation called for discontinuation of "health supplements" claim for some other products including kale powder, fruit extracts of cashew, passion fruit, and kiwi, broccoli, and enzymes pectinase and xylanase. Recently a Guidance Note on Food for Special Medical Purpose of FSSAI (28/Aug/2020) categorizes the foods for medical purposes as (a) health supplements, (b) nutraceuticals, (c) foods for special dietary uses (FSDU), and (d) foods for special medical purposes (FSMP). Further, the note delineates the applicable age groups, target population, format/matrix requirements, requirements of medical supervision, formulations allowed, and relevant applicable ingredient schedules, etc. (https://fssai.gov.in/upload/uploadfiles/files/Guidance_Note_FSMP_28_08_2020.pdf). In light of these viewpoints, Santini et al. 2018 have proposed a differentiation of nutraceuticals and food supplements based on the availability of clinical evidences, however, stressing the needs of efficacy/safety of these products. It further calls for necessary steps including prior identification of target health condition to address, appropriate food matrix selection, biological and functional activity assays, metabolic profiling, proper dose assessment, and safety in clinical trials to consider while developing a novel nutraceutical product (Santini et al. 2018). It is also reasonable for the national agencies to demand the suppliers or manufacturers of nutraceuticals to provide data on safety, clinical trials, and data supporting mechanisms of actions so that informed decision could be arrived at. Further stricter guidelines are mandatory at the international level considering the ramifications of large transnational movement of goods and services.

4.6 Concluding Remarks

Nutraceuticals are source of natural remedies which besides preventing the serious diseases cure the life-threatening disorders. The physiological effects of some of the nutraceuticals and their beneficial role in the field of human nutrition and disease management warrant long-term investigations. In addition, the effect of nutraceuticals on the pathogenesis, disease progression, or alternatively remission requires scientific advances. It is also pertinent to assess the interaction effects of food and nutraceuticals so as to improve the bioefficacy and bioavailability of the latter in the context of our improved comprehension on food matrices and their interactive physiological effects. As stated above, appropriate delivery mechanisms have to be formulated to improve the efficiency of nutraceuticals along with physical attributes such as flavor, color, and texture. The preclinical and clinical trials of nutraceuticals should have adequate sample size, and information on toxicological effect has to be generated. Lastly, the commerce and regulatory regimen pertaining to nutraceuticals are required to be streamlined to ward off spurious products and to promote the overall well-being of masses.

References

Abbas S, Bashari M, Akhtar W, Li WW, Zhang X (2014) Process optimization of ultrasound-assisted curcumin nanoemulsions stabilized by OSA-modified starch. Ultrason Sonochem 21: 1265–1274

Aceituno-Medina M, Mendoza S, Rodríguez BA, Lagaron JM, López-Rubio A (2015) Improved antioxidant capacity of quercetin and ferulic acid during in-vitro digestion through encapsulation within food-grade electrospun fibers. J Funct Foods 12:332–341

Ahmad B, Rehman MU, Amin I, Arif A, Rasool S, Bhat SA, Afzal I, Hussain I, Bilal S (2015) A review on pharmacological properties of zingerone (4-(4-Hydroxy-3-methoxyphenyl)-2-butanone). ScientificWorldJournal 2015:816364. https://doi.org/10.1155/2015/816364

Alissa EM, Ferns GA (2017) Dietary fruits and vegetables and cardiovascular diseases risk. Critic Rev Food Sci Nutr 57:1950–1962

Ameen AM, Elkazaz AY, Mohammad HMF (2017) Anti-inflammatory and neuroprotective activity of boswellic acids in rotenone parkinsonian rats. Can J Physiol Pharmacol 95(7):819–829

Amjad Khan W, Chun-Mei H, Khan N, Iqbal A, Lyu SW, Shah F (2017) Bioengineered plants can be a useful source of omega-3 fatty acids. Biomed Res Int 2017:7348919. https://doi.org/10.1155/2017/7348919

Anantharaju PG, Reddy BD, Padukudru MA, Kumari Chitturi CM, Vimalambike MG, Madhunapantula SV (2017) Naturally occurring benzoic acid derivatives retard cancer cell growth by inhibiting histone deacetylases (HDAC). Cancer Biol Ther 18(7):492–504

Angelino D, Godos J, Ghelfi F, Tieri M, Titta L, Lafranconi A, Marventano S, Alonzo E, Gambera A, Sciacca S, Buscemi S (2019) Fruit and vegetable consumption and health outcomes: an umbrella review of observational studies. Int J Food Sci Nutr 70(6):652–667

Aqil F, Gupta A, Munagala R, Jeyabalan J, Kausar H, Sharma RJ, Singh IP, Gupta RC (2012) Antioxidant and antiproliferative activities of anthocyanin/ellagitannins-enriched extracts from *Syzygium cumini* L. (Jamun, the Indian blackberry). Nutr Cancer 64(3):428–438

Assadpour E, Jafari SM (2019) A systematic review on nanoencapsulation of food bioactive ingredients and nutraceuticals by various nanocarriers. Crit Rev Food Sci Nutr 59(19): 3129–3151. https://doi.org/10.1080/10408398.2018.1484687

Bacanlı M, Aydın S, Başaran AA, Başaran N (2017) Are all phytochemicals useful in the preventing of DNA damage? Food Chem Toxicol 109:210–217

Bharti VK, Malik JK, Gupta RC (2016) Ashwagandha: multiple health benefits. In: Gupta RC (ed) Nutraceuticals: efficacy, safety and toxicity. Academic Press/Elsevier, Amsterdam, pp 717–733

Bonechi C, Donati A, Tamasi G, Pardini A, Rostom H, Leone G, Lamponi S, Consumi M, Magnani A, Rossi C (2019) Chemical characterization of liposomes containing nutraceutical compounds: Tyrosol, hydroxytyrosol and oleuropein. Biophys Chem 246:25–34

Bopage NS, Kamal Bandara Gunaherath GM, Jayawardena KH, Wijeyaratne SC, Abeysekera AM, Somaratne S (2018) Dual function of active constituents from bark of *Ficus racemosa* L in wound healing. BMC Complement Altern Med 18:29. https://doi.org/10.1186/s12906-018-2089-9

Cao L, Liu X, Qian T, Sun G, Guo Y, Chang F, Zhou S, Sun X (2011) Antitumor and immunomodulatory activity of arabinoxylans: a major constituent of wheat bran. Int J Biol Macromol 48:160–164

Capetti F, Cagliero C, Marengo A, Bicchi C, Rubiolo P, Sgorbini B (2020) Bio-guided fractionation driven by in vitro α-amylase inhibition assays of essential oils bearing specialized metabolites with potential hypoglycemic activity. Plan Theory 9(9):1242. https://doi.org/10.3390/plants9091242

Chakrabarti S, Guha S, Majumder K (2018) Food-derived bioactive peptides in human health: challenges and opportunities. Nutrients 10(11):1738. https://doi.org/10.3390/nu10111738

Chan JY, Yuen AC, Chan RY, Chan SW (2013) A review of the cardiovascular benefits and antioxidant properties of allicin. Phytother Res 27(5):637–646

Chin YW, Chai HB, Keller WJ, Kinghorn AD (2008) Lignans and other constituents of the fruits of *Euterpe oleracea* (Açai) with antioxidant and cytoprotective activities. J Agric Food Chem 56: 7759–7764

Choubey S, Goyal S, Varughese LR, Kumar V, Sharma AK, Beniwal V (2018) Probing gallic acid for its broad spectrum applications. Mini Rev Med Chem 18(15):1283–1293

Cruz LF, de Figueiredo GF, Pedro LP, Amorin YM, Andrade JT, Passos TF, Rodrigues FF, Souza IL, Gonçalves TP, dos Santos Lima LA, Ferreira JM (2020) Umbelliferone (7-hydroxycoumarin): a non-toxic antidiarrheal and antiulcerogenic coumarin. Biomed Pharmacother 129:110432. https://doi.org/10.1016/j.biopha.2020.110432

Cutillas AB, Carrasco A, Martinez-Gutierrez R, Tomas V, Tudela J (2017) Composition and antioxidant, antienzymatic and antimicrobial activities of volatile molecules from Spanish *Salvia lavandulifolia* (Vahl) essential oils. Molecules 22(8):1382. https://doi.org/10.3390/molecules22081382

Dang TT, Onoyovwi A, Farrow SC et al (2012) Biochemical genomics for gene discovery in benzylisoquinoline alkaloid biosynthesis in opium poppy and related species. Methods Enzymol 515:231–266

de Lima RM, Dos Reis AC, de Menezes AA, Santos JV, Filho JW, Ferreira JR, de Alencar MV, da Mata AM, Khan IN, Islam A, Uddin SJ (2018) Protective and therapeutic potential of ginger (*Zingiber officinale*) extract and [6]-gingerol in cancer: a comprehensive review. Phytother Res 32(10):1885–1907

Decker EA, Akoh CC, Wilkes RS (2012) Incorporation of (n-3) fatty acids in foods: challenges and opportunities. J Nutr 142:S610–S613

Demirci M, Caglar MY, Cakir B, Gülseren İ (2017) Encapsulation by nanoliposomes. In: Jafari SM (ed) Nanoencapsulation technologies for the food and nutraceutical industries. Academic Press, San Diego, pp 74–113

Dey A, Nandy S, Mukherjee A, Pandey DK (2020) Plant natural products as neuroprotective nutraceuticals: preclinical and clinical studies and future implications. Proc Natl Acad Sci India B Biol Sci 90:929–943. https://doi.org/10.1007/s40011-020-01170-6

Dinkova-Kostova AT, Fahey JW, Kostov RV, Kensler TW (2017) KEAP1 and done? Targeting the NRF2 pathway with sulforaphane. Trends Food Sci Technol 69:257–269

Fleck A, Gupta RC, Goad JT, Lasher MA, Canerdy TD, Kalidindi SR (2013) Anti-arthritic efficacy and safety of Crominex®+ (trivalent chromium, *Phyllanthus emblica* extract, and Shilajit) in moderately arthritic dogs. J Vet Sci Anim Husb 1(4):1–8. https://doi.org/10.15744/2348-9790.1.401

Garg RC (2016) Fenugreek: multiple health benefits. In: Gupta RC (ed) Nutraceuticals: efficacy, safety and toxicity. Academic Press/Elsevier, Amsterdam, pp 599–617

Ghosh S, More P, Derle A, Patil AB, Markad P, Asok A, Kumbhar N, Shaikh ML, Ramanamurthy B, Shinde VS, Dhavale D, Chopade BA (2014) Diosgenin from *Dioscorea bulbifera*: novel hit for treatment of type II diabetes mellitus with inhibitory activity against α-amylase and α-glucosidase. PLoS One 9(9):e106039

Gu W, Kavanagh JM, McClure DD (2021) Photoautotrophic production of eicosapentaenoic acid. Crit Rev Biotechnol 41(5):731–748. https://doi.org/10.1080/07388551.2021.1888065

Gul K, Singh AK, Jabeen R (2016) Nutraceuticals and functional foods: the foods for the future world. Crit Rev Food Sci Nutr 56(16):2617–2627. https://doi.org/10.1080/10408398.2014.903384

Gupta B, Ghosh KK, Gupta RC (2016) Thymoquinone. In: Gupta RC (ed) Nutraceuticals: efficacy, safety and toxicity. Academic Press/Elsevier, Amsterdam, pp 541–550

Gupta RC, Srivastava A, Sinha A, Lall R (2019) Biomarkers of foods and Nutraceuticals: applications in efficacy, safety, and toxicity. In: Nutraceuticals in veterinary medicine. Springer, Cham, pp 693–710. https://doi.org/10.1007/978-3-030-04624-8_50

Ho HV, Sievenpiper JL, Zurbau A, Mejia SB, Jovanovski E, Au-Yeung F, Jenkins AL, Vuksan V (2016) The effect of oat β-glucan on LDL-cholesterol, non-HDL-cholesterol and apoB for CVD risk reduction: a systematic review and meta-analysis of randomised-controlled trials. Br J Nutr 116(8):1369–1382

Hoshyar R, Mollaei H (2017) A comprehensive review on anticancer mechanisms of the main carotenoid of saffron, crocin. J Pharm Pharmacol 69(11):1419–1427

Imran M, Rauf A, Shah ZA, Saeed F, Imran A, Arshad MU, Ahmad B, Bawazeer S, Atif M, Peters DG, Mubarak MS (2019) Chemo-preventive and therapeutic effect of the dietary flavonoid kaempferol: a comprehensive review. Phytother Res 33(2):263–275

Islam A, Islam MS, Uddin MN, Hasan MM, Akanda MR (2020) The potential health benefits of the isoflavone glycoside genistin. Arch Pharm Res 43(4):395–408

Katouzian I, Jafari SM (2016) Nano-encapsulation as a promising approach for targeted delivery and controlled release of vitamins. Trends Food Sci Technol 53:34–48

Kim SH, Hong JH, Lee JE, Lee YC (2017) 18β-Glycyrrhetinic acid, the major bioactive component of Glycyrrhizae radix, attenuates airway inflammation by modulating Th2 cytokines, GATA-3,

STAT6, and Foxp3 transcription factors in an asthmatic mouse model. Environ Toxicol Pharmacol 52:99–113

Kumar N, Goel N (2019) Phenolic acids: natural versatile molecules with promising therapeutic applications. Biotechnol Rep 24:e00370. https://doi.org/10.1016/j.btre.2019.e00370

Kumar A, Chopra K, Mukherjee M, Pottabathini R, Dhull DK (2015) Current knowledge and pharmacological profile of berberine: an update. Eur J Pharmacol 761:288–297

Kumar A, Agarwal DK, Kumar S, Reddy YM, Chintagunta AD, Saritha KV, Pal G, Kumar SJ (2019) Nutraceuticals derived from seed storage proteins: implications for health wellness. Biocatal Agric Biotechnol 17:710–719

Lee W, Hwang MH, Lee Y, Bae JS (2018) Protective effects of zingerone on lipopolysaccharide-induced hepatic failure through the modulation of inflammatory pathways. Chem Biol Interact 281:106–110

Li M, Zhu L, Zhang T, Liu B, Du L, Jin Y (2017) Pulmonary delivery of tea tree oil-beta-cyclodextrin inclusion complexes for the treatment of fungal and bacterial pneumonia. J Pharm Pharmacol 69(11):1458–1467

Liu MW, Wei R, Su MX, Li H, Fang TW, Zhang W (2018) Effects of *Panax notoginseng* saponins on severe acute pancreatitis through the regulation of mTOR/Akt and caspase-3 signaling pathway by upregulating miR-181b expression in rats. BMC Complement Altern Med 18(51):18. https://doi.org/10.1186/s12906-018-2118-8

Lu QY, Ma JQ, Duan YY, Sun Y, Yu S, Li B, Zhang GM (2019) Carthamin yellow protects the heart against ischemia/reperfusion injury with reduced reactive oxygen species release and inflammatory response. J Cardiovasc Pharmacol 74(3):228–234

Maltsev Y, Maltseva K (2021) Fatty acids of microalgae: diversity and applications. Rev Environ Sci Biotechnol 20:515–547. https://doi.org/10.1007/s11157-021-09571-3

Martinez SE, Chen Y, Ho EA, Martinez SA, Davies NM (2015) Pharmacological effects of a c-phycocyanin-based multicomponent nutraceutical in an *in-vitro* canine chondrocyte model of osteoarthritis. Can J Vet Res 79:241–249

Mohanty C, Sahoo SK (2017) Curcumin and its topical formulations for wound healing applications. Drug Discov Today 22(10):1582–1592

Moses JA, Dutta S, Anandharamakrishnan C (2019) Encapsulation of nutraceutical ingredients in liposomes and their potential for cancer treatment. Nutr Cancer 70(8):1184–1198. https://doi.org/10.1080/01635581.2018.1557212

Murdock N, Gupta CR, Vega N, Kotora K, Miller J, Goad TJ, Lasher AM, Canerdy DT, Kalidindi SR (2016) Evaluation of *Terminalia chebula* extract for anti-arthritic efficacy and safety in osteoarthritic dogs. J Vet Sci Technol 7(1):290. https://doi.org/10.4172/2157-7579.1000290

Musial C, Kuban-Jankowska A, Gorska-Ponikowska M (2020) Beneficial properties of green tea catechins. Int J Mol Sci 21(5):1744

Oda K, Murakami T (2017) Pharmacokinetic interaction of green tea beverage containing cyclodextrins and high concentration catechins with p-glycoprotein substrates in LLC-GA5-COL150 cells in vitro and in the small intestine of rats in vivo. J Pharm Pharmacol 69:1736–1744

Oiram Filho F, Alcântra DB, Rodrigues TH, Alexandre E Silva LM, de Oliveira Silva E, Zocolo GJ, de Brito ES (2018) Development and validation of a reversed phase HPLC method for determination of anacardic acids in cashew (*Anacardium occidentale*) nut shell liquid. J Chromatogr Sci 56(4):300–306

Ovalle-Magallanes B, Eugenio-Perez D, PedrazaCharerri J (2017) Medicinal properties of Mangosteen (*Garcinia mangostana* L.): a comprehensive update. Food Chem Toxicol 109:102–122

Patel RV, Mistry BM, Shinde SK, Syed R, Singh V, Shin HS (2018) Therapeutic potential of quercetin as a cardiovascular agent. Eur J Med Chem 155:889–904

Ramesh SV, Pandiselvam R, Hebbar KB, Manikantan MR, Shameena Beegum PP, Praveen P, Sruthi NU (2020) Antiviral potential of coconut (Cocos nucifera L.) oil and COVID-19. Coronaviruses 2(4):405–410. https://doi.org/10.2174/2666796701999201104164010

Ramesh SV, Krishnan V, Praveen S, Hebbar KB (2021) Dietary prospects of coconut oil for the prevention and treatment of Alzheimer's disease (AD): a review of recent evidences. Trends Food Sci Technol 112:201–211

Ranasinghe P, Jayawardena R, Pigera S, Wathurapatha WS, Weeratunga HD, Premakumara GS, Katulanda P, Constantine GR, Galappaththy P (2017) Evaluation of pharmacodynamic properties and safety of *Cinnamomum zeylanicum* (Ceylon cinnamon) in healthy adults: a phase I clinical trial. BMC Complement Altern Med 17:550. https://doi.org/10.1186/s12906-017-2067-7

Rastogi A, Shukla S (2013) Amaranth: a new millennium crop of nutraceutical values. Crit Rev Food Sci Nutr 53(2):109–125

Razzaghi-Asl N, Garrido J, Khazraei H, Borges F, Firuzi O (2013) Antioxidant properties of hydroxycinnamic acids: a review of structure-activity relationships. Curr Med Chem 20(36): 4436–4450

Ríos JL, Giner RM, Marín M, Recio MC (2018) A pharmacological update of ellagic acid. Planta Med 84(15):1068–1093

Risuleo G (2016) Resveratrol: multiple activities on the biological functionality of the cell. In: Gupta RC (ed) Nutraceuticals: efficacy, safety and toxicity. Academic Press/Elsevier, Amsterdam, pp 453–464

Sachdeva V, Roy A, Bharadvaja N (2020) Current prospects of nutraceuticals: a review. Curr Pharm Biotechnol 21(10):884–896

Saini RK, Rengasamy KR, Mahomoodally FM, Keum YS (2020) Protective effects of lycopene in cancer, cardiovascular, and neurodegenerative diseases: an update on epidemiological and mechanistic perspectives. Pharmacol Res 155:104730. https://doi.org/10.1016/j.phrs.2020.104730

Salehi B, Venditti A, Sharifi-Rad M, Kręgiel D, Sharifi-Rad J, Durazzo A, Lucarini M, Santini A, Souto EB, Novellino E, Antolak H (2019) The therapeutic potential of apigenin. Int J Mol Sci 20(6):1305. https://doi.org/10.3390/ijms20061305

Salem MZ, Elansary HO, Ali HM, El-Settawy AA, Elshikh MS, Abdel-Salam EM, Skalicka-Woźniak K (2018) Bioactivity of essential oils extracted from *Cupressus macrocarpa* branchlets and *Corymbia citriodora* leaves grown in Egypt. BMC Complement Altern Med 18:23. https://doi.org/10.1186/s12906-018-2085-0

Santini A, Cammarata SM, Capone G, Ianaro A, Tenore GC, Pani L, Novellino E (2018) Nutraceuticals: opening the debate for a regulatory framework. Br J Clin Pharmacol 84(4): 659–672

Satoh T (2016) Astaxanthin: health benefits and toxicity. In: Gupta RC (ed) Nutraceuticals: efficacy, safety and toxicity. Academic Press/Elsevier, Amsterdam, pp 531–539

Serrilli AM, Frasca G, Rizza L, Bonina FP, Bianco A (2013) Nocellaralactone, a new monoterpenoid with anti-inflammatory activity, from *Olea europaea* L., cultivar Nocellara del Belice. Nat Prod Res 27(24):2311–2319

Sudha P, Saikat H, Fayaj M, Smita Z, Hirekodathakallu T, Ameeta R (2015) Gedunin and azadiradione: human pancreatic alpha-amylase inhibiting limonoids from neem (*Azadirachta indica*) as anti-diabetic agents. PLoS One 10(10):e0140113. https://doi.org/10.1371/journal.pone.0140113

Sun F, Xiong S, Zhu Z (2016) Dietary capsaicin protects cardiometabolic organs from dysfunction. Nutrients 8(5):174. https://doi.org/10.3390/nu8050174

Taroncher M, Vila-Donat P, Tolosa J, Ruiz MJ, Rodríguez-Carrasco Y (2021) Biological activity and toxicity of plant nutraceuticals: an overview. Curr Opin Food Sci 42:113–118. https://doi.org/10.1016/j.cofs.2021.05.008

Testai L, Calderone V (2017) Nutraceutical value of citrus flavanones and their implications in cardiovascular disease. Nutrients 9(5):502. https://doi.org/10.3390/nu9050502

Thaipong K, Boonprakob U, Crosby K, Cisneros-Zevallos L, Byrne DH (2006) Comparison of ABTS, DPPH, FRAP, and ORAC assays for estimating antioxidant activity from guava fruit extracts. J Food Compos Anal 19:669–675

Thrane M, Paulsen PV, Orcutt MW, Krieger TM (2017) Soy protein: impacts, production, and applications. In: Sustainable protein sources. Academic Press, London, pp 23–45. https://doi.org/10.1016/B978-0-12-802778-3.00002-0

Wang S, Noh SK, Koo SI (2006) Green tea catechins inhibit pancreatic phospholipase A2 and intestinal absorption of lipids in ovariectomized rats. J Nutr Biochem 17(7):492–498

Wang J, Zhang X, Lan H, Wang W (2017a) Effect of garlic supplement in the management of type 2 diabetes mellitus (T2DM): a meta-analysis of randomized controlled trials. Food Nutr Res 61: 1377571. https://doi.org/10.1080/16546628.2017.1377571

Wang L, Lin Q, Yang T, Liang Y, Nie Y, Luo Y, Shen J, Fu X, Tang Y, Luo F (2017b) Oryzanol modifies high fat diet-induced obesity, liver gene expression profile, and inflammation response in mice. J Agric Food Chem 65(38):8374–8385

Woo YJ, Joo YB, Jung YO, Ju JH, La Cho M, Oh HJ, Jhun JY, Park MK, Park JS, Kang CM, Sung MS (2011) Grape seed proanthocyanidin extract ameliorates monosodium iodoacetate-induced osteoarthritis. Exp Mol Med 43:561–570

Wulan DR, Utomo EP, Mahdi C (2015) Antidiabetic activity of *Ruellia tuberosa* L., role of α-amylase inhibitor: *in silico*, *in vitro*., and *in vivo* approaches. Biochem Res Int 2015: 349261. https://doi.org/10.1155/2015/349261

Xiang CP, Han JX, Li XC, Li YH, Zhang Y, Chen L, Qu Y, Hao CY, Li HZ, Yang CR, Zhao SJ (2017) Chemical composition and acetylcholinesterase inhibitory activity of essential oils from Piper species. J Agric Food Chem 65:3702–3710

Xiao J, Capanoglu E, Jassbi AR, Miron A (2016) Advance on the flavonoid C-glycosides and health benefits. Crit Rev Food Sci Nutr 56(sup1):S29–S45. https://doi.org/10.1080/10408398.2015.1067595

Yu W, Simmons-Menchaca M, Gapor A, Sanders BG, Kline K (1999) Induction of apoptosis in human breast cancer cells by tocopherols and tocotrienols. Nutr Cancer 33(1):26–32

Yu X, Tang YH, Liu PY (2017) Flaxseed oil alleviates chronic HFD-induced insulin resistance through remodeling lipid homeostasis in obese adipose tissue. J Agric Food Chem 65(44): 9635–9645

Zhai J, Bo Y, Lu Y, Liu C, Zhang L (2017) Effects of coenzyme Q10 on markers of inflammation: a systematic review and meta-analysis. PLoS One 12(1):e0170172. https://doi.org/10.1371/journal.pone.0170172

Zou Y, Kim AR, Kim JE, Choi JS, Chung HY (2002) Peroxynitrite scavenging activity of sinapic acid (3, 5-dimethoxy-4-hydroxycinnamic acid) isolated from *Brassica juncea*. J Agric Food Chem 50:5884–5890

Chapter 5
Plant-Based Milk Alternatives: Nutritional Potential and Challenges

Ramesh S. V., P. P. Shameena Beegum, R. Pandiselvam, M. R. Manikantan, and K. B. Hebbar

Abstract Beverage industry has significantly evolved in formulating diverse products to meet the requirements of nutraceutical or functional food category. In this context, plant-based extracts from diverse sources such as soybean, almond, coconut, oat, pulses, and rice called plant-based milk alternatives (PBMAs) or analogs form an integral component of beverage industry. The growth in the PBMA industry could be attributed to various reasons, namely, dietary preferences, and nutritional needs. Additionally, the plant-based milk products are rich sources of health-promoting bioactives and are devoid of cholesterol and ecologically require less energy input per unit of milk production and thus are much appreciated. Nevertheless, there are technological bottlenecks in developing a wholesome substitute for cow's milk owing to different physicochemical properties of PBMAs. This chapter discusses various sources of PBMAs, their nutritional composition, blending of PBMAs for nutritional complementation effect and to improve the sensory profile of the product and the need for post-harvest technological intervention, alternate strategies, and challenges ahead in the production process of PBMAs.

Keywords Biochemical composition · Beverages · Food processing · Functional foods · Milk analogs · Plant milk

5.1 Introduction

Plant-based milk alternatives (PBMAs) or analogs are water-soluble extracts of diverse plants such as legumes, cereals, nuts, pseudocereals, and oil seeds that mimic the physical and biochemical qualities of bovine milk (Yadav et al. 2017).

R. S. V. (✉) · P. P. Shameena Beegum · R. Pandiselvam · M. R. Manikantan · K. B. Hebbar
Physiology, Biochemistry and Post-Harvest Technology Division, ICAR-Central Plantation Crops Research Institute, Kasaragod, Kerala, India
e-mail: ramesh.sv@icar.gov.in

R. S. V., S. Praveen (eds.), *Conceptualizing Plant-Based Nutrition*,
https://doi.org/10.1007/978-981-19-4590-8_5

These PBMAs are called as beverages, drinks, or dairy alternatives to distinguish it from the widely consumed cow's milk. Among these, the most common milk alternatives include soybean, coconut, and almond (Cornucopia Institute 2019). The ingredients of these milk alternatives include water extractants of nuts, cereals, endosperm, and oilseeds of diverse plant sources, emulsifier, and additives. One of the most widely consumed PBMA is soy milk, and the product was successfully launched in Hong Kong in 1940 since then the market share of plant-based milk analogs has grown rapidly due to technological improvements in the production of soy milk. Despite the large share of soybean milk in this segment, the emerging milk alternatives derived from other plants such as coconut, oats, almond, and peanut have also witnessed a huge growth. The large-scale production and marketing of plant-based milk analogs have led to its exponential growth worldwide (Sethi et al. 2016). Europe has witnessed a growth of 9% market share in these plant-based beverages. In the United States, a remarkable increase in the demand for non-dairy alternatives and concurrently a considerable decrease in dairy milk consumption are documented (Singhal et al. 2017). However, the market for plant-based milk substitutes is still in infancy and soybean milk is greatest contributor to this segment due to its nutrient profile (Vanga and Raghavan 2018).

These plant-based milk substitutes are considered as food products that would replace bovine milk for various reasons including lactose intolerance, allergic to cow's milk, or as a lifestyle choice (Mäkinen et al. 2015). Around 68% of the global population suffers from lactose malabsorption (NIDDK 2022), and in Indian context, almost 60–65% of population are lactose-intolerant (Economic Times 2020). In addition, increased demand for non-dairy products also has come mainly due to vegetarianism and the cholesterol content in bovine milk. It is also important to observe that for lactose-intolerant individuals other alternatives such as products free of lactose and utilization of lactase enzyme are available; however, for individuals suffering from allergenicity and vegans, plant-based milk remains the only choice. The controversy surrounding the β-casein variants of dairy milk (A1 and A2 milk) and consumption of A1 dairy milk (which has A1 β-casein) potentially predisposes humans to various diseases such as inflammation, type 1 diabetes, heart ailments, and autism which warrants a healthy alternative (Kaskous 2020). The production process of these beverages essentially remains the same. It involves the soaking of raw materials followed by processing with water. The extract is filtered to remove any insoluble residues; then, flavoring agents, sugar, emulsifier, or stabilizers may be added depending upon the requirement. In general, processes such as improving the stability, homogenization, and pasteurization to improve the shelf life are completed at the end of production flow, so that the milk extracts remain a stable colloidal suspension or emulsion (Jeske et al. 2017) (Fig. 5.1).

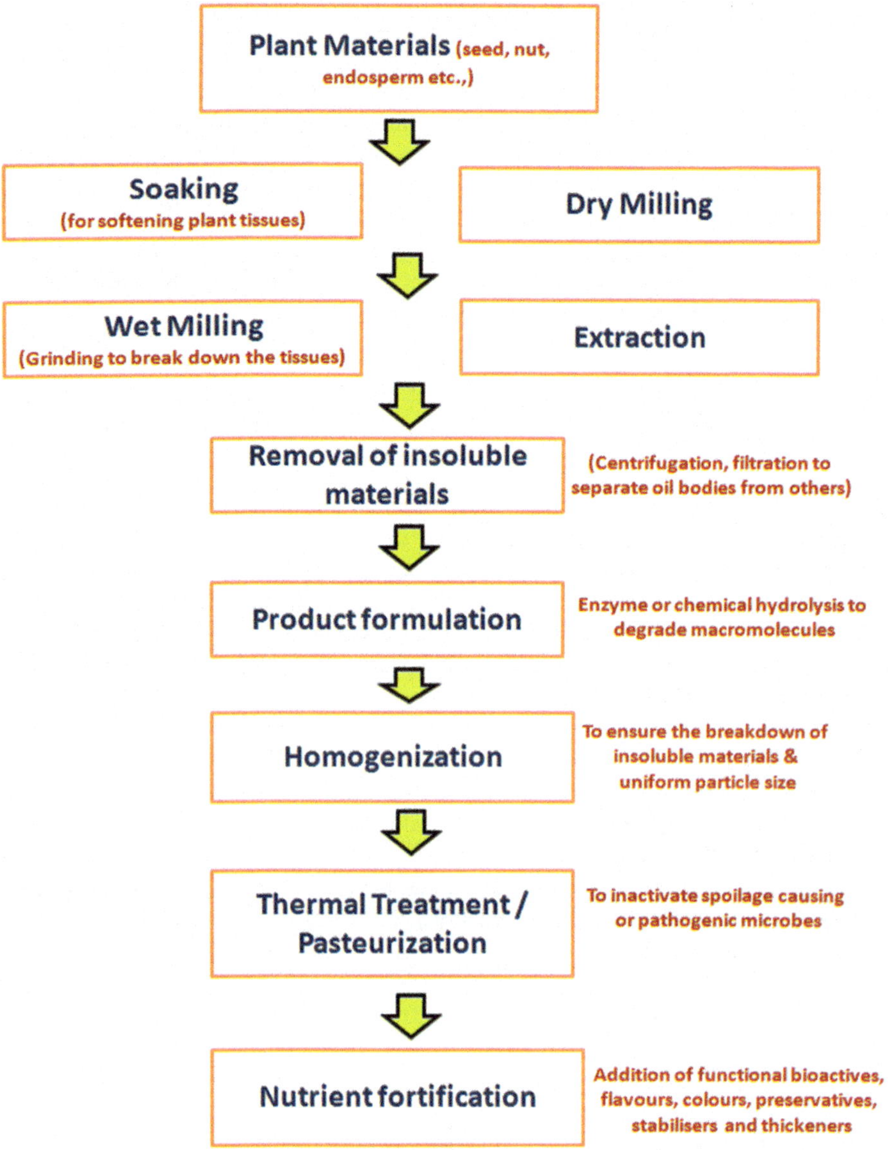

Fig. 5.1 Processing steps involved in the development of plant-based milk alternatives. (Adapted from McClements et al. 2019; Reyes-Jurado et al. 2021)

5.2 Plant-Based Milk Analogs

Plant-based milk substitutes are obtained from multiple sources such as cereals (corn, oats, rice, rye, spelt, etc.), legumes (Bambara groundnut, chickpea, cowpea, kidney bean, lupin, peanut, soybean, pea), nuts (almond, cashew, coconut, pistachio, tiger nut, walnut), oil seeds (sesame, flaxseed, hemp, sunflower), and pseudocereals (amaranth, quinoa, and teff) (Reyes-Jurado et al. 2021). There are other sources of plant milk such as sunflower, melon seed, hazel nut, and quinoa; however, research-based literature on these aspects is very limited. The nutritional composition of PBMAs in comparison with bovine milk is presented in Table 5.1.

5.2.1 *Soymilk*

Soybean (*Glycine max* L.) products have attained nutritional importance and preference among the vegetarians because of its relatively high content of protein (~40%) and other phytochemicals. Soybean seed-derived milk, which is a refreshing nutritional beverage, has ~7 g/236.6 mL of protein comparable to that of dairy milk (Krans 2017). Soy milk is rich in isoflavones (daidzein, genistein, and glycitein) that offer protective effect against multiple ailments such as cancer, cardiovascular disease, and osteoporosis (Rizzo and Baroni 2018). The milk is also rich in fibers, minerals (especially calcium, iron, and zinc), vitamin B, and heart-healthy fatty acids (Rizzo and Baroni 2018). Other bioactives such as phytic acid (1.0–2.2%), sterols (0.23–0.46%), and saponins (0.17–6.16%) offer added health benefits. Nevertheless, the major constituent, isoflavone, mimics mild estrogens and could affect gestation and infancy and other reproductive failures (Katz 2018). The oligosaccharides remain indigestible in human gastrointestinal tract causing production of gas. Furthermore, some degree of allergic reactions in humans was recorded for soy milk (Jeske et al. 2017).

5.2.2 *Almond Milk*

Almonds (*Prunus dulcis*) are rich in vitamin E (25.87 mg α-tocopherol/100 g), vitamin B-complex (B1, B2, B3, B5, and B6), protein (16–23 g/100 g), and MUFA (31 g/100 g) and hence are considered brain foods (Grundy et al. 2016). Almond milk, instead of soy milk, is suggested for people experiencing lactose intolerance (Lee et al. 2018). Almonds, as foods, are known to offer anti-inflammatory, lipid-lowering, tumor-suppressant, and antioxidant ingredients (Barreira et al. 2008). The milk is also known to have prebiotics properties. Further, the seed storage protein components of almonds [amandin, legumin (11S), prunin, and conglutin γ] which cause allergenic reaction are to be removed either by using

Table 5.1 Nutritional composition of various plant-based milk alternatives (values are expressed per 100 mL; for comparison purpose, nutritional information on cow's milk is also provided)

Plant-based milk analogs and bovine milk	Bioactives	Energy (kcal)	Proteins (g)	Carbohydrates (g)	Total sugars (g)	Total fat (g)	Fiber (g)	Calcium (mg)	Iron (mg)	Vitamin A (% daily value)[a]
Almond	α-Tocopherol, folate, niacin (B3), arabinose, flavonoids and phytosterols, (β-sitosterol, campesterol, stigmasterol)	15	0.59	0.58	0	1.10	0	197.00	0.35	10
Cashew	Phytosterols, polyunsaturated fats	47	0.28	9.17	5.28	0.97	0.3	118.00	0.20	–
Coconut	Lauric acid, medium-chain triglycerides, vitamin E	54.17	1.67	10	7.92	4.12	–	145.83	0.75	10
Hemp	Linolenic acid, linoleic acid, c-tocopherol, cannabidiolic acid, and lignanamides	42.10	1.99	3.33	2.5	2.92	0	125.00	1.08	10
Oat	β-Glucan and phytosterols	66	1.9	4.44	1.27	4.65	0.8	8.00	0.76	10
Pea	Resveratrol, niacin, vitamin E, and arginine	42.08	3.33	2.5	2.5	1.88	0	187.90	1.12	–
Rice	Phytosterols, especially β-sitosterol and γ-oryzanol	47–112.00	0.28–1.60	9.41–12.70	7.86	0.97–1.11	0.30–0.65	118–121.00	0.20–0.96	10
Soybean	Isoflavones, phytosterol α-tocopherol (genistein, daidzein, glycitein)	43	2.6	4.92	3.65	1.47	0.2	123.00	0.42	10
Cow milk[b]	Casein, lactoferricin, casoxins, casocidin, casokinins, IgG, IgA	69.0–118.0	2.90–6.40	3.2–5.4	4.58	3.40–6.40	Not reported	122.00–134.00	0.07–0.08	168 μg

Data compiled from multiple sources: U.S. Department of Agriculture (2022), Bridges (2018), Sousa and Kopf-Bolanz (2017) and Sethi et al. (2016)
[a]Vitamin A per serving of 240 mL
[b]Cow milk values per/100 g

mechanical or fermentation treatments while preparing almond milk (Lee et al. 2018). The major bioactives of almond milk with nutritional potential are α-tocopherol, sugar arabinose, flavonoids, and phytosterols (Makinde and Adebile 2018).

5.2.3 *Coconut Milk*

Coconut milk is a natural oil-in-water emulsion, stabilized by proteins such as globulins, albumins, and phospholipids (Manikantan et al. 2019). It is obtained from the endosperm or kernel of the palm through mechanical means or Aqueous Enzymatic Extraction Process (AEEP) Viscozyme L enzyme method (Agarwal and Bosco 2014). Thus, coconut milk is prepared at home from the grated pieces of endosperm or kernel by squeezing, whereas production on industrial scale involves the use of screw press or hydraulic expeller (Patil and Benjakul 2018). Traditionally, coconut milk is used for culinary purposes in the parts of southern India and other Asian nations like Sri Lanka, Thailand, Indonesia, Malaysia etc. Coconut milk is characteristically rich in medium-chain triglycerides (MCTs) and hence could be easily absorbed and metabolized by the liver to produce ketone bodies which provide neuroprotective functions. Consumption of coconut milk increases the HDL (high-density lipoprotein) levels, which help in reducing the harmful LDL (low-density lipoprotein) (Vanga and Raghavan 2018). Further, the relatively good quantity of insoluble and soluble fiber content improves the nutritional value of coconut milk (Fernando et al. 2015). The coconut milk is known to promote the proper brain development besides boosting the immune system. It also helps in the maintenance of elasticity of blood vessels and provides antiageing property due to skin nourishment. Also, the medium-chain triglycerides are linked with weight loss and neuroprotective effects (Ramesh et al. 2021). Comparison of nutrient profiles of coconut milk alternative with bovine milk reveals that the former is rich in fiber content, iron, potassium, and phosphorous contents and comparable energy and fat content (Table 5.2) (Data compiled from Paul et al. 2020; McClements et al. 2019). However, the amino acid profile (histidine, isoleucine, leucine, lysine, methionine, phenylalanine, threonine, tryptophan, and valine) of coconut nondairy milk substitute is found to be poor compared to that of dairy milk (Patil and Benjakul 2018). Vitamin composition of coconut milk is also found to be deficient when compared to cow milk. However, fat-soluble vitamins such as A, D, and folate were found to be in appreciable quantity compared to bovine milk (Table 5.2).

5.2.4 *Oat Milk*

Oat (*Avena sativa* L.) is rich in antioxidant and nutritional contents having phenolics, avenanthramides (2–289 mg/kg), and saponins (avenacoside A—290 mg/kg and

Table 5.2 Nutritional comparison of coconut milk and bovine milk

Nutritional ingredients	Coconut milk	Bovine milk
Carbohydrate (g/100 g)	3.75–9.41	3.20–5.40
Protein (g/100 g)	0.59–2.00	2.90–6.00
Fat (g/100 g)	4.12–6.00	3.40–6.40
Fiber (g/100 g)	5.30–5.98	Not reported
Energy (k cal)	50.00–92.00	69.0–118.0
Minerals (mg/100 g)		
Fe	3.90–4.01	0.07–0.08
K	631.0–639.02	152.0–181.0
P	240.0–256.35	119.0–121.0
Vitamins		
Vitamin C (mg/100 mL)	0.0	1.50
Thiamine (mg/100 mL)	–	0.04
Riboflavin (mg/100 mL)	–	0.16
Niacin (mg/100 mL)	–	0.08
Vitamin B6 (mg/100 mL)	–	0.04
Vitamin E (mg/100 mL)	–	–
Folate (μg/100 mL)	19.2	5.00
Vitamin B-12 (μg/100 mL)	0.75	0.36
Vitamin A (μg/100 mL)	60	33
Vitamin D (μg/100 mL)	2.92	–

avenacoside B—110 mg/kg) (Sang and Chu 2017), phytate and phytosterols, dietary fibers (2.3–8.5), and calcium content (0.54%) (Rasane et al. 2015). The β-glucan of oat is known to have anticancerous properties and also confers reduced blood cholesterol and blood pressure levels in human. Also, the relatively balanced protein composition of oats makes it more nutritious than other widely consumed cereals. The aforesaid nutritional properties make the oats an important healthy milk alternative, and many products are available in the market "Oat Milk"® (Frolich 1996; Onning et al. 1998) and "Pro Viva"® obtained from oat meal following fermentation with *Lactobacillus plantarum* (Bekers et al. 2001). Fermentation process is considered a convenient method of preparation of oats milk which increases the plant phenolics content and glucosamine content, thereby increasing the antioxidant properties of the milk (Bei et al. 2017). However, oat milk is deficient in calcium, and hence, Ca fortification is indispensable (Sethi et al. 2016).

5.2.5 *Rice Milk*

Rice (*Oryza sativa* L.) is a widely consumed cereal not only in Asia but also worldwide. Rice has been utilized as a raw material for the production of milk substituted product mimicking the quality features of bovine milk. The wide acceptability of rice as a non-allergenic cereal ensured production of rice-based milk comparable in physical and nutritional properties of soybean milk. Though rice is rich in starch, its protein composition lacks threonine and lysine. Also, rice bran is rich source of polyphenol, and hence, methodologies have been explored to utilize the whole rice (including the bran) to produce rice bran milk. The processing techniques such as soaking (which enhances mineral and vitamins) and fermentation using lactic acid bacteria will improve the mineral contents (such as Ca, Mg, and Fe) and significantly reduce the antinutritional factors (Sharma and Gayathri 2018). Further, rice bran milk has been known to have low TSS and viscosity compared to soy milk (Issara and Rawdkuen 2014).

5.2.6 Cocoa Milk

Cocoa (*Theobroma cacao* L.) is rich in phytophenolics (18%) and flavonoids that have cardio-protective, anticancer, and neuroprotective functions (Rodríguez-Lagunas et al. 2019). Further cocoa and its products are known to have suppressive effect on lactose intolerance making it a suitable PBMA. The cardiovascular health benefits of consumption of cocoa and products include reduced blood pressure and positive modulations in the metabolism of carbohydrates and lipids. Further, the cocoa-derived flavanols significantly affect the carbohydrate digestion and absorption in the gut, thereby improving the secretion of insulin (Ramos et al. 2017). Also, the bioactives theobromine and caffeine provide antiageing properties (Fonseca Maciel et al. 2017).

5.2.7 Hemp Milk

The seeds of hemp (*Cannabis sativa* L.) are rich in PUFA such as α-linolenic acid and linoleic acid, essential amino acids, insoluble fibers (~15%), vitamin E (90 mg/100 g), and mineral constituents making it a good candidate alternative for dairy milk and other plant-based milks such as soy or nut milk which are high in allergens (Frassinetti et al. 2018). As with other plant-based milk analogs, the milk derived from hemp is an oil-in-water emulsion that is very unstable and flocculates to generate a layer of cream decreasing its shelf life to great extent. In industrial scale, emulsifiers and stabilizers are used to counter this problem; nevertheless, usage of these chemical agents is fraught with other health concerns and is not an economically viable option.

5.2.8 *Kidney Bean Milk*

The seeds of kidney bean (*Phaseolus vulgaris* L.) are soaked in water until it swells and milk is extracted following boiling and grinding processes (Chen et al. 2019). In order to reduce the antinutritional factors and allergen-causing ingredients, fermentation process is followed which not only enhances antioxidant potential of the product but also improves the production of isoflavone aglycones (Limón et al. 2015). In addition, different enzymatic or gaseous treatments along with fermentation processes enhance the content of gamma-aminobutyric acid (GABA) which has many health-improving properties such as suppression of cancer cell proliferation and reduction in blood pressure and blood cholesterol content (Nikmaram et al. 2017).

5.2.9 *Peanut Milk*

Peanut milk and its products are known to have immense health benefits because of its rich protein content, minerals, and linoleic and oleic acids, the essential fatty acids. Peanut milk is extensively consumed in developing nations characterized with low-income starch diets, vegans, and lactose-intolerant children (Diarra et al. 2005). Various methodologies and techniques have been developed to produce peanut milk. In the grinding method, fat content is removed to yield a yellow liquid which is rich in protein, or alternatively, it can be fermented (Arya et al. 2016). Various other physical treatments such as soaking, defatting, steaming, roasting, and heating are performed followed by filtration to obtain the milk with reduced content of antinutritional factors (Adegoke and Falade 2016). Poor stability is one of the main problems associated in the peanut milk production process due to its high-fat content and hence emulsifiers (alginates, gelatin, or vegetable gums 1%) are used.

5.2.10 *Tigernut Milk*

Tigernut milk is obtained from the tigernut plant (*Cyperus esculentus* L.) of Cyperaceae. The grass is cultivated for its small rhizome which is eaten raw or roasted and pressed for its juice to make beverage or milk. It is a healthy and rich source of nutrients such as carbohydrates, vegetable fat, protein, fiber, vitamins, minerals, energy, and some digestive enzymes such as catalase, lipase, and amylase (Adejuyitan 2011; Chima et al. 2013). It is devoid of sodium, lactose sugar, casein protein, gluten, cholesterol, or any allergens and therefore ideal for people who are hypertensive or do not tolerate gluten or lactose and its derivatives present in cow milk (Belewu and Abodunrin 2006).

5.3 Blending of Milk Analogs and Alternative Strategies

Considering the nutritional deficiencies of the individual plant-based milk alternatives, it was proposed to blend two or more non-dairy milk alternatives to develop a wholesome, nutritious beverage and to improve the sensorial properties. Blending of diverse plant-derived milk products of soybean, almond, peanut, tiger nut, and coconut has helped in avoiding or reducing the beany flavor and in improving the nutritional profile of the end product in terms of protein quality, dietary fiber content, etc. (Kundu et al. 2018; Ajala et al. 2013; Adedokun et al. 2014). Further, biochemical and sensory properties of a probiotic beverage prepared from the blends of milks of African yam bean, coconut, and soybean reveal that fermented product (utilizing *Lactobacillus delbrueckii*) of this blend was acceptable in terms of sensory aspects (Ikujenlola et al. 2020). Vegetable milks can act as composite milk to replace cow milk without markedly affecting the quality of ice cream (AboulfAzli et al. 2014).

Pulse protein ingredients have found their application in the development of plant-based milk alternatives. The developments in the field of extraction of high-quality protein from pulses and processing methods have paved way for incorporation of pulse-derived proteins as an important functional and nutritive ingredient in the formulation of superior plant-based milk alternatives. Various methodologies such as dry fractionation techniques (air classification and tribo-electric separation) and aqueous fractionation protocols (isoelectric precipitation, ultrafiltration and salt extraction/micellization) to extract protein concentrates from pulses have been standardized (Vogelsang-O'Dwyer et al. 2021). Several studies have explored the possibility of formulating milk alternatives utilizing pulse protein ingredients. Jacobs et al. (2016) and Jeske et al. (2019) have developed lupin and lentil protein-based milk alternatives, respectively. Lentil-derived protein has shown appreciable potential to develop milk substitutes with high protein content that is similar to cow's milk (Jeske et al. 2019). Rincon et al. (2020) formulated a chickpea and coconut extract-based milk alternative as a potential substitute for cow's milk. Also, some of the pulse protein-based milk alternatives have become commercially available (Vogelsang-O'Dwyer et al. 2021).

Multiple research approaches have been undertaken on plant-based non-dairy products. Shameena Beegum et al. (2021) tapped the potential of utilizing coconut products particularly coconut milk in developing a frozen coconut delicacy. Soy milk and coconut milk (either alone or as blends with cow milk) were found to be a good vehicle for the delivery of probiotic strains such as *Lactobacillus acidophilus* and *Bifidobacterium bifidum* in ice cream (Aboulfazli et al. 2016). Ice creams made of both the soy and coconut milk provide a richer growth medium of amino acids and sugar content for both the microbial strains than cow's milk ice cream. Similarly, improved growth of probiotic bacteria was reported by Mridula and Sharma (2015), while the sprouted wheat, barley, pearl millet, and green gram in combination with oats, and soy milk were utilized in a probiotic drink. Coconut milk-based cottage cheese/*paneer* which consists of 50:50 blend of cow's milk and coconut milk was developed (Sughanya and Ramaswamy (2017). Similarly, the potential of coconut milk as a substitute for cow milk in cheese making was explored (Okon and Ojimelukwe 2017). A European patent (17157951.9) by Iruthayathasan and Lahousse (2018) claims a method of preparing a vegan cheese with various vegetarian sources including coconut milk and soy milk and using calcium chloride, a beneficial bacterial culture and plant rennet. However, dairy alternative yogurts can have structural disadvantages compared to dairy yogurts made with animal milks, because of the nature of the proteins. Sridhar et al. (2015) developed coconut milk and cow milk-based curd using *Lactobacillus lactis* and *L. plantarum.* Study on supplemented milk with quinoa flour revealed that quinoa can be added to dairy products to improve nutrition, while not affecting the probiotic quality (Casarotti et al. 2014). *Kheer* made out of blends of buffalo milk and soy milk along with sugar and rice resulted in sensorially acceptable product (Pariskar et al. 2015). Physicochemical and acid gelation properties of UHT-treated commercial soy, oat, quinoa, rice, and lactose-free bovine milks revealed that particles of plant-based milk substitutes were significantly more polydispersed compared to those of bovine milk (Mäkinen et al. 2015). Upon acidification with glucono-D-lactone (GDL), bovine, soy, and quinoa milks formed structured gels, while oat and rice milks did not. Since plant based milks are produced by disintegration of plant materials the resulting particle sizes and composition are not as uniform as in bovine milk.

5.4 Challenges in the Production of Milk Analogs

The major challenges encountered during the production of plant-based milk substitutes include nutrient imbalances (especially protein quality compared to bovine milk), presence of antinutritional compounds, and physical properties such as its appearance and texture profile (Pontonio and Rizzello 2021). From the nutrition point of view, the presence of antinutritional factors severely affects the sensory profile of the product and influences the bioavailability of other nutrients (Munekata et al. 2020). Production of PBMAs encounters various technological problems including poor stability as this feature is influenced by particle size (fat globules of milk), emulsion formation, starch, and protein solubility. Hence, to overcome this instability, emulsifiers, food stabilizers (oleosins, microgels, etc.), and processing changes such as ultrahigh-pressure homogenization (UHPH) and ultrasonic homogenization high-intensity ultrasound irradiation are proposed. Further, plant-based milk products are considered to have off-flavor which is due to the presence of enzymes, lipoxygenases, and unsaturated fatty acids. To remove the off-flavor, enzyme inactivation strategies, namely rapid hydration grinding, high-pressure processing, ohmic heating, and cold plasma, are suggested. Also, artificial or natural flavoring agents could be added to mask the off-flavor. Similarly, physical treatments such as boiling, sprouting, soaking, steam treatment, blanching, and enzyme-based bioprocessing biotechnology operations are suggested to remove or inactivate the inhibitors. Combination of germination and fermentation is a successful way to improve nutritional quality by reducing the content of sugars while enhancing the levels of thiamine, niacin, lysine, and soluble dietary fiber of plant-based (wheat, barley, soy, etc.) beverages, especially milk and fermented drink (Arora et al. 2010). Since the shelf life of PBMA is very less due to high content of sugars and fatty acids, physical treatment procedures such as UHPH, ultrasound processing, and hurdle technology are proposed (Munekata et al. 2020; Paul et al. 2020).

5.5 Concluding Remarks

One of the major advantages with plant-based milk substitutes compared to conventional or bovine milk is its reduced carbon footprint (i.e., less energy input) to produce per unit quantity. Further, market dynamics and forecast for dairy alternatives state that at the global level the market for this segment is valued at 22.6 billion USD in the year 2020 which is projected to scale 40.6 billion USD by 2026. Thus, a compound annual growth rate of 10.3% in its value is forecasted owing to numerous health benefits (Markets and Markets 2021) changing lifestyles and increasing health awareness. In addition, diverse phytochemicals, absence of cholesterol, preference for vegan foods, and limited milk availability are some of the factors contributing to the expansion of nondairy, plant-based milk substitute industry. On the other hand, major challenges include improving its sensory profile, removal of antinutritional factors or undesirable beany flavor and poor protein quality. Among these, poor protein quality could be manipulated by sourcing the proteins from pulses or other legumes. To address other challenges, there is a need for concerted effort from the researchers and industries to develop technologically feasible, functional, and nutritionally superior beverage with an appreciable economics of operations. Conclusive research evidences are also required to understand the complete health benefits of plant-based milks in human nutrition so that it paves way for development of novel, nutritionally superior products of plant sources. It can be safely concluded that this arena of research offers ample scope for plant biochemists, nutritionists, and food technologists to develop superior food products.

References

AboulfAzli F, Ahmad Salihin Baba AS, Misran M (2014) Effect of vegetable milks on the physical and rheological properties of ice cream. Food Sci Technol Res 20(5):987–996

Aboulfazli F, Shori BA, Baba AS (2016) Effects of the replacement of cow milk with vegetable milk on probiotics and nutritional profile of fermented ice cream. LWT Food Sci Technol 70: 261–270

Adedokun II, Okorie SU, Batu B (2014) Evaluation of proximate, fibre qualities and consumer acceptability of bambaranut-tigernut-coconut milk beverage blends. Inter J Nutr Food Sci 3(5): 430–437

Adegoke GO, Falade AT (2016) Effect of Aframomum danielli on peanut milk characteristics and flavor. Nutr Food Technol: Open Access 3:1–5. https://doi.org/10.16966/2470-6086.136

Adejuyitan JA (2011) Tigernut processing: its food uses and health benefits. Am J Food Technol 6(3):197–201. https://doi.org/10.3923/ajft.2011.197.201

Agarwal RK, Bosco S (2014) Optimization of viscozyme-l assisted extraction of coconut milk and virgin coconut oil. Asian J Dairy Food Res 33:276–284. https://doi.org/10.5958/0976-0563.2014.00617.4

Ajala L, Ologunde MO, Adetuyi FO (2013) Physicochemical and sensory qualities of spiced soy-corn milk. Afr J Biotechnol 12(17):2262–2265

Arora S, Jood S, Khetarpaul N (2010) Effect of germination and probiotic fermentation on nutrient composition of barley based food mixtures. Food Chem 119(2):779–784. https://doi.org/10.1016/j.foodchem.2009.07.035

Arya SS, Salve AR, Chauhan S (2016) Peanuts as functional food: a review. J Food Sci Technol 53(1):31–41. https://doi.org/10.1007/s13197-015-2007-9

Barreira JCI, Ferreira C, Oliveira MBP, Pereira JA (2008) Antioxidant activity and bioactive compounds of ten Portuguese regional and commercial almond cultivars. Food Chem Toxicol 46(6):2230–2235. https://doi.org/10.1016/j.fct.2008.02.024

Bei Q, Liu Y, Wang L, Chen G, Wu Z (2017) Improving free, conjugated, and bound phenolic fractions in fermented oats (*Avena sativa* L.) with *Monascus anka* and their antioxidant activity. J Funct Foods 32:185–194. https://doi.org/10.1016/j.jff.2017.02.028

Bekers M, Marauska M, Laukevics J, Grube M, Vigants A, Karklina D, Skudra L, Viesturs U (2001) Oats and fat-free milk based functional food product. Food Biotechnol 15(1):1–12

Belewu MA, Abodunrin OA (2006) Preparation of kunnu from unexploited rich food source: tigernut (*Cyperus esculentus*). World J Dairy Food Sci 21:19–21

Bridges M (2018) Moo-ove over, cow's milk: the rise of plant-based dairy alternatives. Pract Gastroenterol 21:20–27

Casarotti SN, Carneiro BM, Penna ALB (2014) Evaluation of the effect of supplementing fermented milk with quinoa flour on probiotic activity. J Dairy Sci 97(10):6027–6035

Chen Y, Zhang H, Liu R, Mats L, Zhu H, Pauls KP et al (2019) Antioxidant and anti-inflammatory polyphenols and peptides of common bean (*Phaseolus vulgaris* L.) milk and yogurt in Caco-2 and HT-29 cell models. J Funct Foods 53:125–135. https://doi.org/10.1016/j.jff.2018.12.013

Chima OA, Abuajah Izuchukwu C, Utuk Afonabasi R (2013) Tigernut milk: a nutritious under-utilized food ingredient. Food Biol 2(2):14–17

Cornucopia Institute (2019) "Pouring" over plant-based beverages a consumer's guide to identifying the best non-milk alternatives. Cornucopia Institute, Cornucopia, WI

Diarra K, Nong ZG, Jie C (2005) Peanut milk and peanut milk based products production: a review. Crit Rev Food Sci Nutr 45(5):405–423

Economic Times (2020) Lactose intolerance. https://timesofindia.indiatimes.com/life-style/health-fitness/diet/60-per-cent-of-indians-suffer-from-milk-intolerance-and-many-dont-even-realise-it/photostory/75807121.cms. Accessed 8 Mar 2022

Fernando WMADB, Martins IJ, Goozee KG, Brennan CS, Jayasena V, Martins RN (2015) The role of dietary coconut for the prevention and treatment of Alzheimer's disease: potential mechanisms of action. Br J Nutr 114(1):1–14

Fonseca Maciel L, Felício ALDSM, Hirooka EY (2017) Bioactive compounds by UPLC-PDA in different cocoa clones (*Theobroma cacao* L.) developed in the southern region of Bahia, Brazil. Br Food J 119(9):2117–2127. https://doi.org/10.1108/BFJ-09-2016-0423

Frassinetti S, Moccia E, Caltavuturo L, Gabriele M, Longo V, Bellani L, Giorgi G, Giorgetti L (2018) Nutraceutical potential of hemp (*Cannabis sativa* L.) seeds and sprouts. Food Chem 262:56–66. https://doi.org/10.1016/j.foodchem.2018.04.078

Frolich W (1996) Novel food – is there a market for barley and oat. In: Scoles G, Rossnagel B (eds) Proc. V International Oat Conference & VII International Barley Genetics Symposium. 1996, Canada, pp 65–71

Grundy MML, Lapsley K, Ellis PR (2016) A review of the impact of processing on nutrient bioaccessibility and digestion of almonds. Int J Food Sci Technol 51:1937–1946. https://doi.org/10.1111/ijfs.13192

Ikujenlola AV, Adurotoye EA, Adeniran HA (2020) Chemical and sensory properties of probioticated drinks from blends of African yam bean, soybean and coconut milk analogues. Acta Univ Cibiniensis Ser E Food Technol 23:147–156

Iruthayathasan EE, Lahousse B (2018) Patent: method of preparing a vegan cheese. PCT/EP2018/054618

Issara U, Rawdkuen S (2014) Organic rice bran milk: production and its natural quality attributes. In: Proceeding of 1st joint ACS AGFD-ACS ICSCT symposium on agricultural and food chemistry. Academia, San Francisco, pp 82–88

Jacobs D, Stephany M, Eisner P, Toelstede S (2016) Sensory quality of lupin protein based milk alternatives. Agro Food Ind Hi-Tech 27(2):12–15

Jeske S, Zannini E, Arendt EK (2017) Evaluation of physicochemical and glycaemic properties of commercial plant-based milk substitutes. Plant Foods Hum Nutr 72(1):26–33

Jeske S, Bez J, Arendt EK, Zannini E (2019) Formation, stability, and sensory characteristics of a lentil-based milk substitute as affected by homogenisation and pasteurisation. Eur Food Res Technol 245(7):1519–1531

Kaskous S (2020) A1-and A2-milk and their effect on human health. J Food Eng Technol 9(1): 15–21. https://doi.org/10.32732/jfet.2020.9.1.15

Katz AC (2018) Milk nutrition and perceptions. Submitted in partial fulfillment of the requirements for the university honors scholar designation at Johnson & Wales University, pp 4–12. http://scholarsarchive.jwu.edu/student_scholarship/29

Krans B (2017) Comparing milks: almond, dairy, soy, rice, and coconut. Healthline.com. www.healthline.com/health/milk-almond-cow-soy-rice. Accessed 27 Feb 2022

Kundu P, Dhankhar J, Sharma A (2018) Development of non dairy milk alternative using soymilk and almond milk. Curr Res Nutr Food Sci 6(1):203–210

Lee J, Townsend JA, Thompson T, Garitty T, De A, Yu Q, Peters BM, Wen ZT (2018) Analysis of the cariogenic potential of various almond milk beverages using a *Streptococcus mutans* biofilm model in vitro. Caries Res 52(1–2):51–57. https://doi.org/10.1159/000479936

Limón RI, Peñas E, Torino MI, Martínez-Villaluenga C, Dueñas M, Frias J (2015) Fermentation enhances the content of bioactive compounds in kidney bean extracts. Food Chem 172:343–352

Makinde FM, Adebile TV (2018) Influence of processing treatments on quality of vegetable milk from almond (*Terminalia catappa*) kernels. ACTA Sci Nutr Health 2(6):37–42

Mäkinen OE, Thérèse Uniacke-Lowe T, O'Mahony JA, Arendt EK (2015) Physicochemical and acid gelation properties of commercial UHT-treated plant-based milk substitutes and lactose free bovine milk. Food Chem 168:630–638

Manikantan MR, Pandiselvam R, Beegum S, Mathew AC (2019) Harvest and postharvest technology. In: Nampoothiri K, Krishnakumar V, Thampan P, Nair M (eds) The coconut palm (*Cocos nucifera* L.)—research and development perspectives. Springer, Singapore. https://doi.org/10.1007/978-981-13-2754-4_13

Markets and Markets (2021) Dairy alternatives market by source (soy, almond, coconut, oats, rice, hemp), application (milk, yogurt, ice creams, cheese, creamers), distribution channel (supermarkets, health food stores, pharmacies), formulation, and region—Global Forecast to 2026. https://www.marketsandmarkets.com/Market-Reports/dairy-alternative-plant-milk-beverages-market-677.html. Accessed 14 Feb 2022

McClements DJ, Newman E, McClements IF (2019) Plant-based milks: a review of the science underpinning their design, fabrication, and performance. Compr Rev Food Sci Food Saf 18(6): 2047–2067. https://doi.org/10.1111/1541-4337.12505

Mridula D, Sharma M (2015) Development of non-dairy probiotic drink utilizing sprouted cereals, legume and soymilk. LWT Food Sci Technol 62(1):482–487. https://doi.org/10.1016/j.lwt.2014.07.011

Munekata PES, Domínguez R, Budaraju S, Roselló-Soto E, Barba FJ, Mallikarjunan K, Roohinejad S, Lorenzo JM (2020) Effect of innovative food processing technologies on the physicochemical and nutritional properties and quality of non-dairy plant-based beverages. Foods 9:288

NIDDK (National Institute of Diabetes and Digestive and Kidney Disease) (2022) Definition and facts for lactose intolerance. https://www.niddk.nih.gov/health-information/digestive-diseases/lactose-intolerance/definition-facts. Accessed 8 Mar 2022

Nikmaram NB, Dar N, Roohinejad S, Koubaa M, Barba FJ, Greiner R, Johnson SK (2017) Recent advances in c-aminobutyric acid (GABA) properties in pulses: an overview. J Sci Food Agric 97(9):2681–2689. https://doi.org/10.1002/jsfa.8283

Okon EG, Ojimelukwe PC (2017) Potentials of coconut milk as a substitute for cow milk in cheese making. J Adv Microbiol 4(2):1–9

Onning G, Akesson B, Oste R, Lundquist I (1998) Effects of consumption of oat milk, soya milk, or cow's milk on plasma lipids and antioxidative capacity in healthy subjects. Ann Nutr Metab 42: 211–220

Pariskar JR, Patil RA, Padghan PV, Londheand GK, Bhosale KS (2015) Studies on chemical composition of *kheer* prepared from soy milk blended with buffalo milk. Asian J Dairy Food Res 34(2):109–112

Patil U, Benjakul S (2018) Coconut milk and coconut oil: their manufacture associated with protein functionality. J Food Sci 83(8):2019–2027

Paul AA, Kumar S, Kumar V, Sharma R (2020) Plant based alternatives to conventional milk, production, potential and health concerns. Crit Rev Food Sci Nutr 60(18):3005–3023

Pontonio E, Rizzello CG (2021) Milk alternatives and non-dairy fermented products: trends and challenges. Foods 10(2):222

Ramesh SV, Krishnan V, Praveen S, Hebbar KB (2021) Dietary prospects of coconut oil for the prevention and treatment of Alzheimer's disease (AD): a review of recent evidences. Trends Food Sci Technol 112:201–211

Ramos S, Martın M, Goya L (2017) Effects of cocoa antioxidants in type 2 diabetes mellitus. Antioxidants 6(4):84. https://doi.org/10.3390/antiox6040084

Rasane P, Jha A, Sabikhi L, Kumar A, Unnikrishnan VS (2015) Nutritional advantages of oats and opportunities for its processing as value added foods—a review. J Food Sci Technol 52(2): 662–675. https://doi.org/10.1007/s13197-013-1072-1

Reyes-Jurado F, Soto-Reyes N, Dávila-Rodríguez M, Lorenzo-Leal AC, Jiménez-Munguía MT, Mani-López E, López-Malo A (2021) Plant-based milk alternatives: types, processes, benefits, and characteristics. Food Rev Int 2021:1952421. https://doi.org/10.1080/87559129.2021.1952421

Rincon L, Botelho RB, de Alencar ER (2020) Development of novel plant-based milk based on chickpea and coconut. LWT 128:109479. https://doi.org/10.1016/j.lwt.2020.109479

Rizzo G, Baroni L (2018) Soy, soy foods and their role in vegetarian diets. Nutrients 10(1):43. https://doi.org/10.3390/nu10010043

Rodríguez-Lagunas MJ, Vicente F, Pereira P, Castell M, Pérez-Cano FJ (2019) Relationship between cocoa intake and healthy status: a pilot study in university students. Molecules 24(4): 812. https://doi.org/10.3390/molecules24040812

Sang S, Chu Y (2017) Whole grain oats, more than just a fiber: role of unique phytochemicals. Mol Nutr Food Res 61(7):1600715

Sethi S, Tyagi SK, Anurag RK (2016) Plant-based milk alternatives an emerging segment of functional beverages: a review. J Food Sci Technol 53(9):3408–3423

Shameena Beegum PP, Nair JP, Manikantan MR, Pandiselvam R, Shil S, Neenu S, Hebbar KB (2021) Effect of coconut milk, tender coconut and coconut sugar on the physico-chemical and sensory attributes in ice cream. J Food Sci Technol 59(7):2605–2616. https://doi.org/10.1007/s13197-021-05279-y

Sharma N, Gayathri R (2018) Assessment of nutritional value of overnight soaked cooked rice over un-soaked cooked rice. Int J Res Pharm Sci 9:616–619

Singhal S, Baker RD, Baker SS (2017) A comparison of the nutritional value of cow's milk and nondairy beverages. J Pediatr Gastroenterol Nutr 64(5):799–805

Sousa A, Kopf-Bolanz KAK (2017) Nutritional implications of an increasing consumption of non-dairy plant-based beverages instead of cow's milk in Switzerland. Adv Dairy Res 5(4): 1000197. https://doi.org/10.4172/2329-888X.1000197
Sridhar R, Roopa BS, Varadaraj MC, Vijayendra SV (2015) Optimization of a novel coconut milk supplemented dahi—a fermented milk product of Indian subcontinent. J Food Sci Technol 52(11):7486–7492. https://doi.org/10.1007/s13197-015-1825-0
Sughanya R, Ramaswamy L (2017) Preparation of paneer from coconut milk, its quality characteristics and shelf life. Int J Recent Sci Res 8(3):16053–16057
U.S. Department of Agriculture (2022) Food data central. https://fdc.nal.usda.gov/
Vanga SK, Raghavan V (2018) How well do plant based alternatives fare nutritionally compared to cow's milk? J Food Sci Technol 55(1):10–20
Vogelsang-O'Dwyer M, Zannini E, Arendt EK (2021) Production of pulse protein ingredients and their application in plant-based milk alternatives. Trends Food Sci Technol 110:364–374
Yadav DN, Bansal S, Jaiswal AK, Singh R (2017) Plant based dairy analogues: an emerging food. Agric Res Technol 10:23–26. https://doi.org/10.19080/ARTOAJ.2017.10.555781

Chapter 6
Legumes and Pulses: Ways and Means to Enhance the Protein Quality

T. Vinutha, Ranjeet Ranjan Kumar, Navita Bansal, G. Rama Prashat, Suneha Goswami, Gyan P. Mishra, and Chellapilla Bharadwaj

Abstract Leguminous crops such as peas, beans, pigeon pea, lentils, and chickpea are also called as pulses. Pulses constitute one of the paramount sources of dietary proteins for major parts of the world's population, especially in those regions wherein consumption of animal protein is limited due to higher cost, nonaccessibility, and religious or cultural beliefs. In general, quality protein is mostly derived from animal source. The essential amino acids can also be obtained from plant proteins especially legume proteins by pairing them with cereal grains/ proteins. Since, pulses have twofold high-protein content, compared with cereal grains, pulses can make an excellent complementary food source of protein for infants, children, and adults. In order to cater to the consumer's demand for plant proteins, various processing techniques have been employed to enhance the protein quality including protein digestibility. Thermal processing (cooking, autoclaving, heating, and microwave), germination, irradiation, fermentation, extrusion, and spray- and freeze-drying methods have been adopted for improving the protein quality, especially protein digestibility, in pulses. Biofortification and genetic engineering approaches could also contribute as viable options to enhance essential amino acids or quality protein in mature seeds. Adoption of economically feasible options like processing methods discussed in this chapter and genetic enhancement of essential amino acids as well as protein quality in pulses and legumes can greatly help in alleviating malnutrition.

Keywords Essential amino acids · Legumes · Malnutrition · Plant proteins · Protein quality

T. Vinutha and Ranjeet Ranjan Kumar contributed equally with all other contributors.

T. Vinutha (✉) · R. R. Kumar · N. Bansal · S. Goswami
Division of Biochemistry, ICAR-Indian Agricultural Research Institute, New Delhi, India
e-mail: vinutha.t@icar.gov.in; ranjeet.ranjan@icar.gov.in

G. Rama Prashat · G. P. Mishra · C. Bharadwaj
Division of Genetics, ICAR-Indian Agricultural Research Institute, New Delhi, India

R. S. V., S. Praveen (eds.), *Conceptualizing Plant-Based Nutrition*,
https://doi.org/10.1007/978-981-19-4590-8_6

6.1 Introduction

Leguminous crops such as beans, peas, lentils, pigeon pea, and chickpea are also called as pulses. Pulses constitute one of the principal sources of dietary proteins for major parts of the world, especially in those regions wherein utilization of animal protein is limited due to higher cost, non-accessibility, and religious or cultural beliefs. In general, pulses contain crude protein in the range of 21–40% by weight and are excellent source of protein than cereals like wheat, rice, barley, and quinoa (Nosworthy and House 2017). The amino acid composition of various pulses is presented in Table 6.1. Proteins are indispensable component of human nutrition and play an essential role in biological and cellular processes. These processes regulate the structural and functional role in living systems right from building tissues, muscles, immunity, synthesis of hormones, enzymes, and energy. Proteins are made of amino acids—among them, nine amino acids (histidine, isoleucine, leucine, lysine, methionine, phenylalanine, threonine, tryptophan, and valine) are considered as essential and are indispensable. Humans including other vertebrates cannot synthesize these amino acids in their body using metabolic intermediates and hence are required from daily dietary sources. Fundamentally, these essential amino acids can be obtained from single complete protein or quality protein which is generally derived from animal source. Protein quality is determined by taking into account of composition of essential amino acids, and its digestibility and bioavailability, and those proteins which satisfy the metabolic demands of these three components are called as quality food proteins. The essential amino acids can be obtained from incomplete proteins, especially plant-based proteins, wherein they are limited by one or two essential amino acids; for example, methionine and tryptophan are limited in pulses and lysine in cereals. In general, plant protein have digestibility rate of 75–80% compared to animal proteins (90–95%) (Sa et al. 2019). If pulses are paired with cereal grains/proteins, plant proteins can fulfill the daily requirement of essential amino acids at affordable price. Globally, plant-based proteins are in high demand not only because of its affordability, but most plant-based proteins contain a negligible amount of saturated fat, are cholesterol-free, and have heme iron and higher fiber; above all, they are an excellent source of antioxidants and other phytochemicals, which help in reducing risk of heart, and obesity related diseases. Several other studies have shown the advantages of daily intake of plant-based protein compared with animal proteins for minimizing the blood pressure (Elliott et al. 2006; Altorf-van der Kuil et al. 2012) and the risk of type 2 diabetes (Pounis et al. 2010; Sluijs et al. 2010). Pulses hold double the quantity of protein, compared with cereals, and hence, pulses can make an excellent complementary food source of protein for infants, children, and adults to meet their daily protein requirement in the diet.

In order to cater the consumer's demand for plant-based proteins, several processing techniques have been employed to enhance the protein quality, especially the trait protein digestibility. Thermal processing (cooking, autoclaving, heating, and

Table 6.1 Amino acid content in the various legumes reported in g/100 g protein

Amino acids (g/100 g)	Peas[a]	Faba beans[a]	Sweet lupines[a]	Soybeans[a]	Chickpea[b,c,d]	Pigeonpea[e]	Lentils[c]	Mung bean[d,e,f]
Lysine	1.68	1.67	1.54	2.39	6.68	6.99	1.720	6.95
Methionine	0.23	0.22	0.22	0.53	1.30	1.12	0.210	1.20
Cysteine	0.32	0.35	0.45	0.57	1.34	1.15	0.322	0.87
Threonine	0.97	0.95	1.18	1.44	3.71	3.53	0.882	3.28
Leucine	1.6	2.00	2.27	2.89	7.12	7.13	1.786	7.75
Isoleucine	0.97	1.13	1.38	1.63	4.30	3.60	1.06	4.23
Valine	1.04	1.22	1.28	1.82	4.19	4.31	1.22	5.18
Phenylalanine + tyrosine	1.80	2.03	2.53	2.26	7.83	11.04	1.88	9.02
Tryptophan	0.21	0.24	0.26	0.49	0.96	0.97	0.22	1.90
Arginine	2.02	2.40	3.26	2.85	9.42	5.98	1.90	6.99
Histidine	0.56	0.73	0.83	0.99	2.75	3.57	0.69	2.93
Sum of indispensable amino acids	11.40	12.94	15.20	17.86	49.6	49.39	11.89	50.33
Alanine	0.95	1.05	1.14	1.59	4.29	4.47	1.03	4.39
Aspartic acid	2.56	2.80	3.26	3.89	11.65	9.88	2.72	11.52
Glutamic acid	3.87	4.40	7.00	6.05	17.48	23.15	3.18	17.83
Glycine	0.95	1.09	1.38	1.32	4.14	3.70	1.00	3.98
Proline	0.94	0.99	1.37	1.65	4.13	4.38	1.03	4.57
Serine	1.05	1.22	1.61	1.67	5.04	4.71	1.14	4.92
Sum of dispensable amino acids	10.32	11.55	15.76	16.17	46.73	50.29	10.1	47.21
AA score	100	91	91	100	137	–	–	135
True digestibility (%)	95.9	90.8	89.4	90.7	85.2	57	71	80.2
PDCAA score	95.9	82.6	81.4	90.7	83.6	–	63	–

[a]From Erbersdobler and Jahreis (2017)
[b]From Alajaji and El-Adawy (2006)
[c]https://nutritiondata.self.com/facts/legumes-and-legume-products/4326/2
[d]From Han et al. (2020)
[e]From https://www.medindia.net/nutrition-data/pigeon-peas-red-gram-mature-seeds-raw.htm and https://www.medindia.net/nutrition-data/mung-beans-mature-seeds-raw.htm
[f]From Mubarak (2005)

microwave) is adopted for improving the protein quality though other processing techniques like germination, irradiation, fermentation, extrusion, spray-drying and freeze-drying methods are in vogue. The major challenge in utilizing plant proteins is to develop novel food processing techniques that could successfully blend two or more plant proteins to yield a complete protein and simultaneously enhances the protein quality and functional properties. Furthermore, the developed plant protein products must satisfy consumer's acceptance in terms of taste, texture, flavor, nutrition, and affordability. Protein quality enhancement is also been addressed by genetic manipulation of seed storage proteins and engineering of synthetic proteins which are tailored to meet the market specifications and consumer's demand (Young and Pellet 1994; Jiang et al. 2016). This chapter majorly focuses on strategies like supplementation, processing techniques, and genetic tools that help in improving the quality of plant proteins.

6.2 Protein Quality Assessment

The protein quality depends on the types of amino acids particularly the dietary indispensable amino acids, the physiological utilization of specific amino acids after digestion (or protein digestibility), as well as their bioavailability (Friedman 1996; Butts et al. 2012). The digestibility of protein starts with hydration and solubilization in the mouth. Once the food reaches the stomach, HCl denatures the proteins and enables proteolytic digestive enzymes to act upon the peptide bond. The pepsinogen produced in the stomach is converted into the pepsin (a type of protease enzyme) by HCl, which helps in cleavage of food-derived proteins into peptides. The proteolytic enzymes such as trypsin, chymotrypsin, carboxypeptidases, collagenase, and elastase secreted by pancreas enter into the duodenum and further catalyze cleavage of peptides into smaller peptides. The aminopeptidases and tripeptidases present in the small intestine further cleave shorter peptides into amino acids or dipeptides and tripeptides, which facilitates its absorption by the mucosal cells of intestine. Unabsorbed or undigested peptide/nitrogenous residues are transported to the large intestine (colon), wherein possibility of exposure of these substances into microbial modifications within the large intestine can occur, prior to fecal excretion.

The nutritional quality of the dietary proteins can be assessed using a variety of different markers and approaches such as amino acid score (AAS), nitrogen balance (NB), protein efficiency ratio (PER), net protein ratio (or retention) (NPR), net protein utilization (NPU), protein digestibility, biological value (BV), and protein digestibility corrected amino acid score (PDCAAS) (Boye et al. 2012). These bioassays (PER, NPR, NPU), mostly performed on animal models such as laboratory mice, are questionable as the amino acid requirements of these animals are quite different from humans and also entail time and are expensive (Schaafsma 2012). The in vitro protein digestibility (IVPD) methodology can be adopted to quickly evaluate protein digestibility as compared to in vivo methods. The in vitro assays are simple, inexpensive, reliable, and rapid. In vitro methods also provide information on protein stability and quality and can be used for quick profiling of large number of samples (Coda et al. 2017). The PDCAAS method, which was approved and recommended by Food and Agriculture Organization (FAO) in 1991 to determine protein quality, is most widely used method which considers two factors into account such as availability of essential (indispensable) amino acids and protein digestibility (Butts et al. 2012; Tavano et al. 2016). In PDCAAS, amino acid profile of a food protein is compared to a reference value, and an amino acid score is determined by the ratio of the limiting amino acid content in the test protein to that of the reference protein. The amino acid score is then corrected by multiplying with digestibility (true digestibility, fecal digestibility or in vitro digestibility) of the protein to generate a PDCAAS value (Schaafsma 2012; Hughes et al. 2011). There are different recommended patterns given by FAO or World Health Organization (WHO). For infants under 1 year of age, the recommended reference protein is human milk protein and the reference pattern used for other age groups is the amino acid scoring pattern recommended by FAO/WHO (1991) for children in the age group of 2–5 years, since at this age the requirement of the essential amino acids by human body is the maximum, and further, it decreases slightly with advancing age (Schaafsma 2012).

6.3 Processing Techniques to Improve the Protein Digestibility

6.3.1 Germination

Germination is also called as a bioprocess involving a series of biochemical reactions that facilitates changes in protein content by activating the transcriptional machinery of seeds (Ohanenye et al. 2020; Weitbrecht et al. 2011). Seed protein quality is determined by seed structure, primary structure of proteins, and antinutritional compounds (phytic acids, polyphenols, trypsin–chymotrypsin inhibitors, and tannins). Therefore, germination helps in improving protein digestibility in legume seeds by disintegrating cell wall, stored proteins in the seed, and antinutrients. Germination of lentil and faba bean favored protein digestibility causing reduced content of antinutrients (phytic acid and tannins) (Expósito et al. 2021). Enhanced true protein digestibility (TPD) in cooked black bean products was reported by Kannan et al. (2011), and they observed no correlation between TDS and PDCAAS due to limiting amino acid score. However, highest TPD and PDCAAS values were observed for cooked germinated beans in combination with rice. Little effect of germination on amino acid profile of cowpea was documented; however, increased in vitro starch and protein digestibility with higher PDCAAS score were documented in germinated cowpea flour-based weaning food (Jirapa et al. 2001). Germinated mung bean, chickpea, and cowpea not only showed increased IVPD in the order of 15–25, 6–17, and 6–17%, but also influenced the higher protein content in the order of 9–11, 11–16, and 8–11% (Uppal and Bains 2012). A sixth day after germination caused increased protein content in chickpea (*Cicer aretinium* L.), lentil (*Lens culinaris* Merr.), and yellow pea (*Pisum sativum* L.) (Xu et al. 2019). Indian bean (*Dolichos lablab* var. *lignosus*) was found to have increased IVPD and PER after 32 h of germination and was comparable with that of reference protein casein (Ramakrishna et al. 2008). In addition to protein, germination of green gram (*Vigna radiata* (L.) R. Wilczek), cowpea (*Vigna unguiculata* (L.) Walp.), lentil (*Lens culinaris* Medik.), and chickpea (*Cicer arietinum* L.) caused a significant increase in in vitro iron, calcium bioavailability, thiamine content, and in vitro protein digestibility (Ghavide and Prakash 2007). Increased methionine content was reported in germinated soybean and lupin seeds (Escobedo et al. 2014; Chilomer et al. 2010; Martínez-Villaluenga et al. 2010). Enhanced digestibility of protein was due to germination and is majorly attributed to increased enzymatic hydrolysis of protein that causes compositional changes in the constituents like phytic acid, polyphenols, and protease inhibitors (Chitra et al. 1996; Mbithi-Mwikya et al. 2000; Bau et al. 1997).

6.3.2 Infrared Heating and Wet/Heat Moisture Treatment

Depending on the degree of processing and its types, protein digestibility and compositions of amino acid can be modified to improve the protein quality or nutritional value of the food grains/flours. Significant increase in the PDCAAS value from 0.65 to 0.71 was only found in *desi* chickpea when the sample was subjected to tempering (20% moisture) and heating at 135 °C (Bai et al. 2018). Enrichment of protein quality and digestibility of starch in navy bean and chickpea seeds was reported utilizing infrared heating with tempering (Guldiken et al. 2022). Total essential amino acid content increased in cowpea, pea, and kidney beans following soaking, boiling, microwave cooking, and autoclaving treatments (Khattab et al. 2009). The sulfur-containing amino acids were also increased, and the autoclaving was found to be highly efficient in improving the protein quality in terms of PER and amino acid scores. IVPD and PER improved by all cooking treatments from 84 to 90% and 2.3 to approximately 2.5, respectively. The improved IVPD was due to decreased antinutritional compounds (phytic acid, tannins, trypsin inhibitor, hemagglutinin activity, and saponins) in chickpea (Saleh and El-Adawy 2006). Soaking followed by cooking was found to be highly effective in reducing trypsin inhibitor activity in *Dolichos lablab* beans, and improved IVPD was observed in mung bean, chickpea, and cowpea sprouts upon pressure cooking and microwaving (Osman 2007; Uppal and Bains 2012). These processing treatments cause partial denaturation of protein, thereby providing easy accessibility to the action of protease digestive enzymes. It also destroys protease inhibitors at different levels of seed moisture and surface temperatures which in turn affects the protein quality, functional, physicochemical, and nutritional properties of the flours.

6.3.3 *Extrusion*

Extrusion is thermomechanical process which involves subjecting the food ingredient to high-temperature and high-shearing processes and is predominantly used in food texturization, commercially being used for the production of various snacks. It is effective in reducing the activity of antinutritive compounds (Cotacallapa-Sucapuca et al. 2021). The high temperature and shear pressure in the process induce chemical and structural changes and cause denaturation of protein which in turn affects protein digestibility. The impact of extrusion process on the protein or amino acid content of various pulses was documented (Batista et al. 2010; Kelkar et al. 2012; Simons et al. 2015). Although the process of extrusion does not facilitate alteration in protein content in beans (Batista et al. 2010; Simons et al. 2015), reduced sulfur-containing amino acid like cysteine and methionine was observed due to high temperatures and disruptive forces of the extruding process (Arija et al. 2006). Increased IVPD was reported in faba bean, pea, chickpea, and kidney beans at extrusion conditions of 140–180 °C (El-Hady and Habiba 2003; Nosworthy et al. 2018; Batista et al. 2010). Slight increase in protein recovery with decreased trypsin inhibitory activity was observed in extruded pea seeds. Significant decrease in valine, phenylalanine, and lysine content was reported at 129 °C, and decreased trypsin content was observed at 142 °C (Frias et al. 2011). Enhanced protein digestibility by 56% was observed in cooked cowpea flour subjected to extrusion at 120 °C (Batista et al. 2010). It was reported that extrusion did not impact the protein digestibility of soybean; however, it helped to reduce trypsin inhibitors (Bertipaglia et al. 2008).

6.3.4 *Irradiation*

Food irradiation is a kind of processing technique, wherein food is exposed to ionizing radiation (alpha, beta, gamma, X-ray, or energetic electrons), to destroy pathogens of microbial origin and insects which influences food quality as well as safety. Depending upon the purpose, different doses of irradiation are being used; for instance, <1 kGy is used to achieve insect disinfection, delayed sprouting, and ripening; 1–10 kGy is being employed to kill microorganisms and to change the functional properties of food, whereas 10–50 kGy is utilized for commercial sterilization like virus elimination (Ehlermann 2016; Lima et al. 2019). Food irradiation is not allowed to employ for nutritional profile modification; nevertheless, its impact on protein quality has been evaluated. The dry common beans showed improved protein digestibility when irradiated with 1, 5, and 10 kGy doses of γ-radiation using ^{60}Co as source (Lima et al. 2019). Electron beam-irradiated lotus seeds showed higher content of essential amino acid like threonine, valine, leucine, tyrosine, tryptophan, and lysine; however, decreased PDCAAS from 43 to 24% was reported when the samples were subjected to 30 kGy irradiation (Bhat and Sridhar 2008). Irradiation at 0.5–1 kGy improved protein digestibility (79.9%) and decreased phytic acid in Sudanese faba bean (Osman et al. 2014).

6.3.5 Fermentation

Fermentation is a type of processing technique, wherein desirable biochemical changes in food matrix are brought by microorganisms (bacteria, molds, and yeasts) particularly through enzymatic action (Kahajdova and Karovicova 2007). It is being adopted to improve the nutrient bioaccessibility as well as bioavailability from various food sources (Hotz and Gibson 2007) and improves shelf life and organoleptic properties of food (Chaves-Lopez et al. 2014). Fermentation aids in hydrolysis process which could contribute to decreased antinutritional compounds and thus helps in nutritional quality enhancement in the food. Fermented chickpea seeds (soaked chickpeas subjected to cooking at 90 °C for 30 min and inoculated with *Rhizopus oligosporus* and allowed for fermentation at 34.9 °C for 51.3 h followed by drying at 52 °C for 12 h followed by milling) showed improved IVPD of 83% compared to unfermented seeds (72%). Further, improved PER, NPR, and PDCAAS from 1.6 to 2.3, 2.7 to 3, and 73 to 92%, respectively, were reported (Angulo-Bejarano et al. 2008). A fermented product of common beans (tempeh-type) prepared using *R. oligosporus* showed decreased trypsin inhibitor, phytic acid content, and improved protein quality (Paredes-López and Harry 1989). Increased protein digestibility was attributed to increased proteolytic enzymes, wherein fermentation process not only degrades antinutritional compounds but also helps in breaking down complex proteins into simpler and smaller peptides, thereby facilitating release of peptides and amino acids (Nkhata et al. 2018). However, Kannan et al. (2011) found no significant increase in PDCAAS scores in fermented black bean products. The effects of physical processing methods on protein quality of pulses are summarized in a Fig. 6.1.

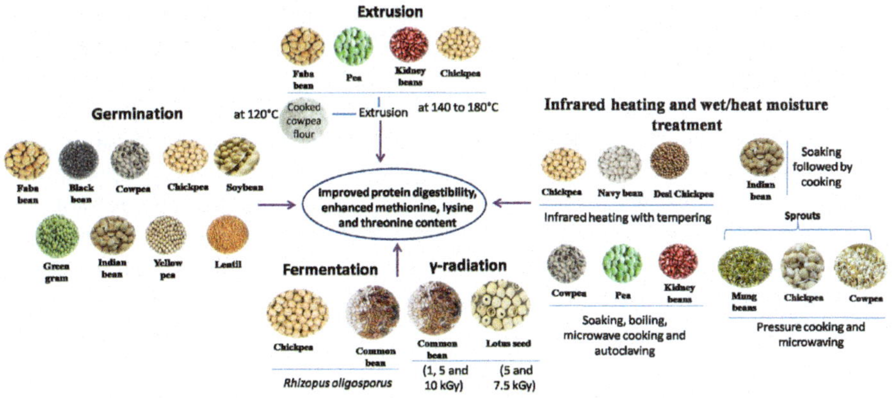

Fig. 6.1 Graphical representation showing the effect of physical processing methods on protein quality of pulses

6.4 Genetic Approaches to Enhance Protein Quality of Pulses

Biofortification of crops with quality protein or essential amino acids through genetic engineering approach has both economic and nutritional significance. Application of genetic approaches to improve protein quality of crop is predominantly restricted to model plants with enhanced essential amino acid (like Lys, Trp, and Met) synthesis. Due to lack of annotated crop genome sequences, this approach has witnessed limited success in crop species. Nevertheless, enhanced methionine content (11.11 mg/g protein) in soybean was reported by overexpressing de novo synthetic protein—MB16 (Zhang et al. 2014). Overexpression of endogenous Met-rich protein is one of the strategies to address the deficiency of sulfur-containing amino acids (SAA) in plants. This approach was used to enhance total methionine content in seeds by 6.8% in transgenic soybean (Yamada et al. 2008). Enrichment of free SAA as well as increased SAA-rich seed proteins was successful in narbon bean (*Vicia narbonensis*)—a close relative of faba bean (Demidov et al. 2003). Overexpression of 2S albumin storage protein and bacterial aspartate kinase gene resulted in enhanced seed methionine content up to 2.4-fold compared to that of wild type. The impact of starch biosynthesis on seed protein content especially albumin fraction (rich in SAA) was reported, wherein mutation in genetic loci of pea plants showed lower levels of starch content and enhanced protein content with relatively high content of the albumin fraction of seed protein (Casey et al. 1998; Hughes et al. 2001). *Glycine max* 2S-1 (post-translationally processed 2S-albumin) was reported as a candidate gene for overexpression approach to enhance protein quality in legumes including soybean (Galvez et al. 2008). Modification of nucleotide sequence in an endogenous gene has also found to be promising approach to enhance SAA; for instance, a part of gene (45 bp sequence) that encodes Met-rich region was isolated from maize and incorporated into a β-*phaseolin* gene from *Phaseolus vulgaris* for overexpression (Hoffman et al. 1988). Several Met-rich proteins were detected in soybean which helps in utilizing these proteins in enhancing protein quality (George and De Lumen 1991). Transgenic soybean and canola plants were developed by overexpressing bacterial DHPS (dihydrodipicolinate synthase) gene and observed elevated levels of free lysine in mature seeds (Falco et al. 1995). Protein quality of rice was enhanced by overexpression of synthetically designed fusion proteins and observed higher lysine and threonine content (Jiang et al. 2016). Gibbon and Larkins (2005) developed "quality protein maize" and showed two fold increase in lysine content in maize seeds, and it was achieved by using high lysine maize mutant *opaque2* (Mertz et al. 1964) as a parent line. Higher lysine content (14%) in rice plants was achieved through regeneration from calli (Schaeffer and Sharpe 1987). Through modification of biosynthetic and catabolic fluxes, increased essential amino acid content, especially free lysine and methionine, was reported in tobacco (Shaul and Galili 1992), canola (Falco et al. 1995), and Arabidopsis (Ben-Tzvi Tzchori et al. 1996). Slight increase in free lysine was observed in rice and barley through overexpression of bacterial *DHPS* (Lee et al. 2001; Brinch-Pedersen et al. 1996). Improved amino acid contents like Lys and Thr in rice were reported through silencing of *LKR/SDH* by RNA interference (RNAi) (Frizzi et al. 2008; Houmard et al. 2007). Increased free lysine (~60-fold) in rice seeds was reported by overexpression of *AK* and *DHPS* as well as silencing *LKR/SDH* genes by RNAi (Long et al. 2013). Transgenic maize and rice seeds with 10–65% and 20.6% lysine, respectively, were achieved through overexpression of 3 lysine-rich genes in maize (Yue et al. 2014) and RLRH1 and RLRH2 in rice (Wong et al. 2015). The salient achievements in the field of protein quality improvement in pulses and other crops are summarized in Table 6.2.

6.5 Concluding Remarks

As the world population, especially developing countries, is suffering from protein malnutrition (hidden hunger), attaining nutritional security has become a major challenge for the countries. The protein digestibility is determined by an amount of protein absorbed by an organism relative to the total protein consumed; it depends on the structure of proteins, processing methods, and the prevalence of antinutritional compounds in the food that limit the digestion. Thus, the application of suitable processing method to inactivate antinutritional factors and to modulate the protein structure in favor of its digestibility can bring practical application of plant protein as a animal protein substitution.

Table 6.2 The list of genes and proteins exploited for enhancing protein quality in pulses and other crop plants using genetic engineering approach

Genetic tools	Crop	Protein quality	Genes involved	References
Transgenic	Soybean	Enhanced methionine content	Synthetic protein (MB16)	Zhang et al. (2014)
Transgenic	Soybean	Methionine enhanced by 6.8%	Gene encoding methionine-rich protein	Yamada et al. (2008)
Transgenic	Narbon bean	Enhanced SAA	2S Albumin storage protein and bacterial aspartate kinase gene	Demidov et al. (2003)
Transgenic	Pea	Enhanced protein	Gene encoding albumin fraction of seed protein	Casey et al. (1998) and Hughes et al. (2001)
Transgenic	Soybean	Enhanced methionine-rich protein	Gm2S-1 (posttranslationally processed 2S-albumin)	Galvez et al. (2008)
Transgenic	Common bean	Enhanced SAA	Fused protein of 45 bp sequence encoding Met-rich region from maize and gene encoding β-phaseolin	Hoffman et al. (1988)
Transgenic	Soybean	Elevated levels of lysine	Bacterial *DHPS*	Falco et al. (1995)
Transgenic	Rice	Higher lysine and methionine	Synthetic fusion proteins	Jiang et al. (2016)
Plant breeding	Maize	Higher lysine	–	Gibbon and Larkins (2005)
Transgenic	Tobacco	High lysine and methionine	Bacterial *DHPS*	Shaul and Galili (1992)
Transgenic	Canola	High lysine and methionine	Bacterial *DHPS*	Falco et al. (1995)
Transgenic	*Arabidopsis*	High lysine and methionine	Bacterial *DHPS*	Ben-Tzvi Tzchori et al. (1996)
Transgenic	Rice	Slight increase in lysine	Bacterial *DHPS*	Lee et al. (2001)
Transgenic	Barley	Slight increase in lysine	Bacterial *DHPS*	Brinch-Pedersen et al. (1996)
Transgenic	Rice	High lysine and threonine	Silencing of *LKR/SDH*	Frizzi et al. (2008) and Houmard et al. (2007)
Transgenic	Rice	Higher lysine (60-fold)	*AK* and *DHPS*	Long et al. (2013)

References

Alajaji SA, El-Adawy TA (2006) Nutritional composition of chickpea (*Cicer arietinum* L.) as affected by microwave cooking and other traditional cooking methods. J Food Compos Anal 19: 806–812

Altorf-van der Kuil W, Engberink MF, Vedder MM et al (2012) Sources of dietary protein in relation to blood pressure in a general Dutch population. PLoS One 7:e30582

Angulo-Bejarano PI, Verdugo-Montoya NM, Cuevas-Rodríguez EO et al (2008) Tempeh flour from chickpea (*Cicer arietinum* L.) nutritional and physicochemical properties. Food Chem 106(1):106–112

Arija I, Centeno C, Viveros A, Brenes A, Marzo F, Illera JC, Silvan G (2006) Nutritional evaluation of raw and extruded kidney bean (*Phaseolus vulgaris* L. var. Pinto) in chicken diets. Poult Sci 85(4):635–644

Bai T, Nosworthy MG, House JD, Nickerson MT (2018) Effect of tempering moisture and infrared heating temperature on the nutritional properties of desi chickpea and hull-less barley flours, and their blends. Int Food Res J 108:430–439

Batista KA, Prudencio SH, Fernandes KF (2010) Changes in the functional properties and antinutritional factors of extruded hard-to-cook common beans (*Phaseolus vulgaris*, L.). J Food Sci 75:286–290

Bau H et al (1997) Effect of germination on chemical composition, biochemical constituents and antinutritional factors of soya bean (*Glycine max*) seeds. J Sci Food Agric 73:1

Ben-Tzvi Tzchori I, Perl A, Galili G (1996) Lysine and threonine metabolism are subject to complex patterns of regulation in Arabidopsis. Plant Mol Biol 32:727–734

Bertipaglia LMA, DeMelo GMP, Sugohara A et al (2008) Chemical changes in soybean and corn processed by extrusion. Rev Bras Zootec 37(11):2003–2010

Bhat R, Sridhar KR (2008) Nutritional quality evaluation of electron beam-irradiated lotus (*Nelumbo nucifera*) seeds. Food Chem 107:174–184

Boye J, Wijesinha-Bettoni R, Burlingame B (2012) Protein quality evaluation twenty years after the introduction of the protein digestibility corrected amino acid score method. Br J Nutr 108:S183–S211

Brinch-Pedersen H, Galili G, Knudsen S, Holm PB (1996) Engineering of the aspartate family biosynthetic pathway in barley (*Hordeum vulgare* L.) by transformation with heterologous genes encoding feed-back-insensitive aspartate kinase and dihydrodipicolinate synthase. Plant Mol Biol 32:611–620

Butts CA, Monro JA, Moughan PJ (2012) In vitro determination of dietary protein and amino acid digestibility for humans. Br J Nutr 108:S282–S287

Casey R, Domoney C, Forster C et al (1998) The effect of modifying carbohydrate metabolism on seed protein gene expression in peas. J Plant Physiol 152:636–640

Chaves-Lopez C, Serio A, Grande-Tovar CD, Cuervo-Mulet R, Delgado-Ospina J, Paparella A (2014) Traditional fermented foods and beverages from a microbiological and nutritional perspective: the Colombian heritage. Compr Rev Food Sci Food Saf 13:1031–1048

Chilomer K, Zaleska K, Ciesiolka D, Gulewicz P, Frankiewicz A, Gulewcz K (2010) Changes in the alkaloid, α-galactoside and protein fractions content during germination of different lupin species. Acta Soc Bot Pol Pol 79(1):11–20

Chitra O et al (1996) Phytic acid, in vitro protein digestibility, dietary fiber, and minerals of pulses as influenced by processing methods. Plant Foods Hum Nutr 49:307

Coda R, Varis JM, Verni CG, Rizzello KK (2017) Improvement of the protein quality of wheat bread through faba bean sourdough addition. LWT Food Sci Technol 82:296–302

Cotacallapa-Sucapuca M, Vega EN, Maieves HA, Berrios JDJ, Morales P, Fernández-Ruiz V, Cámara M (2021) Extrusion process as an alternative to improve pulses products consumption. A review. Foods 10:1096

Demidov D, Horstmann C, Meixner M et al (2003) Additive effects of the feed-back insensitive bacterial aspartate kinase and the Brazil nut 2S albumin on the methionine content of transgenic narbon bean (*Vicia narbonensis* L.). Mol Breed 11:187–201

Ehlermann DAE (2016) Wholesomeness of irradiated food. Radiat Phys Chem 129:24–29

El-Hady EAA, Habiba RA (2003) Effect of soaking and extrusion conditions on antinutrients and protein digestibility of legume seeds. LWT 36:285–293

Elliott P, Stamler J, Dyer AR et al (2006) Association between protein intake and blood pressure: the INTERMAP study. Arch Intern Med 166:79–87

Erbersdobler FH, Jahreis G (2017) Legumes in human nutrition nutrient content and protein quality of pulses. Ernahrungs Umschau 64(9):134–139

Escobedo RM, Berrios JDJ, Gutiérrez-López GF (2014) Seeds as functional foods and nutraceuticals: new frontiers in food science. Nova Science Publishers, Inc, New York, pp 127–142

Expósito SB, Vandenberg A, Peñas E, Frias J, Villaluenga CM (2021) Lentil and fava bean with contrasting germination kinetics: a focus on digestion of proteins and bioactivity of resistant peptides. Front Plant Sci 12:754287

Falco SC, Guida T, Locke M, Mauvais J, Sandres C, Ward RT, Webber P (1995) Transgenic canola and soybean seeds with increased lysine. Nat Biotechnol 13:577–582

Frias J, Giacomino S, Peñas E et al (2011) Assessment of the nutritional quality of raw and extruded *Pisum sativum* L. var. laguna seeds. LWT Food Sci Technol 44:1303–1308

Friedman M (1996) Food browning and its prevention: an overview. J Agric Food Chem 44:631–653

Frizzi A et al (2008) Modifying lysine biosynthesis and catabolism in corn with a single bifunctional expression/silencing transgene cassette. Plant Biotechnol J 6:13–21

Galvez AF, Revilleza MJ, de Lumen BO, Krenz DC (2008) Enhancing the biosynthesis of endogenous methionine-rich proteins (MRP) to improve the protein quality of legumes via genetic engineering. Food for health in the Pacific rim. Food & Nutrition Press, Trumbull, pp 540–552

George AA, De Lumen BO (1991) A novel methionine-rich protein in soybean seed: identification, amino acid composition, and N-terminal sequence. J Agric Food Chem 39:224–227

Ghavide RA, Prakash J (2007) The impact of germination and dehulling on nutrients, antinutrients, in vitro iron and calcium bioavailability and in vitro starch and protein digestibility of some legume seeds. LWT Food Sci Technol 40:1292–1299

Gibbon BC, Larkins BA (2005) Molecular genetic approaches to developing quality protein maize. Trends Genet 21:227–233

Guldiken B, Konieczny D, Franczyk A et al (2022) Impacts of infrared heating and tempering on the chemical composition, morphological, functional properties of navy bean and chickpea flours. Eur Food Res Technol 248(3):767–781

Han F, Moughan PJ, Li J, Pang S (2020) Digestible Indispensable Amino Acid Scores (DIAAS) of six cooked Chinese pulses. Nutrients 12(12):3831

Hoffman LM, Donaldson DD, Herman EM (1988) A modified storage protein is synthesized, processed, and degraded in the seeds of transgenic plants. Plant Mol Biol 11(6):717–729

Hotz C, Gibson RS (2007) Traditional food-processing and preparation practices to enhance the bioavailability of micronutrients in plants-based diets. J Nutr 137:1097–1100

Houmard NM et al (2007) High-lysine corn generated by endosperm-specific suppression of lysine catabolism using RNAi. Plant Biotechnol J 5:605–614

Hughes RK, Desforges N, Selwood C et al (2001) Genes affecting starch biosynthesis exert pleiotropic effects on the protein content and composition of pea seeds. J Sci Food Agric 81: 877–882

Hughes GJ, Ryan DJ, Mukherjea R, Schasteen CS (2011) Protein digestibility-corrected amino acid scores (PDCAAS) for soy protein isolates and concentrate: criteria for evaluation. J Agric Food Chem 59(23):12707–12712

Jiang S, Ma A, Xie L et al (2016) Improving protein content and quality by over-expressing artificially synthetic fusion proteins with high lysine and threonine constituent in rice plants. Sci Rep 6:34427

Jirapa P, Normah H, Zamaliah MM, Asmah R, Mohamad K (2001) Nutritional quality of germinated cowpea flour (*Vigna unguiculata*) and its application in home prepared powdered weaning foods. Plant Foods Hum Nutr 56:203–216

Kahajdova Z, Karovicova J (2007) Fermentation of cereals for specific purpose. J Food Nutr Res 46:51–57

Kannan S, Nielsen SS, Mason AC (2011) Protein digestibility-corrected amino acid scores for bean and bean—rice infant weaning food products. J Agric Food Chem 49:5070–5074

Kelkar S, Siddiq M, Harte J, Dolan K, Nyombaire G, Suniaga H (2012) Use of low-temperature extrusion for reducing phytohemagglutinin activity (PHA) and oligosaccharides in beans (*Phaseolus vulgaris* L.) cv. Navy and Pinto. Food Chem 133:1636–1639

Khattab RY, Arntfield SD, Nyachoti CM (2009) Nutritional quality of legume seeds as affected by some physical treatments. Part 1: protein quality evaluation. LWT- Food Sci Technol 42:1107–1112

Lee SI et al (2001) Constitutive and seed-specific expression of a maize lysine-feedback insensitive dihydrodipicolinate synthase gene leads to increased free lysine levels in rice seeds. Mol Breed 8:75–84

Lima DC, Miano AC, Augusto PED, Arthur V (2019) Gamma irradiation of common beans: effect on nutritional and technological properties. LWT 116:108539

Long X, Liu Q, Chan M, Wang Q, Sun SS (2013) Metabolic engineering and profiling of rice with increased lysine. Plant Biotechnol J 11:490–501

Martínez-Villaluenga C, Torres A, Frias J, Vidal-Valverde C (2010) Semolina supplementation with processed lupin and pigeon pea flours improve protein quality of pasta. LWT Food Sci Technol 43(4):617–622

Mbithi-Mwikya S et al (2000) Nutrient and antinutrient changes in finger millet (*Eleusine coracan*) during sprouting. LWT Food Sci Technol 33:9

Mertz ET, Bates LS, Nelson OE (1964) Mutant gene that changes protein composition and increases lysine content of maize endosperm. Science 145:279–280

Mubarak AE (2005) Nutritional composition and antinutritional factors of mung bean seeds: the effect of cooking on in vitro digestibility of selected legumes 17 (*Phaseolus aureus*) as affected by some home traditional processes. Food Chem 89:489–495

Nkhata SG, Ayua E, Kamau EH, Shingiro JB (2018) Fermentation and germination improve nutritional value of cereals and legumes through activation of endogenous enzymes. Food Sci Nutr 6(8):2446–2458

Nosworthy MG, House JD (2017) Factors influencing the quality of dietary proteins: implications for pulses. Cereal Chem 94:49–57

Nosworthy MG, Medina G, Franczyk AJ, Neufeld J, Appah P, Utioh A, Frohlich P, House JD (2018) Effect of processing on the in vitro and in vivo protein quality of beans (*Phaseolus vulgaris* and *Vicia faba*). Nutrients 10:671

Ohanenye I, Tsopmo A, Ejike C, Udenigwe C (2020) Germination as a bioprocess for enhancing the quality and nutritional prospects of legume proteins. Trends Food Sci Technol 101:213–222

Osman MA (2007) Effect of different processing methods, on nutrient composition, antinutritional factors, and in vitro protein digestibility of dolichos lablab bean [*Lablab purpureus* (L) sweet]. Pak J Nutr 6:299–303

Osman AMA, Hassan AB, Osman GAM, Mohammed N, Rushdi MAH, Diab EE et al (2014) Effects of gamma irradiation and/or cooking on nutritional quality of faba bean (*Vicia faba* L.) cultivars seeds. Int J Food Sci 51(8):1554–1560

Paredes-López O, Harry GI (1989) Changes in selected chemical and antinutritional components during tempeh preparation using fresh and hardened common beans. J Food Sci 54:968–970

Pounis GD, Tyrovolas S, Antonopoulou M et al (2010) Long-term animal-protein consumption is associated with an increased prevalence of diabetes among the elderly: the Mediterranean Islands (MEDIS) study. Diabetes Metab 36:484–490

Ramakrishna V, Rani PJ, Rao PR (2008) Nutritional quality of storage proteins during germination of Indian bean (*Dolichos lablab.* var. *lignosus*) seeds. Int J Food Sci Technol 43:944–949

Sa AGA, Moreno YMF, Carciofi BAM (2019) Food processing for the improvement of plant proteins digestibility. Crit Rev Food Sci Nutr 60(20):3367–3386. https://doi.org/10.1080/10408398.2019.1688249

Saleh AA, El-Adawy TA (2006) Nutritional composition of chickpea (*Cicer arietinum* L.) as affected by microwave cooking and other traditional cooking methods. J Food Compos Anal 19:806–812

Schaafsma G (2012) Advantages and limitations of the protein digestibility-corrected amino 17 acid score (PDCAAS) as a method for evaluating protein quality in human diets. Br J Nutr 108: S333–S336

Schaeffer GW, Sharpe FT (1987) Increased lysine and seed storage protein in rice plants recovered from calli selected with inhibitory levels of lysine plus threonine and S-(2-aminoethyl) cysteine. Plant Physiol 84:509–515

Shaul O, Galili G (1992) Increased lysine synthesis in transgenic tobacco plants expressing a bacterial dihydrodipicolinate synthase in their chloroplasts. Plant J 2:203–209

Simons CW, Hall C, Tulbek M, Mendis M, Heck T, Ogunyemi S (2015) Acceptability and characterization of extruded pinto, navy and black beans. J Sci Food Agric 95(11):2287–2291

Sluijs I, Beulens JW, van der Daphne AL et al (2010) Dietary intake of total, animal, and vegetable protein and risk of type 2 diabetes in the European Prospective Investigation into Cancer and Nutrition (EPIC)-NL study. Diabetes Care 33:43–48

Tavano OL, Neves VA, da Silver Júnior SI (2016) In vitro versus in vivo protein digestibility techniques for calculating PDCAAS (protein digestibility-corrected amino acid score) applied to chickpea fractions. Food Res Int 89:756–763

Uppal V, Bains K (2012) Effect of germination periods and hydrothermal treatments on in vitro protein and starch digestibility of germinated legumes. J Food Sci Technol 49:184–191

Weitbrecht K, Müller K, Leubner-Metzger G (2011) First off the mark: early seed germination. J Exp Bot 62:3289–3309

Wong HW, Liu Q, Sun SS (2015) Biofortification of rice with lysine using endogenous histones. Plant Mol Biol 87:235–248

Xu M, Jin Z, Simsek S, Hall C, Rao J, Chen B (2019) Effect of germination on the chemical composition, thermal, pasting, and moisture sorption properties of flours from chickpea, lentil, and yellow pea. Food Chem 295:579–587

Yamada T, Matsuda F, Kasai K, Fukuoka S, Kitamura K, Tozawa Y, Miyagawa H, Wakasa K (2008) Mutation of a rice gene encoding a phenylalanine biosynthetic enzyme results in accumulation of phenylalanine and tryptophan. Plant Cell 20(5):1316–1329

Young VR, Pellet PL (1994) Plant proteins in relation to human protein and amino acid nutrition. Am J Clin Nutr 59:1203S–1212S

Yue J, Li C, Zhao Q, Zhu D, Yu J (2014) Seed-specific expression of a lysine-rich protein gene, GhLRP from cotton significantly increases the lysine content in maize seeds. Int J Mol Sci 15: 5350–5365

Zhang Y, Schernthaner J, Labbé N, Hefford MA, Zhao J, Simmonds DH (2014) Improved protein quality in transgenic soybean expressing a de novo synthetic protein, MB-16. Transgenic Res 23(3):455–467

Chapter 7
Microgreens: A Novel Food for Nutritional Security

Gyan P. Mishra, Priti, H. K. Dikshit, Muraleedhar Aski, Seema Sangwan, Tsering Stobdan, Ajeet Singh, Ranjeet Ranjan Kumar, and Shelly Praveen

Abstract Microgreens are 7–21-day-old seedlings of certain crop species which are harvested at first true leave stage manually or mechanically cutting the seedlings 5–10 mm above the growing media surface. Microgreens are considered as high-value functional foods as these are the storehouse of various antioxidants and certain minerals like K, Ca, Fe, and Zn. Microgreens have gained a lot of attention and popularity over last few years as a novel food, mainly due to their unique flavor, color, texture, and nutritional profiles. Recent studies have revealed that microgreens are richer than mature greens in some vitamins, sugars, and antioxidants, including carotenoids. The consumption of microgreens also appears to be associated with multiple health benefits like reduced risk of cardiovascular disease, possibly due to prevention of hypercholesterolemia, and also provides protection against inflammatory processes, oxidative stress, and chronic diseases. Until now, microgreens have gained market mostly in the western countries; however, in other parts of the world, this is gaining foothold, especially in the urban and peri-urban settings. Rapid growth cycle, limited space requirement, rich flavor, diverse color, and highly economic produce make microgreens a dietary alternative that may contribute to the nutritional security of a large population. Success of microgreens technology will largely depend on the collective and collaborative efforts from the industry and researchers in the food chemistry, biochemistry, genetics, and human nutrition

---

G. P. Mishra (✉) · Priti · H. K. Dikshit · M. Aski
Division of Genetics, Indian Agricultural Research Institute, New Delhi, India
e-mail: gyan_mishra@icar.gov.in

S. Sangwan
Division of Microbiology, Indian Agricultural Research Institute, New Delhi, India

T. Stobdan
Defence Institute of High Altitude Research, DRDO, Leh, Ladakh, India

A. Singh · R. R. Kumar
Division of Biochemistry, Indian Agricultural Research Institute, New Delhi, India

S. Praveen
Division of Biochemistry, ICAR-Indian Agricultural Research Institute, New Delhi, Delhi, India

R. S. V., S. Praveen (eds.), *Conceptualizing Plant-Based Nutrition*,
https://doi.org/10.1007/978-981-19-4590-8_7

working to enhance the production of secondary metabolites. In this chapter, we have comprehensively covered various functional and nutritional aspects of a number of microgreens which are popularly being grown and consumed across the globe.

Keywords Biofortification · Functional foods · Lighting · Microgreens · Novel foods

7.1 Introduction

In an era of fast-paced lifestyle, humans require easily available, and healthy food options at affordable prices (Cohen and Garrett 2010). In this context, microgreens are nutrient-rich food crops which can be produced from a number of crops like vegetables, herbs, grains, or even some wild species. The term "microgreens" signify the very small ("micro") and delicate seedlings (mostly of "green" color) of certain crop species which are consumed either raw or partially cooked. Microgreens are also called "vegetable confetti" which are generally 7–21-day-old tender immature greens of 5–10 cm height (Fig. 7.1) having three major parts, viz. stem, cotyledonary leaf, and a pair of true leaves (Xiao et al. 2012; Sun et al. 2013). The global market of microgreens can be segmented mainly into four broad categories, viz. (1) green types like Brassicaceae (cabbage, broccoli, etc.), Asteraceae (lettuce, chicory, etc.), Amaranthaceae (amaranth, spinach, etc.), Cucurbitaceae (cucumber, melons, etc.), Lamiaceae (basil, mint, etc.), and others (lentils, mung bean, leeks, etc.); (2) farm

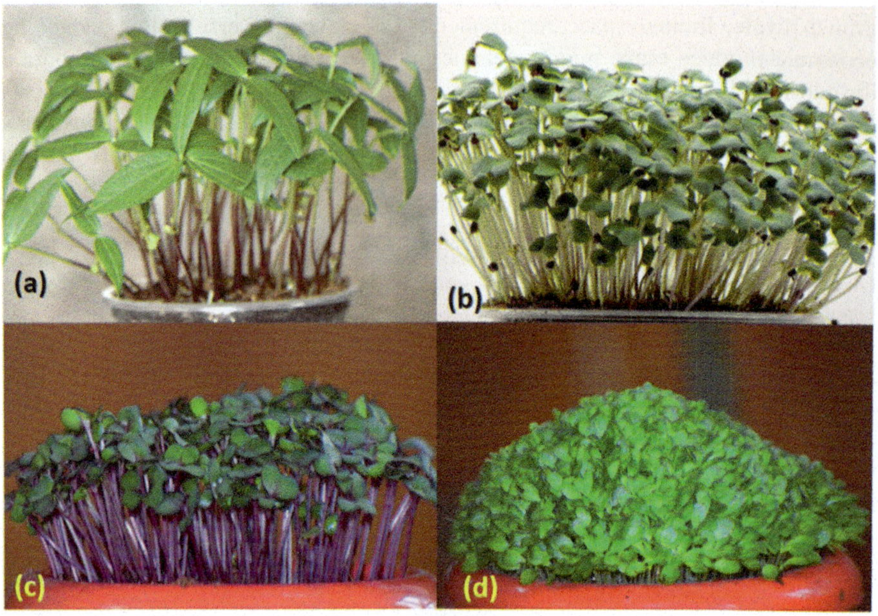

Fig. 7.1 Microgreens of (**a**) mungbean, (**b**) mustard, (**c**) red cabbage, and (**d**) lettuce

types (outdoor farming, greenhouse farming, vertical farming); (3) end uses (food and beverages, cosmetics, etc.); and (4) geographical region-based (North America, Latin America, Europe, Asia Pacific, Middle East, and Africa) (Globe Newswire Europe 2018; Samuolienė et al. 2013a).

The United States of America (U.S.A.) is a major producer of microgreens in the global market which is followed by Canada and Mexico. In terms of geography, North America is leading the microgreens market with a share of nearly 50% in terms of dollar sales in 2019. The large-scale microgreens farming and consumption (mostly in the restaurants) in the U.S.A. are supporting the microgreens market in this region (https://www.datamintelligence.com). During the 5-year period of 2020–2025, the global microgreens market is anticipated to grow at a CAGR (compound annual growth rate) of 7.5–8.0% (www.researchandmarkets.com), while in U.S.A. it is projected to register a CAGR of 10.1% (www.reportlinker.com). Overall, the market of indoor farming, including the hydroponic system kits for microgreens, was assessed to have a worth of nearly 25.40 billion US dollars in the year 2017 and is expected to reach the value of 40.25 billion US dollars (Globe Newswire Europe 2018).

Microgreens, as a culinary delight, were first reported in late 1980s by the chefs of some restaurants in San Francisco, California (USA), especially in imparting color and flavor to the cuisines. It has then gained attention during last decade as an innovative cooking constituent (Treadwell et al. 2010). The popularity of microgreens is also due to their uniquely varied colors, delicate structures, textures, and flavors, which are required for the garnishing of salads, sandwiches, soups, etc. (www.agresearchmag.ars.usda.gov). In addition, microgreens are loaded with an array of phytonutrient constituents possessing potential bioactive functions (Sun et al. 2013; Mishra et al. 2022; Xiao et al. 2012).

Microgreens are sometimes misconstrued as sprouts and baby greens or baby leaf. However, sprouts, microgreens, and baby leaf are of different food categories which are of special interest due to their unique sensorial and nutritional properties. According to definition of European Union (2013), "sprouts" are the "product obtained from the germination of seeds and their development in water or another medium, harvested before the development of true leaves and which is intended to be eaten whole, including the seed" (EU/208/2013), while "baby leaf" is the "young leaves and petioles of any crops (including Brassica) harvested up to 8 true leaf stage" (EU 752/2014). However, till now there is no "legal definition" for "microgreens," and it is still a marketing or a commercial term (Treadwell et al. 2010). The fine differences between these terminologies are presented in the Table 7.1.

Microgreens differ from sprouts as the former requires light, a growing medium (both soil or soilless), more growth period, and shoots are the edible portion. Nevertheless, compared to baby greens, microgreens need less growth period, do not necessitate any agrochemicals, and may be marketed without cutting of the seedlings (with growing media), which extends their shelf life window (www.botanicalinterests.com). However, all the three are preferably consumed as raw (Di Gioia et al. 2017a). When microgreens are grown in some solid medium (soil,

Table 7.1 Key characteristics of sprouts, microgreens, and baby leaf or baby greens

Features	Sprouts	Microgreens	Baby leaf/baby greens
Growth period (day)	4–10	7–21	20–40
Edible portion	Sprout	Shoots (cotyledons and first pair of true leaves, but no roots)	True leaves (no roots)
Growth system	Soilless (only water)	Mainly soilless (require some growing medium)	Soil or soilless (as growing medium)
Light requirement	No	Yes	Yes
Nutrient requirement	No	Yes (if growing medium is devoid of nutrients)	Yes
Agrochemicals requirements	No	No	Yes
Plant harvest stage	After germination but before full cotyledonary leaves stage	Generally, between full cotyledonary leaf and first true leaves stage	Between first to eighth true leaves stage
Harvesting (cutting)	No	Yes	Yes

Adapted from Di Gioia et al. (2015, 2017a)

peat, vermiculite, etc.), they pose very little risk of microbial contamination compared to that of sprouts (Di Gioia et al. 2017a).

Microgreens can be comfortably grown either at home or at commercial scale under controlled environmental conditions (greenhouses) or even under open conditions, irrespective of the season (Ebert et al. 2015, 2017) in a variety of growing medium (soil, soilless), depending on the scale of production. The growing media is very crucial for the proper germination and growth of microgreens. The desired physical properties of the solid growing media include nearly 85% porosity, water holding capacity between 55 and 70% of the total volume, and aeration to the extent of 20–30% of total volume for the roots (Abad et al. 2001). The growing media can be organic (peat, coir, etc.) or inorganic (like perlite and vermiculite). The most commonly used growing substrates for the microgreens production are vermiculite, peat, sand, and perlite either individually or in combination depending on the species grown (Di Gioia et al. 2015). Desired chemical properties of the media include a pH range of 5.5–6.5 and electrical conductivity below 500 μS/cm and should be free of any heavy metal and microbial contamination such as *Salmonella* and *E. coli* (Di Gioia et al. 2015, 2017a). Microgreens are generally grown in the plastic trays, of various sizes having depth of 3–5 cm, which is required for placing the ample growing medium to support the microgreens till it reaches the harvesting stage. Based on the type of microgreens grown, the base of the tray can be with or without holes, more often with holes for facilitation of the drainage (Di Gioia et al. 2015).

The trays should be placed on a leveled surface on the benches (movable or static) (Di Gioia et al. 2017a).

Special attention is required while harvesting the microgreens to avoid the sticking of any growing media particles and seed integuments which in certain species tend to remain attached (Di Gioia et al. 2015). Immediately after the harvest, microgreens are washed and cooled (1–5 °C) (Kyriacou et al. 2016) or alternatively marketed in trays or growing plants are packed with the growing media (Di Gioia et al. 2017a). Thus, postharvest handling is very crucial for extending the shelf life of the microgreens which otherwise are highly perishable. A method of shelf life extension of microgreens, to at least 10 days, has been patented by Sasuga (2014). The most important parameters for the storage of microgreens are temperature (18–24 °C) and relative humidity (40–60%) (Hodges and Toivonen 2008) as these factors significantly affect the tissue electrolytic leakage and influence microbial contamination (Kou et al. 2013).

Phytonutrient content is reportedly varying with the changing growth stage of the plants, and a decrease has been observed from the seedling (sprout/microgreen) to the fully grown stage. Seed germination enhances the nutritive value of the plants by activation of the enzymes which reduces or even eliminates the antinutritional factors, especially in the legumes (Bau et al. 1997; Mubarak 2005). During germination, there is breakdown of fibrous components which are bound to vitamins, minerals, and amino acids, and thus, the availability of these desired phytochemicals including micronutrients like Fe and Zn increases. In addition, germination also eliminates the flatulence-causing agents (Bird 2014).

Considering a few days of photosynthesis, microgreens are reported to contain much higher contents of various antioxidants, vitamins, and minerals than the sprouts. In general, microgreens contain nearly 4–6 times more nutrients than that of their mature leaves. Microgreens contain relatively high phytonutrients (ascorbic acid, β-carotene, α-tocopherol, and phylloquinone) and minerals (Ca, Mg, Fe, Mn, Zn, Se, and Mo) and less nitrate contents than their mature counterparts (Pinto et al. 2015; Xiao et al. 2012). In this context, microgreens are one of the novel food products which could also be considered as functional and nutraceutical foods for the health-conscious consumers (Kyriacou et al. 2016). Microgreens offer a great potential to become a food of choice to achieve nutritional security of a broad range of settlements due to their ease in the cultivation under varied environmental conditions.

7.2 Crop Species Suitable for Microgreens Cultivation

The crop species used for the production of microgreens are generally of intense color and flavor and rich in various phytochemicals such as antioxidants and vitamins. In addition, the selected crop species are of such type which can be consumed raw as seedlings. A range of crops can be used for the production of microgreens which include beet, broccoli, flax, kale, peas, and radish. The most

Table 7.2 List of commonly grown microgreens belonging to nine crop families

S. no.	Family/species	Species
1.	Amaranthaceae	Amaranth, beet, chard, quinoa, spinach
2.	Amaryllidaceae	Chive, garlic, leeks, onion
3.	Apiaceae	Carrot, celery, dill, fennel
4.	Asteraceae	Chicory, endive, lettuce, radicchio
5.	Brassicaceae	Arugula, broccoli, cabbage, cauliflower, Chinese cabbage, kale, mustard, radish, radish, savoy cabbage, tatsoi, watercress
6.	Cucurbitaceae	Cucumber, melon, squash
7.	Fabaceae	Alfalfa, beans, chickpea, clover, fenugreek, fava bean, lentil, mung bean, pea
8.	Lamiaceae	Mint, basil, rosemary, sage, oregano
9.	Poaceae	Barley, corn, rice, oat, pearl millet, wheatgrass
10.	Aromatic species	Basil, chives, cilantro, cumin
11.	Wild edible plants	Amaranth, *Beta vulgaris*, borage, common dandelion, *Diplotaxis erucoides*, goatsbeard, *Portulaca oleracea*, prickly golden fleece, pigweed, salicornia, sea fennel, wild chicory, wild fennel, wild radish, white mustard

Source: https://grocycle.com/types-of-microgreens/; Turner et al. (2020) and Di Gioia et al. (2015)

commonly used species are from the crop families like Amaranthaceae, Amaryllidaceae, Apiaceae, Asteraceae, Brassicaceae, Chenopodiaceae, Cucurbitaceae, Fabaceae, and Lamiaceae.

Some members of the solanaceous family (tomato, brinjal, and pepper) are not considered edible as they contain various antinutrients (Di Gioia et al. 2015) and thus cannot be grown as the microgreens. Even among the edible species, there are various other factors like palatability, flavor, smell, texture, and color that are key traits for the consumer acceptability, while companies/producers of the microgreens look for attractive colors, shapes, flavor, and shelf life (Di Gioia et al. 2015). From the commercial perspective, the selection of microgreens species should be based on the availability of good quality untreated seeds with high and homogeneous germination and have least unit cost of the seeds (Di Gioia et al. 2017a). A comprehensive list of microgreens under cultivation across different countries is presented in Tables 7.2 and 7.3.

7.3 Growth Conditions and Quality of Microgreens

A number of factors that regulate the overall quality of microgreens and phytochemical contents are (1) genetic variability (between and within the taxa), (2) environmental impact (temperature, light quality, and quantity, photoperiod, etc.), and (3) genotype and environmental interaction. However, these factors have not yet been investigated very critically for a large number of species used in the production

Table 7.3 List of most commonly grown microgreens, their growth, harvest, and nutritive properties

S. no.	Crop species	Soaking/presoak (h)	Suitable growth medium	Germ time (day)	Harvest time (day)	Color	Flavor	Nutrients
1.	Amaranth	No	S/H	2–3	8–12	Red/pink	Mild and sweet	Vitamin (K, E, C), Ca, Fe, beta carotenes
2.	Arugula	No	S/H	1–2	6–8	Green	Peppery and slightly buttery	Vitamin (A, C), Ca, Fe, P
3.	Barley	8–12	S/H	2–3	6–9	Bright green	Sweet	–
4.	Basil	No	H	3–4	8–12	Purple or green	Intense basil type	–
5.	Beets	4–10	S	3–4	11–21	Red stems and green top	Sweet and earthy	Vitamin (A, B, C, E, K), Ca, Mg, K, Fe, Zn, protein
6.	Broccoli	No	S/H	2–3	8–12	Green	Strong broccoli type	Vitamin (A and C), Ca, Fe, P
7.	Brussel sprouts	No	S/H	2–3	7–14	White/pink/purple	Like broccoli and cabbage	Vitamin (B, C, K), folic acid, fiber
8.	Cabbage	No	S/H	2–3	6–14	Green	Strong brassica type	Vitamin (C, K, E), beta carotenes, Fe
9.	Cauliflower	No	S/H	2–3	8–14	Deep green	Strong brassica type	Vitamin (C, K, E), beta carotenes, Fe
10.	Chives	No	S/H	7–14	21–25	Green	Onion type	–
11.	Coriander	8–10	S/H	2–3	21–28	Green	Cilantro type	Vitamin (A, C), Ca, Fe, P
12.	Clover	No	S/H	1–2	8–12	Green	Mild, fresh	–
13.	Corn	12–16	H/S	2–3	12–16	Bright yellow to light green	Sugary and sweet	Vitamin (A, B, C, E), Ca, Mg
14.	Cress	No	S/H	2–3	7–14	Green	Intense peppery	Vitamin (B, C, K), folic acid, fiber
15.	Dill	No	S/H	1–2	10–14	Green	Sweet like dill	–
16.	Fennel	No	S/H	3–4	12–14	Green	Mild, anise like	–
17.	Kale	No	S/H	2–3	8–12	Pale green	Broccoli like, nutty, and rich	Antioxidants, fiber, vitamin (A, C, K), Fe, Cu
18.	Lettuce	No	S/H	3–4	14–16	Green	Lettuce like	Vitamin (B, C, K), folic acid, fiber
19.	Mustard	No	S/H	2–3	8–12	Green	Mustard like	Antioxidants, fiber, vitamin (A, C, E, K)
20.	Oat	1–4	S/H	2–3	6–9	Bright green	Fresh and mild	–

(continued)

Table 7.3 (continued)

S. no.	Crop species	Soaking/ presoak (h)	Suitable growth medium	Germ time (day)	Harvest time (day)	Color	Flavor	Nutrients
21.	Onion/leek	No	S/H	3–4	12	Green	Onion	–
22.	Oregano	No	S/H	7–14	20–22	Light pink to deep red	Oregano like	–
23.	Parsley	No	S/H	4–7	20–22	Light pink to deep red	Oregano like	–
24.	Pea	4–12	H/S	2–3	12–16	Green	Crunchy, sweet (like peas)	Vitamin (A, C), folic acid, fiber
25.	Radish	4–6	S/H	1–2	6–12	Red stem and deep green top	Spicy and slightly floral	Vitamin (A, B, C, E, K), folic acid, niacin, K, Fe, Zn, P, Ca, Mg, pantothenic acid, carotenes
26.	Rye	8–10	S/H	1–2	5–9	Green	Slightly bitter, like barley	Vitamin (B, C, K), folic acid, fiber
27.	Sunflower	8–12	S	2–3	8–12	Green	Crunchy, nutty, fresh	Vitamin (A, B, D, E), Ca, Fe, Mg, K, P
28.	Swiss chard	4–10	S	3–4	11–21	Dark red	Sweet and earthy, like Swiss chard microgreens	Vitamin (A, B, C, E, K), Ca, Mg, K, Fe, Zn, protein
29.	Turnip	No	S/H	2–3	8–12	Deep green	Fresh turnip and radish-like	Vitamin (C, K, E), beta carotenes, Fe
30.	Wheat	6–12	S/H	2–3	6–9	Bright green	Sweet with little or no bitterness	–
31.	Pearl millet	No	S/H	2–3	6–9	Bright green	Sweet with little or no bitterness	–
32.	Lentil	8–12	S/H	2–3	8–10	Green	Mild bitter, pea-like	Vitamin (A, B, C, E), low fat, folate, K, Fe, protein, beta carotenes
33.	Mung bean	8–12	S/H	1–2	6–8	Green	Mild beany taste, slight buttery	Vitamin (C, K, E), Fe, beta carotenes
34.	Chickpea	8–10	S/H	2–3	8–10	Bright green	Sweet and nut-like	Protein, fiber, folate, vitamin (A, C, K, B6)
35.	Fenugreek	No	S/H	2–3	10–14	Green	Subtle bitter taste, mild spicy, nutty	Vitamin C, protein, fibers, antioxidant, K, Fe

S soil, *H* hydroponic, *h* hour, *d* days
Source: https://www.hydrocentre.com.au/blog/types-of-microgreens/; https://microveggy.com/types-of-microgreens/

of microgreens. Very high variations in the bioactive contents largely depend upon both the genetics of the trait and also on the prevailing environmental conditions (Kader 2008). Hitherto, the effect of light quality and quantity is one of the most investigated parameters which is known to regulate the overall biochemical composition of the microgreens.

7.3.1 Light Spectra and the Biochemical Composition of Microgreens

The morphophysiology of microgreens is highly influenced by the light conditions as it significantly regulates the biosynthesis and accumulation of various phytochemicals (Delian et al. 2015). Light quality has more definite effects over light intensity or photoperiod in the regulation of growth and physiology of the microgreens (Bian et al. 2015). Instead of natural lighting, growers prefer to use high-pressure sodium (HPS) lamps (~150 μmol/m^2/s) (Vaštakaitė and Viršilė 2015). However, research is exploring the utility of light-emitting diode (LED)-based illumination for the optimal microgreens cultivation (Agarwal and Gupta 2016), as these can be matched with the plant photoreceptors to optimize the production of various phytochemicals (Morrow 2008). LED-based systems are environment friendly over HPS, and they allow even light dispersal over any conventional lighting systems (Agarwal and Gupta 2016; Morrow 2008).

Moreover, the light quality in terms of photon flux and photoperiod (wavelength) can help in the improvement of some biochemicals, thereby regulating the functional quality of microgreens (Kyriacou et al. 2016). Supplementation with green light and standard LED illumination (blue/red/far-red) has shown the improvement in the carotenoid content of the mustard microgreens and red pak choi/tatsoi microgreens, respectively (Brazaitytė et al. 2015a). Three-day application of supplementary red light (pre-harvest) has recorded better antioxidant levels in some microgreens (Samuolienė et al. 2012). Red, blue, or mix of theses lights were found more effective over white or yellow light alone in reducing the undesirable nitrates contents in the microgreens (Ohashi-Kaneko et al. 2007; Qi et al. 2007). Nevertheless, the precise molecular or biochemical mechanisms regulating the spectral quality-induced variations in the bioactive compounds of the microgreens have not been uncovered yet (Kyriacou et al. 2017).

Light quality is known to affect various plant growth, color, flavor, and nutrition-related parameters (Kyriacou et al. 2016). Alrifai et al. (2019) found red, blue, and combined lights are more effective than the white light for better photosynthesis and metabolism. Better antioxidant profile of lentil and wheat was recorded when supplemented with green light (510 nm) (Samuolienė et al. 2011), while better mineral profile was observed in beet microgreens (Brazaitytė et al. 2018). Green LED lighting produced different anthocyanin levels in the microgreens produced from the green and red genotypes of the same species (Carvalho and Folta 2016).

However, red and blue lights showed improved phenolic content and free radical scavenging activity in the green and red ocimum cultivars, respectively (Lobiuc et al. 2017). Amber light (595 nm) supplementation enhanced antioxidants in radish sprouts (Samuolienė et al. 2011), while supplementation of short-term red LED lighting could alter the antioxidant composition in some of the microgreens including ocimum, amaranth, brassica, spinach, broccoli, beetroot, and green peas (Samuolienė et al. 2012). In general, supplemental light wavelengths are reported to cause enhanced production of various bioactive compounds, which could play protective role against mild photooxidative stress, in a number of microgreens species.

Vaštakaitė et al. (2015b) imposed photostress by both insufficient and an excess of blue light, which has resulted in the biosynthesis of various protective antioxidants. Differential synthesis of various phytochemicals and antioxidant activity under similar supplemental lighting is dependent on genotype and the season of cultivation (Turner et al. 2020). The presence of relative cloud cover, day length of the microgreen growing period, and incident light angle are some of the key factors affecting both light quality and quantity which suggests the importance of the supplemental light while growing microgreens (Turner et al. 2020).

Ultraviolet (UV) spectra, which fall beyond the visible spectra, are also reported to influence the physiological responses of the plants, and UV-A (320–400 nm) spectrum is considered least harmful (Brazaitytė et al. 2015b). A number of studies have shown that by changing the spectral composition, certain targeted phytochemicals content of the microgreens can be modified (Table 7.4).

Besides the wavelength, even changes in the light pulse frequency can also influence the overall plant developmental and photosynthetic activities (Ani et al. 2014; Vaštakaitė et al. 2017, 2018). Same light quality with varying irradiance levels may cause differential effects on overall nutritional quality of microgreens. High-light conditions cause increased photosynthesis in the growing microgreens, which in turn reduces the susceptibility to photodamage. However, low-light conditions increase the number of light-harvesting complexes for the optimized light utilization (Walters 2005).

Photoperiod also affects the accumulation of various phytochemicals in the microgreens, and it interacts with both quality and intensity of the light used for growth and development of microgreens. Effect of light intensity on the growth and nutrition of microgreens is well known, but the effect of photoperiod has not been thoroughly investigated. However, the effect of photoperiod on the nutrient composition of baby spinach was reported by Lester et al. (2010, 2013). In case of pea-derived microgreens, Wu et al. (2007) studied the effects of 96-h continuous illumination based on blue, red, and white LEDs on biosynthesis and accumulation of various phytochemicals. In-depth research is required to unravel the mechanism regulating the induction of secondary metabolites synthesis and light-associated signal transduction pathways in different microgreens species (Kyriacou et al. 2016).

Environmental conditions of high-altitude regions (Leh, India), especially regions having wide temperature amplitude, PAR, and UV-B content, cause differential nutrient profile of the lentil and mung bean microgreens when compared to that of

Table 7.4 Effect of light quality and quantity on the growth and nutritional composition of various microgreens

S. no.	Microgreens species	Lighting	Effect	References
1.	Kale, broccoli, pea	Red (638 nm)	Increased (ascorbic acid, phenolics, anthocyanins)	Samuolienė et al. (2012)
2.	Mustard, borage, beet, parsley	Red (638 nm)	Reduced (anthocyanins)	Samuolienė et al. (2012)
3.	Mustard	463 μmol/m^2/s	Reduced (β-carotene) Increased (zeaxanthin)	Kopsell et al. (2012)
4.	Purple mint (*Perilla frutescens*)	Red (638 nm)	Increased (anthocyanins, ascorbic acid) Decreased (nitrate content)	Brazaitytė et al. (2013)
5.	Broccoli	Blue (470 nm; 41 μmol/m^2/s)	Increased (β-carotene, violaxanthin, glucoraphanin, K, Mg, Fe)	Kopsell and Sams (2013)
6.	Broccoli	Red (627 nm; 88%) + blue (470 nm; 12%); 350 μmol/m^2/s	Decreased (β-carotene, violaxanthin, glucoraphanin, K, Mg, Fe)	Kopsell and Sams (2013)
7.	Kohlrabi, mustard, red pak choi, tatsoi	330–440 μmol/m^2/s	Increased (leaf area, anthocyanins, phenolics, DPPH activity) Decreased (nitrate content)	Samuolienė et al. (2013b)
8.	Tatsoi, red pak choi	110–220 μmol/m^2/s	Increased (ascorbic acid, α-tocopherol)	Samuolienė et al. (2013b)
9.	Lettuce	Red + blue + white; 400–600 μmol/m^2/s	Increased (biomass)	Lin et al. (2013)
10.	Red pak choi, tatsoi, basil	Blue (447 nm) + red (638, 665 nm) + far-red (731 nm)	Increased (ascorbic acid, phenols, anthocyanins, flavanols, DPPH scavenging, leaf area) Decreased (hypocotyl length, plant height)	Vaštakaitė et al. (2015a)
11.	Mustard, red pak choi	Basal light (447, 638, 665, 731 nm), green (520 nm), yellow (595 nm), or orange (622 nm)	Increased (carotenoids in mustard) Decreased (carotenoids in red pak choi)	Brazaitytė et al. (2015a)
12.	Tatsoi	Supplemental yellow	Increased (violaxanthin, carotenoid)	Brazaitytė et al. (2015a)
13.	Basil, beet, pak choi	UV-A + basal lighting (12.4 μmol/m^2/s)	Increased (antioxidants)	Brazaitytė et al. (2015b)
14.	Pak choi	UV-A	Increased (leaf area, FW, DPPH activity, phenols, anthocyanins, ascorbic acid, α-tocopherol)	Brazaitytė et al. (2015b)

(continued)

Table 7.4 (continued)

S. no.	Microgreens species	Lighting	Effect	References
15.	Basil	UV-A (1, 7 or 14 days before harvest)	Increased (antioxidant contents)	Vaštakaitė et al. (2015a)
16.	Mustard, beet, parsley	Blue (33%)	Increased (chlorophylls, carotenoid)	Samuolienė et al. (2017)
17.	Mustard, beet, parsley	Blue (16%)	Increased (tocopherols)	Samuolienė et al. (2017)
18.	Ocimum	Blue	Increased (growth, chlorophyll *a*, anthocyanin)	Lobiuc et al. (2017)
19.	Pak choi, tatsoi	32 Hz, 455 nm, 627 nm	Increased (TPC in pak choi, red pak choi, tatsoi)	Vaštakaitė et al. (2017)
20.	Mustard	256, 1024 Hz and 470, 590 nm	Increased (phenolics content)	Vaštakaitė et al. (2017)
21.	Wild rocket	272 μmol/m^2/s	Increased (polyphenols, resveratrol, catechin, epicatechin)	Loedolff et al. (2017)
22.	Beet	Blue (455 nm)	Increased (P, K, Ca, Mg, S, and Mn) Decreased (Na, Fe, Zn, Cu, and B)	Brazaitytė et al. (2018)
23.	Kohlrabi	Blue (455 nm)	Increased (P, K, Ca, Mg, S, and Mn) No effect (Fe, Zn, Cu, or B)	Brazaitytė et al. (2018)
24.	Red pak choi, mustard, tatsoi, basil	Pulse of LEDs at specific frequencies or supplementing HPS lights of specific wavelength	Increased [phenols, anthocyanins, ascorbic acid (in basil), antiradical activity in all]	Vaštakaitė et al. (2017, 2018)
25.	Basil	(1) Blue (470 nm) + red (627 nm) at 1024 Hz (2) Blue (455 nm) at 256 Hz	(1) Increased (TPC, anthocyanins) (2) Increased (TPC)	Vaštakaitė et al. (2018)
26.	Basil	(1) 256 Hz for all wavelengths except 627 nm (2) 32 and 256 Hz	(1) Increased (DPPH activity) (2) Increased (ascorbic acid)	Vaštakaitė et al. (2018)
27.	Tatsoi	Blue	Decreased (nitrate, ascorbic acid)	Simanavičius and Viršilė (2018)
28.	Brassica species	600 μmol/m^2/s; blue: red (15:85)	Increased (FW, DW)	Jones-Baumgardt et al. (2019)
29.	Cabbage	Blue (15%)	Increased (yield, visual quality)	Ying et al. (2020)
30.	Kale, arugula, mustard	Blue (5%)	Increased (yield, visual quality)	Ying et al. (2020)

FW fresh weight, *DW* dry weight, *TPC* total phenolics content microgreens grown in plains (Delhi, India) (Priti et al. 2021). In general, better antioxidant profiles were recorded from the samples grown in Leh. Various enterprises have entered into the venture of growing the microgreens under indoor conditions, in a multilayer system, under artificial lighting having desired level of radiation (nearly 100 μmol/m^2/s of photosynthetically active radiation) for photosynthesis. At times, natural sunlight is integrated with supplemental lighting, with control on light intensity and quality, for the production of microgreens having enhanced nutritional composition (Kopsell and Sams 2013; Samuolienė et al. 2013b).

7.4 Biochemical Composition of Microgreens

Different microgreens species have varied flavor and are also quite rich in different bioactive contents, and hence, there is a need to identify the genotypes which can fulfill both the taste and nutritional priorities (Xiao et al. 2015a). Sprouts and microgreens are also used as dietary supplements (Kovacs 1996) and functional foods which can minimize the risk of various diet-related diseases (Tang et al. 2014). In this section, the details of biochemical composition of microgreens including vitamins, carotenoids, total sugars, minerals, and antioxidants are presented (Table 7.5).

7.4.1 Antioxidants and Vitamins

A study of 25 diverse microgreens species at USDA and University of Maryland revealed nearly 10 times more antioxidant contents over their mature counterparts (Xiao et al. 2012). The total antioxidant capacity (TAC) in radish microgreens increased nearly 1.7 times under high light (HL) (4.6 ± 0.6 mg/g DW) over normal light (NL) (2.6 ± 0.7 mg/g DW), while in kale the increase was nearly 2.5 times under HL (9.2 ± 1.8 mg/g DW) over NL (3.6 ± 0.5 mg/g DW) (Goble 2018). A set of 20 mung bean and lentil genotypes each, when grown as microgreens under plain-altitude (Delhi) and high-altitude (Leh) conditions, showed significant genotypic variations for ascorbic acid, tocopherol, carotenoids, flavonoid, total phenolics, antioxidant activities (DPPH, FRAP), peroxide activity, proteins, enzymes (peroxidase and catalase), micronutrients, and macronutrients contents (Priti et al. 2021).

The dark-green microgreens such as those derived from spinach, kale, and broccoli are known to possess relatively high phylloquinone (or vitamin K1), which is an essential component required for the coagulation of blood (Olson 1984). Xiao et al. (2012) have reported the phylloquinone content in the range of 0.6 (spinach) to 4.1 (amaranth) μg/g fresh weight (FW) among 25 microgreens species. The phylloquinone content in the mature amaranth, basil, and red cabbage was reported as 1.14, 0.41, and 0.04 μg/g FW, respectively (Haytowitz et al. 2002).

Table 7.5 Nutritional composition of some commonly grown microgreens

S. no.	Microgreens	Nutrient	Quantification	Light conditions	Duration (h)	References
1.	Amaranth	Lipophilic AoA	52.63–80.60 mmol TE/100 g DW	$B_{400–500}$, $R_{600–700}$, B-R	12.0	Kyriacou et al. (2019)
2.	Cress	Lipophilic AoA	87.76–99.13 mmol TE 100 g DW	$B_{400–500}$, $R_{600–700}$, B-R	12.0	Kyriacou et al. (2019)
3.	Mizuna	Lipophilic AoA	77.69–94.62 mmol TE/100 g DW	$B_{400–500}$, $R_{600–700}$, B-R	12.0	Kyriacou et al. (2019)
4.	Purslane	Lipophilic AoA	77.72–94.49 mmol TE 100 g DW	$B_{400–500}$, $R_{600–700}$, B-R	12.0	Kyriacou et al. (2019)
5.	Amaranth	Lutein	76.0–135.9 mg/kg DW	$B_{400–500}$, $R_{600–700}$, B-R	12.0	Kyriacou et al. (2019)
6.	Cress	Lutein	73.9–123.1 mg/kg DW	$B_{400–500}$, $R_{600–700}$, B-R	12.0	Kyriacou et al. (2019)
7.	Mizuna	Lutein	54.4–87 mg/kg DW	$B_{400–500}$, $R_{600–700}$, B-R	12.0	Kyriacou et al. (2019)
8.	Purslane	Lutein	91.5–135.2 mg/kg DW	$B_{400–500}$, $R_{600–700}$, B-R	12.0	Kyriacou et al. (2019)
9.	Mustard	Lutein	0.39–0.56 mg/g DW	R:G:B (74:18:8); R:FR:B (84:7:9); 105, 210, and 315 mmol/m^2/s	16.0	Craver et al. (2017)
10.	Basil	Lutein	47.80–74.40 μg/g	B_{455}, R_{638}, R_{665}, FR_{731}; 210 and 300 μmol/m^2/s	16.0	Samuolienė et al. (2016)
11.	Parsley	Lutein	76.31–106.62 μg/g	B_{455}, R_{638}, R_{665}, FR_{731}; 210 and 300 μmol/m^2/s	16.0	Samuolienė et al. (2016)
12.	Mustard	Lutein	3.13–3.44 mg/100 g FW	275 and 463 μmol/m^2/s	–	Kopsell et al. (2012)
13.	Kohlrabi	Lutein	0.52–0.63 mg/g DW	R:G:B (74:18:8), R:FR:B (84:7:9 and 84:7:9); 315, 210 and 105 mmol/m^2/s	16.0	Craver et al. (2017)
14.	Mizuna	Lutein	0.46–0.64 mg/g DW	R:G:B (74:18:8), R:FR:B (84:7:9 and 84:7:9); 315, 210, and 105 mmol/m^2/s	16.0	Craver et al. (2017)
15.	Golden pea tendrils	Lutein	2.7 mg/100 g FW	No light	–	Xiao et al. (2012)
16.	Popcorn shoots	Lutein	1.3 mg/100 g FW	No light	–	Xiao et al. (2012)

17.	Carrot	β-Carotene	5.8 mg/100 g FW	2500–4400 lux	11.5	Ghoora et al. (2020)
18.	Fennel	β-Carotene	9.1 mg/100 g FW	2500–4400 lux	11.5	Ghoora et al. (2020)
19.	Fenugreek	β-Carotene	3.1 mg/100 g FW	2500–4400 lux	11.5	Ghoora et al. (2020)
20.	French basil	β-Carotene	6.8 mg/100 g FW	2500–4400 lux	11.5	Ghoora et al. (2020)
21.	Mustard	β-Carotene	7.4 mg/100 g FW	2500–4400 lux	11.5	Ghoora et al. (2020)
22.	Onion	β-Carotene	3.8 mg/100 g FW	2500–4400 lux	11.5	Ghoora et al. (2020)
23.	Radish	β-Carotene	7.6 mg/100 g FW	2500–4400 lux	11.5	Ghoora et al. (2020)
24.	Roselle	β-Carotene	6.4 mg/100 g FW	2500–4400 lux	11.5	Ghoora et al. (2020)
25.	Spinach	β-Carotene	6.1 mg/100 g FW	2500–4400 lux	11.5	Ghoora et al. (2020)
26.	Sunflower	β-Carotene	4.5 mg/100 g FW	2500–4400 lux	11.5	Ghoora et al. (2020)
27.	Parsley	β-Carotene	43.54–53.45 μg/g	B_{455}, R_{638}, R_{665}, FR_{731}; 210 and 300 μmol/m^2/s	16.0	Samuolienė et al. (2016)
28.	Kohlrabi	β-Carotene	0.28–0.34 mg/g DW	R:G:B (74:18:8), R:FR:B (84:7:9 and 84:7:9); 315, 210, and 105 mmol/m^2/s	16.0	Craver et al. (2017)
29.	Mizuna	β-Carotene	0.22–0.35 mg/g DW	R:G:B (74:18:8), R:FR:B (84:7:9 and 84:7:9); 315, 210, and 105 mmol/m^2/s	16.0	Craver et al. (2017)
30.	Mustard	β-Carotene	0.21–0.34 mg/g DW	R:G:B (74:18:8), R:FR:B (84:7:9 and 84:7:9); 315, 210, and 105 mmol/m^2/s	16.0	Craver et al. (2017)
31.	Golden pea tendrils	β-Carotene	0.6 mg/100 g FW	No light	–	Xiao et al. (2012)
32.	Amaranth	Nitrate	2.1–5.6 mg/g FW	$B_{400–500}$, $R_{600–700}$, B-R	12.0	Kyriacou et al. (2019)
33.	Cress	Nitrate	4.1–5.6 mg/g FW	$B_{400–500}$, $R_{600–700}$, B-R	12.0	Kyriacou et al. 2019
34.	Mizuna	Nitrate	2.3–3.2 mg/g FW	$B_{400–500}$, $R_{600–700}$, B-R	12.0	Kyriacou et al. (2019)
35.	Purslane	Nitrate	2.6–4.1 mg/g FW	$B_{400–500}$, $R_{600–700}$, B-R	12.0	Kyriacou et al. (2019)
36.	Basil	DPPH	9.49–10.04 μmol/g	Basal (B_{447}, R_{638}, DR_{665}, FR_{731}) + UV (366, 390, 402 nm); 6.2 and 12.4 μmol/m^2/s	–	Brazaitytė et al. (2015b)
37.	Beet	DPPH	7.00–10.90 μmol/g	Basal (B_{447}, R_{638}, DR_{665}, FR_{731}) + UV (366, 390, 402 nm); 6.2 and 12.4 μmol/m^2/s	–	Brazaitytė et al. (2015b)

(continued)

Table 7.5 (continued)

S. no.	Microgreens	Nutrient	Quantification	Light conditions	Duration (h)	References
38.	Pak choi	DPPH	7.65–10.20 μmol/g	Basal (B_{447}, R_{638}, DR_{665}, FR_{731} + UV (366,390, 402 nm); 6.2 and 12.4 μmol/m^2/s	–	Brazaitytė et al. (2015b)
39.	Basil	DPPH	7.75–9.85 μmol/g	B_{455}, R_{638}, R_{665}, FR_{731}; 210 and 300 μmol/m^2/s	16.0	Samuolienė et al. (2016)
40.	Parsley	DPPH	5.68–6.83 μmol/g	B_{455}, R_{638}, R_{665}, FR_{731}; 210 and 300 μmol/m^2/s	16.0	Samuolienė et al. (2016)
41.	Basil	Total phenol	1.30–1.93 mg/g	Basal (B_{447}, R_{638}, DR_{665}, FR_{731}) + UV (366, 390, 402 nm)	–	Brazaitytė et al. (2015b)
42.	Beet	Total phenol	0.91–1.28 mg/g	Basal (B_{447}, R_{638}, DR_{665}, FR_{731}) + UV (366, 390, 402 nm); 6.2 and 12.4 μmol/m^2/s	–	Brazaitytė et al. (2015b)
43.	Pak choi	Total phenol	0.62–0.86 mg/g	Basal (B_{447}, R_{638}, DR_{665}, FR_{731}) + UV (366, 390, 402 nm); 6.2 and 12.4 μmol/m^2/s	–	Brazaitytė et al. (2015b)
44.	Basil	Total phenols	0.54–0.64 mg/g	B_{455}, R_{638}, R_{665}, FR_{731}; 210 and 300 μmol/m^2/s	16.0	Samuolienė et al. (2016)
45.	Parsley	Total phenol	0.46–0.57 mg/g	B_{455}, R_{638}, R_{665}, FR_{731}; 210 and 300 μmol/m^2/s	16.0	Samuolienė et al. (2016)
46.	Basil	Total anthocyanins	0.31–0.97 mg/g	Basal (B_{447}, R_{638}, DR_{665}, FR_{731}) + UV (366, 390, 402 nm); 6.2 and 12.4 μmol/m^2/s	–	Brazaitytė et al. (2015b)
47.	Beet	Total anthocyanins	0.28–1.02 mg/g	Basal (B_{447}, R_{638}, DR_{665}, FR_{731}) + UV (366, 390, 402 nm); 6.2 and 12.4 μmol/m^2/s	–	Brazaitytė et al. (2015b)
48.	Pak choi	Total anthocyanins	0.37–0.99 mg/g	Basal (B_{447}, R_{638}, DR_{665}, FR_{731}) + UV (366, 390, 402 nm); 6.2 and 12.4 μmol/m^2/s	–	Brazaitytė et al. (2015b)
49.	Basil	Ascorbic acid	1.31–2.52 mg/g	Basal (B_{447}, R_{638}, DR_{665}, FR_{731}) + UV (366, 390, 402 nm); 6.2 and 12.4 μmol/m^2/s	–	Brazaitytė et al. (2015b)
50.	Beet	Ascorbic acid	0.69–7.49 mg/g	Basal (B_{447}, R_{638}, DR_{665}, FR_{731}) + UV (366, 390, 402 nm); 6.2 and 12.4 μmol/m^2/s	–	Brazaitytė et al. (2015b)

51.	Pak choi	Ascorbic acid	0.30–1.25 mg/g	Basal (B_{447}, R_{638}, DR_{665}, FR_{731}) + UV (366,390, 402 nm); 6.2 and 12.4 µmol/m^2/s	–	Brazaitytė et al. (2015b)
52.	Basil	Ascorbic acid	2.51–5.85 mg/g	B_{455}, R_{638}, R_{665}, FR_{731}; 210 and 300 µmol/m^2/s	16.0	Samuolienė et al. (2016)
53.	Parsley	Ascorbic acid	0.94–13.39 mg/g	B_{455}, R_{638}, R_{665}, FR_{731}; 210 and 300 µmol/m^2/s	16.0	Samuolienė et al. (2016)
54.	Golden pea tendrils	TAA	25.1 mg/100 g FW	No light	–	Xiao et al. (2012)
55.	Popcorn shoots	TAA	31.8 mg/100 g FW	No light	–	Xiao et al. (2012)
56.	Red basil cultivars	Total carotenoids	0.10–0.15 mg/g	R:B (2:1), R:B (1:1), R:B (1:2); 120 µmol/m^2/s	12.0	Lobiuc et al. (2017)
57.	Green basil cultivars	Total carotenoids	0.09–0.11 mg/g	R:B (2:1), R:B (1: 1), R:B (1:2); 120 µmol/m^2/s	12.0	Lobiuc et al. (2017)
58.	Mustard	Total chlorophyll	14.64–20.28 mg/g DW	275 and 463 µmol/m^2/s	12.0	Kopsell et al. (2012)
59.	Kohlrabi	Total chlorophyll	6.21–8.47 mg/g DW	R:G:B (74:18:8), R:FR:B (84:7:9 and 84:7:9); 315, 210, and 105 mmol/m^2/s	16.0	Craver et al. (2017)
60.	Mizuna	Total chlorophyll	5.40–7.89 mg/g DW	R:G:B (74:18:8), R:FR:B (84:7:9 and 84:7:9); 315, 210, and 105 mmol/m^2/s	16.0	Craver et al. (2017)
61.	Mustard	Total chlorophyll	4.37–6.68 mg/g DW	R:G:B (74:18:8), R:FR:B (84:7:9 and 84:7:9); 315, 210, and 105 mmol/m^2/s	16.0	Craver et al. (2017)
62.	Basil	Chlorophyll index	30.5	Basal (B_{447}, R_{638}, DR_{665}, FR_{731}) + UV (366, 390, 7.6.402 nm); 6.2 and 12.4 µmol/m^2/s	–	Brazaitytė et al. (2015b)
63.	Beet	Chlorophyll index	25.2	Basal (B_{447}, R_{638}, DR_{665}, FR_{731}) + UV (366, 390, 402 nm); 6.2 and 12.4 µmol/m^2/s	–	Brazaitytė et al. (2015b)
64.	Pak choi	Chlorophyll index	34.4	Basal (B_{447}, R_{638}, DR_{665}, FR_{731}) + UV (366,390, 402 nm); 6.2 and 12.4 µmol/m^2/s	–	Brazaitytė et al. (2015b)
65.	Red basil cultivar	Anthocyanins	1.44–2.45 mg/g FW	R:B (2:1), R:B (1:1), R:B (1:2); 120 µmol/m^2/s	12.0	Lobiuc et al. (2017)

(continued)

Table 7.5 (continued)

S. no.	Microgreens	Nutrient	Quantification	Light conditions	Duration (h)	References
66.	Red basil cultivar	Caffeic acid	0.62–2.57 mg/g FW	R:B (2:1), R:B (1:1), R:B (1:2); 120 μmol/m^2/s	12.0	Lobiuc et al. (2017)
67.	Red basil cultivar	Rosmarinic acid	0.33–4.99 mg/g FW	R:B (2:1), R:B (1:1), R:B (1:2); 120 μmol/m^2/s	12.0	Lobiuc et al. (2017)
68.	Golden pea tendrils	Phylloquinone	0.7 mg/100 g FW	No light	–	Xiao et al. (2012)
69.	Popcorn shoots	Phylloquinone	0.9 mg/100 g FW	No light	–	Xiao et al. (2012)
70.	Golden pea tendrils	α-Tocopherol	4.9 mg/100 g FW	No light	–	Xiao et al. (2012)
71.	Carrot	α-Tocopherol	15.5 mg/100 g FW	2500–4400 lux	11.5	Ghoora et al. (2020)
72.	Fennel	α-Tocopherol	23.8 mg/100 g FW	2500–4400 lux	11.5	Ghoora et al. (2020)
73.	Fenugreek	α-Tocopherol	5.0 mg/100 g FW	2500–4400 lux	11.5	Ghoora et al. (2020)
74.	French basil	α-Tocopherol	16.5 mg/100 g FW	2500–4400 lux	11.5	Ghoora et al. (2020)
75.	Mustard	α-Tocopherol	31.6 mg/100 g FW	2500–4400 lux	11.5	Ghoora et al. (2020)
76.	Onion	α-Tocopherol	15.2 mg/100 g FW	2500–4400 lux	11.5	Ghoora et al. (2020)
77.	Radish	α-Tocopherol	58.6 mg/100 g FW	2500–4400 lux	11.5	Ghoora et al. (2020)
78.	Roselle	α-Tocopherol	10.3 mg/100 g FW	2500–4400 lux	11.5	Ghoora et al. (2020)
79.	Spinach	α-Tocopherol	17.1 mg/100 g FW	2500–4400 lux	11.5	Ghoora et al. (2020)
80.	Sunflower	α-Tocopherol	48.7 mg/100 g FW	2500–4400 lux	11.5	Ghoora et al. (2020)
81.	Popcorn shoots	α-Tocopherol	7.8 mg/100 g FW	No light	–	Xiao et al. (2012)
82.	Popcorn shoots	γ-Tocopherol	3.5 mg/100 g FW	No light	–	Xiao et al. (2012)
83.	Golden pea tendrils	γ-Tocopherol	3.0 mg/100 g FW	No light	–	Xiao et al. (2012)

AoA antioxidant activity, *B* blue, *DW* dry weight, *FR* far red, *FW* fresh weight, *h* hour, *R* red, *TAA* total ascorbic acid, *UV* ultraviolet

Vitamin C (ascorbic acid) is considered as an essential nutrient (Machlin and Bendich 1987), and the range of total ascorbic acid (TAA) was recorded from 20.4 (sorrel) to 147.0 (red cabbage) mg/100 g FW (Xiao et al. 2012). In mung bean microgreens, the mean vitamin C content was recorded 2.7-fold higher (Ebert et al. 2017) over their mature counterparts.

The vitamin E family includes various isomers of tocopherols (Brigelius-Flohé and Traber 1999) which are present in microgreens. Green daikon radish when grown as microgreen showed maximum tocopherol (α:87.4 and γ:39.4 mg/100 g FW), while golden pea tendrils exhibited minimum (α:4.9; γ:3.9 mg/100 g FW), which are quite higher than those of fully grown spinach (α:2.0; γ:0.2 mg/100 g FW) (USDA-ARS 2018b). β-Carotene acts as a precursor of vitamin A, having key role in the vision (Mayne 1996), and is also having antioxidant function (Sies and Stahl 1995). The β-carotene content varied from 0.6 mg/100 g FW (golden pea tendrils and popcorn shoots) to 12.1 mg/100 g FW (red sorrel), and hence, most of the microgreens are considered as richer source of β-carotene (Choe et al. 2018). Other carotenoids like lutein and zeaxanthin (Bone et al. 1997) act as antioxidants (Sujak et al. 1999). Very high lutein/zeaxanthin content was recorded in cilantro (10.1 mg/100 g FW), while lower values were observed for popcorn-derived microgreens (1.3 mg/100 g FW). Similarly, cilantro microgreens showed higher violaxanthin content (7.7 mg/100 g FW), while popcorn microgreens showed the lower values (0.9 mg/100 g FW) (Xiao et al. 2012).

In red cabbage microgreens, the average vitamin C content was found six folds more (147 and 23.5 mg/100 g FW), a 400-fold more vitamin E (24.1 and 0.06 mg/100 g FW), and nearly 60-fold more vitamin K (2.4 vs 0.04 μg/g FW) over their mature counterpart (Xiao et al. 2012). Thus, the recommended daily intake (European Food Safety Authority) of vitamin C (60 mg), E (13 mg), and vitamin K (70 μg) for a medium weight adult can be met from nearly 41 g red cabbage microgreens, 15 g of green radish microgreens, and 17 g of garnet amaranth, respectively (Di Gioia and Santamaria 2015).

7.4.2 Sugars

Relatively high sugar content (10.3 g/kg) was recorded for the microgreens of China rose radish, while red amaranth recorded 1.7 g/kg of fresh microgreens (Xiao et al. 2012). However, mature vegetables recorded higher sugar content (red amaranth recorded 17 g/kg (USDA-ARS 2018a). High light (HL)-induced biofortification strategy was used for the kale and radish microgreens (Xonti et al. 2020). Radish microgreens accumulated nearly 9 times more total starch under HL (191.9 ± 30.1 mg/g DW) over normal light (NL) conditions (20.9 ± 5.2 mg/g DW), whereas in kale the increase was nearly threefold under HL (106.2 ± 18.2 mg/g DW) over NL (35.7 ± 15.4 mg/g DW) (Goble 2018).

7.4.3 Mineral Content

Microgreens are considered as an excellent source of minerals (Weber 2017; Waterland et al. 2017). Broccoli microgreens have 1–2 times more minerals such as P, K, Mg, Mn, Zn, Fe, Ca, Na, and Cu over their mature counterparts (Weber 2017). Similarly, Waterland et al. (2017) also found more dietary mineral content in kale microgreens on a dry weight basis. Among various minerals, microgreens are considered as a good source of K and Ca (Di Gioia et al. 2017a). Especially, the brassica and basil microgreens contain very high nitrates (over 4000 mg/kg FW) under low sunlight, while Na content is generally very low, which makes microgreens as low-Na food (Di Gioia and Santamaria 2015).

Minerals in the microgreens are also directly related to their abundance in the growth medium or the nutrient solution. Thus, the overall nutritional composition of the microgreens can be enhanced through fortification of growing media with certain micronutrients, while some undesirable elements such as Na and nitrates can be reduced (Di Gioia and Santamaria 2015). The most abundant elements recorded were in the order of K, P, and Ca in mung bean microgreens and K, Ca, and P in the lentil microgreens (Priti et al. 2021).

Agronomic biofortification was attempted for Fe and Zn through enrichment of nutrient media by iron sulfate (0, 10, 20, 40 mg/L) and zinc sulfate (0, 5, 10, 20 mg/L) for Brassicaceae (arugula, red cabbage, and red mustard) microgreens. Application of Zn (10 mg/L) through media had resulted in 281% increase in Zn content over control, while Fe enrichment (20 mg/L) increased its content 278% over control. Thus, for biofortification of microgreens, soilless system or hydroponics is considered the most suitable and handy (Di Gioia et al. 2019). Application of more than 20 mM calcium (as calcium chloride) was found toxic for the cultivation of radish microgreens under hydroponic system. However, application of 5.0 and 10.0 mM Ca gave maximum shoots (%), hypocotyl length and also an increase is observed for the average fresh weight per plant and total Ca accumulation in radish microgreens (Goble 2018). Przybysz et al. (2016) demonstrated that microgreens may be enriched with Mg and Fe.

7.4.4 Others

Microgreens undergo the process of germination and hence are characterized with low phytate levels and more mineral bioavailability (Liang et al. 2009). The bioactive compounds such as polyphenols and glucosinolates which are known to have a role in the prevention of various chronic diseases (Del Rio et al. 2013; Dinkova-Kostova and Kostov 2012) are found more in red cabbage microgreens (71.01 and 17.15 μmol/g, respectively) than the mature ones (50.58 and 8.30 μmol/g, respectively) (Huang et al. 2016a). Despite several studies confirming the superior nutritional content of the microgreens over their mature counterparts, detailed investigations are required to analyze the genotypic and environmental factors regulating their nutritional composition (Choe et al. 2018).

7.5 Diverse Scope of Microgreens

7.5.1 Microgreens as Functional Foods

Microgreens are being used as a functional food in the prevention of diseases like obesity, cancer, cardiovascular diseases (CVD), and type 2 diabetes mellitus (Choe et al. 2018). Health-promoting effect of red cabbage microgreens was reported by Huang et al. (2016a). For the patients ailing with impaired kidney function, the hydroponic nutrient solution (in which microgreens are grown) can be tailored to have low or no potassium so that the resultant microgreens from such a system are low in potassium (Renna et al. 2018). Similarly, Se-supplemented hydroponic solution resulted in the Se fortified basil microgreens which are also having increased antioxidant capacity (Puccinelli et al. 2019). Rocket microgreens are known to be the excessive N accumulator; thus, they can be grown under hydroponic system having limited N content so that their content can be regulated in their produce (Bulgari et al. 2017).

The desulfoglucosinolate content in the red cabbage microgreens (17.15 μmol/g DW) was much higher over their mature counterparts (8.30 μmol/g DW) (Huang et al. 2016a), which can mediate NF-κB signaling pathway. The red cabbage microgreens showed the ability to lower the liver lipids by attenuating the C-reactive protein (CRP) and tumor necrosis factor (TNF-α) (Huang et al. 2016a). NF-κB can induce the pro-inflammatory genes like TNF-α, IL-1β, IL-6, and IL-8 (Tak and Firestein 2001). Polyphenols can interfere with the NF-κB signaling pathways by inhibiting phosphorylation or ubiquitination of kinases (Gupta et al. 2010), and they can also inhibit the interaction of NF-κB subunits with target DNA (Ruiz and Haller 2006). Microgreens contain flavonoids such as kaempferol and quercetin which can suppress the COX-2 activity (Mittal et al. 2014). Thus, microgreens can regulate the process of ROS generation and scavenging, thereby influencing NF-κB and other signaling pathways (Choe et al. 2018). Considerable flavonoids contents are reported in the brassica-based microgreens which may influence *Nrf2* pathway and inflammation (Busbee et al. 2013). Microgreens analyses confirmed them as the rich sources of natural AhR ligands like quercetin and I3C (indole-3-carbinol) which can regulate the AhR-mediated immune pathways. Thus, microgreens do have a significant role in the regulation of inflammation-associated pathways (Choe et al. 2018). Thus, the consumption of microgreens is supposedly having beneficial effect in the prevention of diseases like obesity, CVD, and diabetes via regulation of inflammation. The effects of microgreens could be due to the presence of compounds like I3C and metabolites like β-carotene and retinoic acid which can suppress the adipogenesis and lipid metabolism (Choi et al. 2013; Berry et al. 2012). Microgreens also have the potential to modulate cancer progression via regulation/inhibition of various pathways including modulation of xenobiotic metabolisms (Choe et al. 2018).

The gut microbiome is considered as a key component for the regulation of human health. Flavonoids (kaempferol, quercetin, apigenin, quercetin, catechin, puerarin, etc.) are known to regulate the gut microbiota composition and thus have role in the prevention of disease development (Clemente et al. 2012; Huang et al. 2016b). Microgreens being rich in flavonoids are likely to regulate the gut microbiome, which needs further in-depth studies. Microgreens rich in various bioactive compounds like flavonoids, indoles, and isothiocyanates are known to provide protection against inflammation and oxidative stress and thus prevent the various chronic diseases including cancers through miRNA and/or DNA methylation and histone modification pathways (Choe et al. 2018). Brassica microgreens are rich in compounds like sulforaphane, phenethyl isothiocyanate, and I3C which may regulate promoter and histone methylation and also the activities of different miRNAs (Wagner et al. 2013). Food-derived bioactive compounds like tocopherols, quercetin, curcumin, resveratrol, and lycopene are also known to affect DNA methylation and histone modification (Shankar et al. 2013; Simpkins et al. 1999; Huang et al. 2012) and thereby restore *Nrf2* expression, which impart the protection against prostate cancer (Yu et al. 2010).

7.5.2 Microgreens as Space Food

The extended stay of humans in space requires proper diet to the space travelers with least supply from the earth (Perchonok et al. 2012). A range of stress effects like weight loss, change in the blood composition, and radiation-induced stress are commonly encountered by the space travelers (Vergari et al. 2010; Cohu et al. 2014; Kyriacou et al. 2017). Prevention of such stress calls for the food-based antioxidant supply (Wan et al. 2006), for which microgreens seems an excellent option. Since, microgreens can be grown on board during the mission; therefore, future space missions aim to produce carotenoid-rich food as a part of space life support systems (SLSS) (Perchonok et al. 2012).

A major challenge for adapting agricultural practices in the space is reduced gravity (or microgravity) that impacts fluid and gas distribution around the plants (Kuang et al. 2000); transpiration rates tend to increase (under hypobaric conditions); irradiance levels are low ($\leq$300 μmol/m^2/s) requiring supplemental lighting which is energy demanding for the space farm (Salisbury and Bugbee 1988). Fresh microgreens can be directly harvested by crew members, and their production can be done on any synthetic media with little or no nutrient supplementation (Perchonok et al. 2012; Nyenhuis and Drelich 2015; Kyriacou et al. 2017). Microgreens in general have a low photon flux requirement compared to long-cycle crops. Further, the use of LED lights can reduce the overall power demand per unit of crop area (Poulet et al. 2014, 2016).

7.5.3 Microgreens for the Skin Care Formulation

Microgreens are also used in various skin care formulations due to the abundance of antioxidants and vitamins. The microgreen-enriched formulations provide cleansing, exfoliating and detoxification properties which help in the nourishment, repair, and protection of the skin (https://magazine.lneonline.com/breaking-news-microgreens/).

7.5.4 Microgreens for Nutritional Security

The trans-Himalayan part of cold-arid region covers nearly 80,000 km^2 land area. The Ladakh region of trans-Himalayas harbors more than 90% of the cold desert of India. In such remote areas, due to extreme long winter, the agricultural season is very short for a period from May to September months (Bhoyar et al. 2011a, 2012). In addition, altitudinal variations, seasonal climate, and weather make it very difficult to standardize the package of practices for the year-round cultivation of different crops in such harsh conditions (Bhoyar et al. 2011b; Singh et al. 2009). Among various climatic factors, temperature imposes serious restrictions on the cropping pattern and production techniques of this region (Bhoyar et al. 2010; Mishra et al. 2009). Human settlement in these far-flung areas is even up to 4200 m altitudes, which requires year-round healthy diets at affordable prices (Cohen and Garrett 2010). For enhanced crop production and to ensure the nutritional security in these harsh areas, various comprehensive research programs are required (Bhoyar et al. 2018; Mishra and Singh 2010). One novel but potential strategy is the optimization of nutrient-rich microgreen technology for such conditions (Singh et al. 2020). Although a range of crops such as beet, broccoli, flax, kale, peas, and radish can be used for microgreen lentil, brassica and mung bean may be the cheapest and quickest among all. In addition, growing these crop species is relatively easy for the microgreens purpose over many other crop species.

7.6 Food Safety of Microgreens

During germination, the seeds release a mix of carbohydrates and peptides which attract a number of microbes present in the rhizosphere, thus making microgreens more prone to the microbial contamination than their mature counterparts (Warriner et al. 2003). Microbial load was generally found more for the sprouts over microgreens (Xiao et al. 2014). However, more microbial contamination has been recorded for the hydroponically grown microgreens over soil or media-grown ones (Riggio et al. 2019), which could be due to the constant warm temperature and humid conditions maintained for the hydroponic system. Although studies on the

Table 7.6 Microbial contamination reported for some microgreens

S. no.	Microgreens	Microbial contamination	Inoculation/storage	References
1.	Radish	*E. coli* (O157:H7 and O104:H4)	–	Xiao et al. (2014)
2.	Eight different species	Shiga toxin-producing *E. coli*	Inoculated under hydroponics	Wright and Holden (2018)
3.	Swiss chard	*Salmonella enterica*	Contaminated water irrigation	Reed et al. (2018)
4.	Radish	*E. coli* (O157:H7)	Soil substitute and hydroponics	Xiao et al. (2015b)
5.	Rapini	Lower microbial populations	Recycled fiber mats	Di Gioia et al. (2017b)
6.	Radish	*Listeria monocytogenes*	Soil substitute and hydroponics	Wang et al. (2015)
7.	Kale, mustard	Murine norovirus (MNV)	Hydroponics	Wang and Kniel (2016)
8.	Arugula, kale, lettuce, mizuna	*E. coli* (O157:H7)	Stored in a refrigerator	Park et al. (2013)

survival and growth of pathogens on microgreens are limited (Table 7.6), such studies are abundant for sprouts (Turner et al. 2020).

Microbial contamination can be easily overcome by the use of good agricultural practices like use of uninfected seeds, seed treatment, use of clean utensils, and use of UV for the disinfection of hydroponic system (Riggio et al. 2019). Application of *Trichoderma harzianum* Rifai (strain KRL-AG2 G41) and *T. virens* (strain G-41) (ThTv) to either seed ball or to the growth media was found effective in reducing the damping-off (*Pythium aphanidermatum* (Edson) Fitzp.) in the beet microgreens at 14 days after planting (Pill et al. 2011). Safer microgreens can also be produced deploying blue and UV wavelength lights as these have the antimicrobial properties (Kim et al. 2016; Maclean et al. 2009; McKenzie et al. 2014; Turner et al. 2020). As microgreens are very delicate in nature, it is almost impossible to eliminate the microbial contamination using any sanitization treatment. A recent study revealed that the pathogenic bacteria like *Salmonella* spp. and *Listeria* spp. were not detected in the mungbean, lentil and Indian mustard microgreens when stored for certain duration under 4 °C conditions in the refrigerator. Similarly, total aerobic bacteria (TAB), yeast and mould (Y&M), *Shigella* spp., and *E. coli* were recorded well within the limit to cause any human illness in these microgreens. Washing of the microgreens for 2 min with double distilled water showed some reduction microbial load of these microgreens (Priti et al. 2022).

Although no food-borne outbreak associated with the microgreen consumption is reported, still they are considered as the vehicle of bacterial pathogens (Xiao et al. 2015b). It also warrants more attention to study the survival and proliferation of food-borne pathogens on the microgreens and stored under different conditions for different periods (Di Gioia et al. 2017a).

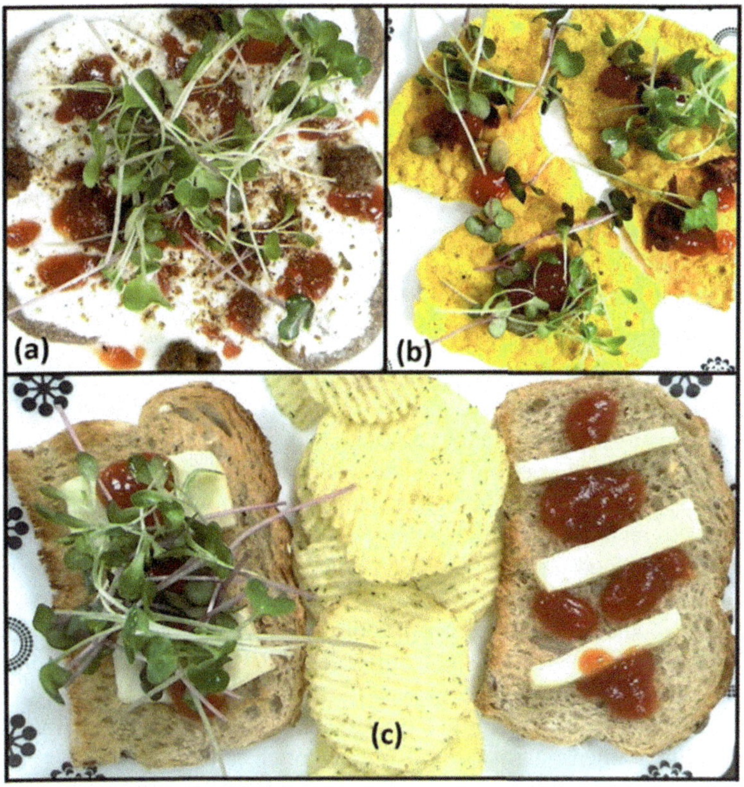

Fig. 7.2 Use of microgreens in various forms (**a**) with *paapdi chaat* (an Indian cuisine), (**b**) with nachos, and (**c**) with garlic bread

7.7 Consumption of Microgreens

Fresh microgreens form an extraordinary ingredient of taste and aesthetics for all kinds of energy drinks. Microgreens can invigorate any liquid creation, raising the bar for freshness, flavor, and overall nutritional composition, especially the antioxidant level. Mung bean and lentil-based microgreens are assumed to be the viable and cheapest option for the novel microgreens-based products. There are a number of ways in which the microgreens can be consumed either raw or after cooking or stir-frying (Fig. 7.2). Some of the most common recipes in which microgreens are used are as follows:

- *Green salads*: Microgreens are best when consumed raw as salads, since these are loaded with antioxidants, minerals, and delicate flavor.
- *Juices/smoothies*: Any microgreen is considered good for juicing or smoothies, but wheatgrass is considered the most used one in 1:3 ratio of microgreens:juice.

- *Sandwiches and wraps*: These are another raw option for consumption (radish, arugula microgreens).
- *Burgers*: Spring onion, radish, lentil, and mung bean microgreens.
- *Pizza*: Sprinkle of peppery microgreens.
- *Pasta* with raw or stir-fried microgreens.
- *Omelette with microgreens*: Any fresh microgreens will work.
- *Dhokla with microgreens*: Any fresh microgreens (preferably brassica) will work.
- *Noodles*: Flavored with microgreens.
- *Cooking with microgreens*: Some microgreens are good for cooking; while some need to be tossed in at the very last second (radish microgreens), others can stand up to a little heat.

The consumption of microgreens is not limited to any specific recipe, but can be consumed in a number of ways as per the regional food preparations (Fig. 7.2).

Microgreens as dry formulation have the ability to contribute to the nutritional security as they can be very easily made available at any part of the world (Ebert et al. 2015, 2017). The dehydration may be performed following cold raw dehydration process to retain full nutritional content of microgreens, and thus, these can be considered a raw food product. The dehydrated microgreens are unique because of their nutritional qualities. It can be used in smoothies, soups, salads, salad dressings, eggs, baked goods, etc. A number of products are now available in the market as dried formulations like tea (broccoli microgreen-based) or dressing. Microgreen-based energy drinks appear an easy way to add more healthy foods into our diet. These dried microgreen-based products are claimed to be packed with nutrients with added benefits of intense taste (https://drinkmicrotea.com).

7.8 Conclusions and Prospects

Balanced nutrition depends on the availability, accessibility, and utilization of quality foods, including microgreens. In recent decades, the consumption of calorie-rich diets which are high in fat and carbohydrates and low in protein has led to increased rates of diabetes, hypertension, and obesity in developing countries, prompting a call for serious changes in dietary patterns. Considering the burgeoning nutritional needs of our population, novel approaches like microgreen-based formulations seem a viable option for nutritional security. It has immense potential to be used as energy drinks and food additives at commercial scale. Thus, enhancing the quality of food using various microgreen-based formulations appears an option to tackle the nutritional security of our population.

The microgreens cultivation is now attracting the greenhouse growers so that the consumer need can be fulfilled especially in the urban settlements (Chandra et al. 2012). As a novel food crop, microgreens cultivation is still in infancy, especially in the developing and underdeveloped countries. However, constantly expanding research data for a number of microgreens species is unfolding their immense potential as superfood (Kyriacou et al. 2016; Xiao et al. 2012).

Currently, microgreens are mainly being used as a fresh flavor ingredient in the cuisines of upscale restaurants. As per the National Restaurant Association, microgreens are going to be considered as a culinary trend across the world. Nearly 51% of the chefs have predicted microgreens as a hot trend in the US eateries (Globe Newswire Report 2020). A few species of microgreens have been explored, and its cost of cultivation or the availability of untreated seeds has not yet been seriously considered. In addition, studies on the varietal or genotypic differences for the nutritional composition or for the shelf life studies have not been focused properly.

Research on postharvest storage should be intensified so as to have crop species-specific storage strategies. Augmentation of phytonutrient content through fortification of growth media should be explored as an alternative strategy of reaping more from same microgreens. Optimization of sanitization and drying techniques should be intensively studied which will help in the formulation of various novel storable food products. In-depth fundamental research for ensuring the food safety of microgreens and microgreens-based products should be done for their quick acceptance by the food industry.

Some of the key researchable areas include the following:

1. Variations in the nutritional composition of microgreens under different altitudinal and environmental conditions and under different drying conditions.
2. Identification of superior genotype(s) of microgreen when grown under different growth conditions (e.g., light, altitude, temperature, photoperiod).
3. Identification of factors responsible for the variations in the nutritional profile of microgreens when grown under different growth conditions using multiple OMICs approaches.
4. Optimization of cold dehydration and raw dehydration process of various microgreens for maximum nutrition retention.
5. Development of storable microgreen-based products such as microgreens powder and microgreen-based energy drink and its nutritional and medicinal characterization.
6. Region or country-specific selection and optimization of microgreens species with added cost economics for their large-scale commercialization.
7. Studies on the bioactive compounds of microgreens for their health-promoting effects in humans and estimation of bioavailability of microgreens bioactive components.

References

Abad M, Noguera P, Bures S (2001) National inventory of organic wastes for use as growing media for ornamental potted plant production: case study in Spain. Bioresour Technol 77:197–200

Agarwal A, Gupta SD (2016) Impact of light-emitting diodes (LEDs) and their potential effects on plant growth and development in controlled-environment plant production systems. Curr Biotechnol 5:28–43. https://doi.org/10.2174/2211550104666151006001126

Alrifai O, Hao X, Marcone MF et al (2019) Current review of the modulatory effects of LED lights on photosynthesis of secondary metabolites and future perspectives of microgreen vegetables. J Agric Food Chem 67:6075–6090. https://doi.org/10.1021/acs.jafc.9b00819

Ani NN, Ahmad R, Zain CM (2014) Effect of RGB LED pulse lights in photomorphogenesis of *Brassica chinensis*. In: Paper presented at 2nd international conference on agriculture and biotechnology, Phuket, Thailand

Bau H, Villaume C, Nicolas JP et al (1997) Effect of germination on chemical composition, biochemical constituents and antinutritional factors of soya bean (*Glycine max*) seeds. J Sci Food Agric 73:1–9

Berry DC, Desantis D, Soltanian H et al (2012) Retinoic acid upregulates preadipocyte genes to block adipogenesis and suppress diet-induced obesity. Diabetes 61(5):1112–1121

Bhoyar M, Mishra GP, Singh R et al (2010) Effects of various dormancy breaking treatments on the germination of wild caper (*Capparis spinosa* L.) seeds from the cold arid desert of trans-Himalayas. Indian J Agric Sci 80(7):620–624

Bhoyar M, Mishra GP, Singh R et al (2011a) Ethno-botany of traditional wild edible plants from cold arid desert of Ladakh-potential source of winter vegetables. Indian Forester 137(8): 1029–1033

Bhoyar MS, Mishra GP, Naik PK et al (2011b) Estimation of antioxidant activity and total phenolics among natural populations of *Capparis spinosa* leaves collected from cold arid desert of trans-Himalayas. Aust J Crop Sci 5(7):912–919

Bhoyar MS, Mishra GP, Naik PK et al (2012) Genetic variability studies among natural populations of *Capparis spinosa* from cold arid desert of trans-Himalayas using DNA markers. Nat Acad Sci Lett 35(6):505–515

Bhoyar MS, Mishra GP, Naik PK et al (2018) Evaluation of antioxidant capacities and total polyphenols in various edible parts of *Capparis spinosa* L. collected from trans-Himalayas. Def Life Sci J 3(3):30–36

Bian ZH, Yang QC, Liu WK (2015) Effects of light quality on the accumulation of phytochemicals in vegetables produced in controlled environments: a review. J Sci Food Agric 95:869–877

Bird E (2014) Lentils: gems in the treasure state. Montana State University, Bozeman

Bone RA, Landrum JT, Friedes LM et al (1997) Distribution of lutein and zeaxanthin stereoisomers in the human retina. Exp Eye Res 64(2):211–218

Brazaitytė A, Jankauskienė J, Novičkovas A (2013) The effects of supplementary short-term red LEDs lighting on nutritional quality of *Perilla frutescens* L. microgreens. Rural Dev 6:54–58

Brazaitytė A, Sakalauskienė S, Samuolienė G et al (2015a) The effects of LED illumination spectra and intensity on carotenoid content in Brassicaceae microgreens. Food Chem 173:600–606. https://doi.org/10.1016/j.foodchem.2014.10.077

Brazaitytė A, Viršilė A, Jankauskienė J et al (2015b) Effect of supplemental UV-A irradiation in solid-state lighting on the growth and phytochemical content of microgreens. Int Agrophys 29: 13–22. https://doi.org/10.1515/intag-2015-0004

Brazaitytė A, Vaštakaitė V, Viršilė A et al (2018) Changes in mineral element content of microgreens cultivated under different lighting conditions in a greenhouse. Acta Hortic 1227: 507–516

Brigelius-Flohé R, Traber MG (1999) Vitamin E: function and metabolism. FASEB J 13(10): 1145–1155

Bulgari R, Baldi A, Ferrante A et al (2017) Yield and quality of basil, Swiss chard, and rocket microgreens grown in a hydroponic system. N Z J Crop Hortic Sci 45:119–129. https://doi.org/10.1080/01140671.2016.1259642

Busbee PB, Rouse M, Nagarkatti M et al (2013) Use of natural AhR ligands as potential therapeutic modalities against inflammatory disorders. Nutr Rev 71(6):353–369

Carvalho SD, Folta KM (2016) Green light control of anthocyanin production in microgreens. In: Currey CJ, Lopez RG, Runkle ES (eds) Proceedings of the VIII international symposium on light in horticulture, vol 1134. ISHS, Leuven, pp 13–18. https://doi.org/10.17660/ActaHortic.2016.1134.2

Chandra D, Kim JG, Kim YP (2012) Changes in microbial population and quality of microgreens treated with different sanitizers and packaging films. Hortic Environ Biotechnol 53(1):32–40
Choe U, Yu LL, Wang TTY (2018) The science behind microgreens as an exciting new food for the 21st century. J Agric Food Chem 66:11519–11530. https://doi.org/10.1021/acs.jafc.8b03096
Choi Y, Um SJ, Park T (2013) Indole-3-carbinol directly targets SIRT1 to inhibit adipocyte differentiation. Int J Obes 37(6):881–884
Clemente JCAC, Ursell LK, Parfrey LW et al (2012) The impact of the gut microbiota on human health: an integrative view. Cell 148(6):1258–1270
Cohen MJ, Garrett JL (2010) The food price crisis and urban food (in) security. Environ Urban 22: 467–482
Cohu CM, Lombardi E, Adams WW III et al (2014) Increased nutritional quality of plants for long-duration spaceflight missions through choice of plant variety and manipulation of growth conditions. Acta Astonaut 94:799–806. https://doi.org/10.1016/j.actaastro.2013.10.009
Craver JK, Gerovac JR, Lopez RG (2017) Light intensity and light quality from sole-source light-emitting diodes impact phytochemical concentrations within Brassica microgreens. J Am Soc Hortic Sci 142(1):3–12. https://doi.org/10.21273/JASHS03830-16
Del Rio D, Rodriguez-Mateos A, Spencer JP et al (2013) Dietary (poly)phenolics in human health: structures, bioavailability, and evidence of protective effects against chronic diseases. Antioxid Redox Signal 18(14):1818–1892
Delian E, Chira A, Badulescu L et al (2015) Insight into microgreens physiology. Sci Pap Ser B Hortic 59:447–454
Di Gioia F, Santamaria P (2015) The nutritional properties of microgreens. In: Di Gioia F, Santamaria P (eds) Microgreens. Eco-logica editore, Bari, pp 41–47
Di Gioia F, Mininni C, Santamaria P (2015) How to grow microgreens. In: Di Gioia F, Santamaria P (eds) Microgreens: microgreens: novel fresh and functional food to explore all the value of biodiversity. ECO-Logica srl, Bari, pp 51–79
Di Gioia F, Renna M, Santamaria P (2017a) Sprouts, microgreens and "baby leaf" vegetables. In: Yildiz F, Wiley R (eds) Minimally processed refrigerated fruits and vegetables. Springer, Boston
Di Gioia F, De Bellis P, Mininni C et al (2017b) Physicochemical, agronomical and microbiological evaluation of alternative growing media for the production of rapini (*Brassica rapa* L.) microgreens. J Sci Food Agric 97:1212–1219. https://doi.org/10.1002/jsfa.7852
Di Gioia F, Petropoulos SA, Ozores-Hampton M et al (2019) Zinc and iron agronomic biofortification of Brassicaceae microgreens. Agronomy 9:677. https://doi.org/10.3390/agronomy9110677
Dinkova-Kostova AT, Kostov RV (2012) Glucosinolates and isothiocyanates in health and disease. Trends Mol Med 18(6):337–347
Ebert AW, Wu TH, Yang RY (2015) Amaranth sprouts and microgreens—a homestead vegetable production option to enhance food and nutrition security in the rural–urban continuum. In: Proceedings of the regional symposium on sustaining small-scale vegetable production and marketing systems for food and nutrition security (SEAVEG 2014), 25–27 February 2014, Bangkok, Thailand, pp 233–244
Ebert AW, Chang CH, Yan MR et al (2017) Nutritional composition of mungbean and soybean sprouts compared to their adult growth stage. Food Chem 237:15–22
Ghoora MD, Haldipur AC, Srividya N (2020) Comparative evaluation of phytochemical content, antioxidant capacities and overall antioxidant potential of select culinary microgreens. J Agric Food Res 2:100046. https://doi.org/10.1016/j.jafr.2020.100046
Globe Newswire Report (2020) United States microgreens market-growth, trends and forecast (2020–2025). https://www.reportlinker.com/p05916379/?utm_source=GNW. https://www.globenewswire.com/news-release/2020/07/02/2057048/0/en/United-States-Microgreens-Market-Growth-Trends-and-Forecast-2020-2025.html. Accessed 31 Dec 2020
Goble CC (2018) Effects of calcium fertilization on growth, yield, and nutrient content of hydroponically grown radish microgreens. MSU graduate theses, vol 3328. https://bearworks.missouristate.edu/theses/3328

Gupta SC, Sundaram C, Reuter S et al (2010) Inhibiting NF-κB activation by small molecules as a therapeutic strategy. Biochim Biophys Acta Gene Regul Mech 1799(10–12):775–787

Haytowitz DB, Peterson J, Booth S, USDA-ARS (2002) Phylloquinone (vitamin K) content of vegetables and vegetable products. https://www.ars.usda.gov/ARSUserFiles/80400525/Articles/ift2002_vitk.pdf

Hodges DM, Toivonen PMA (2008) Quality of fresh-cut fruits and vegetables as affected by exposure to abiotic stress. Postharvest Biol Technol 48:155–162

Huang Y, Khor TO, Shu L et al (2012) A γ-tocopherol-rich mixture of tocopherols maintains *Nrf2* expression in prostate tumors of TRAMP mice via epigenetic inhibition of CpG methylation. J Nutr 142(5):818–823

Huang H, Jiang X, Xiao Z et al (2016a) Red cabbage microgreen lower circulating LDL, liver cholesterol and inflammatory cytokines in mice fed a high fat diet. J Agric Food Chem 64:9161–9171. https://doi.org/10.1021/acs.jafc.6b03805

Huang J, Chen L, Xue B et al (2016b) Different flavonoids can shape unique gut microbiota profile in vitro. J Food Sci 81(9):H2273

Jones-Baumgardt C, Llewellyn D, Ying Q et al (2019) Intensity of sole-source light-emitting diodes affects growth, yield, and quality of Brassicaceae microgreens. HortScience 54:1168–1174

Kader AA (2008) Perspective flavor quality of fruits and vegetables. J Sci Food Agric 88:1863–1868

Kim MJ, Mikš-Krajnik M, Kumar A et al (2016) Inactivation by 405 ± 5 nm light emitting diode on *Escherichia coli* O157:H7, *Salmonella typhimurium*, and *Shigella sonnei* under refrigerated condition might be due to the loss of membrane integrity. Food Control 59:99–107

Kopsell DA, Sams CE (2013) Increases in shoot tissue pigments, glucosinolates, and mineral elements in sprouting broccoli after exposure to short-duration blue light from light emitting diodes. J Am Soc Hortic Sci 138:31–37

Kopsell DA, Pantanizopoulos NI, Sams CE et al (2012) Shoot tissue pigment levels increase in "Florida broadleaf" mustard (*Brassica juncea* L.) microgreens following high light treatment. Sci Hortic 140:96–99. https://doi.org/10.1016/j.scienta.2012.04.004

Kou L, Luo Y, Yang T et al (2013) Postharvest biology, quality and shelf life of buckwheat microgreens. Food Sci Technol 51:73–78

Kovacs J (1996) Composition of dehydrated powdered mung bean sprout and plant fiber for use as dietary supplement in healthcare. U.S. Patent no. 5,487,894. U.S. Patent and Trademark Office, Washington, DC

Kuang A, Xiao Y, McClure G et al (2000) Influence of microgravity on ultrastructure and storage reserves in seeds of *Brassica rapa* L. Ann Bot 85:851–859. https://doi.org/10.1006/anbo.2000.1153

Kyriacou MC, Rouphael Y, Di Gioia F et al (2016) Micro-scale vegetable production and the rise of microgreens. Trends Food Sci Technol 57:103–115. https://doi.org/10.1016/j.tifs.2016.09.005

Kyriacou MC, De Pascale S, Kyratzis A et al (2017) Microgreens as a component of space life support systems: a cornucopia of functional food. Front Plant Sci 8:1587. https://doi.org/10.3389/fpls.2017.01587

Kyriacou MC, El-Nakhel C, Pannico A et al (2019) Genotype-specific modulatory effects of select spectral bandwidths on the nutritive and phytochemical composition of microgreens. Front Plant Sci 10:1501. https://doi.org/10.3389/fpls.2019.01501

Lester GE, Makus DJ, Hodges DM (2010) Relationship between fresh-packaged spinach leaves exposed to continuous light or dark and bioactive contents: effects of cultivar, leaf size, and storage duration. J Agric Food Chem 58:2980–2987. https://doi.org/10.1021/jf401461z

Lester GE, Makus DJ, Hodges DM et al (2013) Summer (subarctic) versus winter (subtropic) production affects spinach (*Spinacia oleracea* L.) leaf bionutrients: vitamins (C, E, folate, K1, provitamin A), lutein, phenolics, and antioxidants. J Agric Food Chem 61:7019–7027. https://doi.org/10.1021/jf401461z

Liang J, Han BZ, Nout MR et al (2009) Effect of soaking and phytase treatment on phytic acid, calcium, iron and zinc in rice fractions. Food Chem 115(3):789–794

Lin KH, Huang MY, Huang WD et al (2013) The effects of red, blue, and white light-emitting diodes on the growth, development, and edible quality of hydroponically grown lettuce (*Lactuca sativa* L. Var. *Capitata*). Sci Hortic 150:86–91. https://doi.org/10.1016/j.scienta.2012.10.002

Lobiuc A, Vasilache V, Oroian M et al (2017) Blue and red LED illumination improves growth and bioactive compounds contents in acyanic and cyanic *Ocimum basilicum* L. microgreens. Molecules 22:2111. https://doi.org/10.3390/molecules22122111

Loedolff B, Brooks J, Stander M et al (2017) High light bio-fortification stimulates de novo synthesis of resveratrol in *Diplotaxis tenuifolia* (wild rocket) microgreens. Funct Foods Health Dis 7:859–872. https://doi.org/10.31989/ffhd.v7i11.380

Machlin LJ, Bendich A (1987) Free radical tissue damage: protective role of antioxidant nutrients. FASEB J 1(6):441–445

Maclean M, MacGregor SJ, Anderson JG et al (2009) Inactivation of bacterial pathogens following exposure to light from a 405-nm light-emitting diode array. Appl Environ Microbiol 75:1932–1937

Mayne ST (1996) Beta-carotene, carotenoids, and disease prevention in humans. FASEB J 10(7):690–701

McKenzie K, Maclean M, Timoshkin IV et al (2014) Enhanced inactivation of *Escherichia coli* and *Listeria monocytogenes* by exposure to 405 nm light under sub-lethal temperature, salt and acid stress conditions. Int J Food Microbiol 170:91–98

Mishra GP, Singh SB (2010) Frozen gene bank at frozen mountain. Curr Sci 98(4):466

Mishra GP, Singh R, Bhoyar M et al (2009) *Capparis spinosa*: unconventional potential food source in cold arid deserts of Ladakh. Curr Sci 96(12):1563–1564

Mishra GP, Ankita, Aski MS et al (2022) Morphological, molecular, and biochemical characterization of a unique lentil (*Lens culinaris* Medik.) genotype showing seed-coat color anomalies due to altered anthocyanin pathway. Plants 11(14):1815. https://doi.org/10.3390/plants11141815

Mittal M, Siddiqui MR, Tran K et al (2014) Reactive oxygen species in inflammation and tissue injury. Antioxid Redox Signal 20(7):1126–1167

Morrow RC (2008) LED lighting in horticulture. HortScience 43:1947–1950

Mubarak AE (2005) Nutritional composition and antinutritional factors of mung bean seeds (*Phaseolus aureus*) as affected by some home traditional processes. Food Chem 89(4):489–495

Nyenhuis J, Drelich JW (2015) Essential micronutrient biofortification of sprouts grown on mineral fortified fiber mats. Int Sch Sci Res Innov 9:981–984

Ohashi-Kaneko K, Takase M, Kon N et al (2007) Effect of light quality on growth and vegetable quality in leaf lettuce, spinach and komatsuna. Environ Cont Biol 45:189–198. https://doi.org/10.2525/ecb.45.189

Olson R (1984) The function and metabolism of vitamin K. Annu Rev Nutr 4(1):281–337

Park HK, Kushad MM, Feng H (2013) Survival of *Escherichia coli* O157:H7 strain 87–23 on arugula, kale, lettuce and mizuna microgreens, and comparison of leaf surface morphology for mature greens and microgreens. In: Presented at poster session, IAFP annual meeting, Charlotte, NC, USA

Perchonok MH, Cooper MR, Catauro PM (2012) Mission to mars: food production and processing for the final frontier. Ann Rev Food Sci Technol 3:311–330. https://doi.org/10.1146/annurev-food-022811-101222

Pill WG, Collins CM, Gregory N et al (2011) Application method and rate of Trichoderma species as a biological control against *Pythium aphanidermatum* (Edson) Fitzp. in the production of microgreen table beets (*Beta vulgaris* L.). Sci Hortic 129:914–918

Pinto E, Almeida AA, Aguiar AA et al (2015) Comparison between the mineral profile and nitrate content of microgreens and mature lettuces. J Food Compos Anal 37:38–43

Poulet L, Massa GD, Morrow RC et al (2014) Significant reduction in energy for plant-growth lighting in space using targeted LED lighting and spectral manipulation. Life Sci Space Res 2:43–53. https://doi.org/10.1016/j.lssr.2014.06.002

Poulet L, Fontaine JP, Dussap CG (2016) Plant's response to space environment: a comprehensive review including mechanistic modelling for future space gardener. Bot Lett 163:337–347. https://doi.org/10.1080/23818107.2016.1194228

Priti, Mishra GP, Dikshit HK et al (2021) Diversity in phytochemical composition, antioxidant capacities, and nutrient contents among mungbean and lentil microgreens when grown at plain-altitude region (Delhi) and high-altitude region (Leh–Ladakh), India. Front Plant Sci 12:812. https://doi.org/10.3389/fpls.2021.710812

Priti, Sangwan S, Kukreja B et al (2022) Yields optimization, microbial load analysis, and sensory evaluation of mungbean (*Vigna radiata* L.), lentil (*Lens culinaris* subsp. *culinaris*), and Indian mustard (*Brassica juncea* L.) microgreens grown under greenhouse conditions. PLoS ONE 17(5):e0268085. https://doi.org/10.1371/journal.pone.0268085

Przybysz A, Wrochna M, Małecka-Przybysz M et al (2016) Vegetable sprouts enriched with iron: effects on yield, ROS generation and antioxidative system. Sci Hortic 203:110–117

Puccinelli M, Malorgio F, Rosellini I et al (2019) Production of selenium biofortified microgreens from selenium-enriched seeds of basil. J Sci Food Agric 99:5601–5605. https://doi.org/10.1002/jsfa.9826

Qi LD, Liu SHQ, Xu L et al (2007) Effects of light qualities on accumulation of oxalate, tannin and nitrate in spinach. Trans Chin Soc Agric Eng 4:201–205. https://doi.org/10.3969/j.issn.1002-6819.2007.4.040

Reed E, Ferreira CM, Bell R et al (2018) Plant-microbe and abiotic factors influencing Salmonella survival and growth on alfalfa sprouts and Swiss chard microgreens. Appl Environ Microbiol 84:1–11. https://doi.org/10.1128/aem.02814-17

Renna M, Castellino M, Leoni B et al (2018) Microgreens production with low potassium content for patients with impaired kidney function. Nutrients 10:675–688. https://doi.org/10.3390/nu10060675

Riggio GM, Wang Q, Kniel KE et al (2019) Microgreens—a review of food safety considerations along the farm to fork continuum. Int J Food Microbiol 290:76–85. https://doi.org/10.1016/j.ijfoodmicro.2018.09.027

Ruiz PA, Haller D (2006) Functional diversity of flavonoids in the inhibition of the proinflammatory NF-kappaB, IRF, and Akt signaling pathways in murine intestinal epithelial cells. J Nutr 136(3):664–771

Salisbury FB, Bugbee B (1988) Plant productivity in controlled environments. HortScience 23:293–299

Samuolienė G, Urbonavičiūtė A, Brazaitytė A et al (2011) The impact of LED illumination on antioxidant properties of sprouted seeds. Cent Eur J Biol 6:68–74. https://doi.org/10.2478/s11535-010-0094-1

Samuolienė G, Brazaitytė A, Sirtautas R et al (2012) The impact of supplementary short-term red LED lighting on the antioxidant properties of microgreens. Acta Hortic 956:649–655. https://doi.org/10.17660/ActaHortic.2012.956.78

Samuolienė G, Brazaitytė A, Sirtautas R et al (2013a) LED illumination affects bioactive compounds in Romaine baby leaf lettuce. J Sci Food Agric 93:3286–3291

Samuolienė G, Brazaitytė A, Jankauskienė J et al (2013b) LED irradiance level affects growth and nutritional quality of *Brassica* microgreens. Cent Eur J Biol 8:1241–1249. https://doi.org/10.2478/s11535-013-0246-1

Samuolienė G, Brazaitytė A, Viršilė A et al (2016) Red light-dose or wavelength dependent photoresponse of antioxidants in herb microgreens. PLoS One 11(9):e0163405. https://doi.org/10.1371/journal.pone.0163405

Samuolienė G, Viršilė A, Brazaitytė A et al (2017) Blue light dosage affects carotenoids and tocopherols in microgreens. Food Chem 228:50–56. https://doi.org/10.1016/j.foodchem.2017.01.144

Sasuga DG (2014) Providing microgreens e.g. celery product with significantly longer shelf life than most other microgreens products. Patent WO2014117034-A2; US2014212549-A1

Shankar S, Kumar D, Srivastava RK (2013) Epigenetic modifications by dietary phytochemicals: implications for personalized nutrition. Pharmacol Ther 138(1):1–17

Sies H, Stahl W (1995) Vitamins E and C, beta-carotene, and other carotenoids as antioxidants. Am J Clin Nutr 62(6):1315S–1321S

Simanavičius L, Viršilė A (2018) The effects of led lighting on nitrates, nitrites and organic acids in tatsoi. Res Rural Dev 2:95–99. https://doi.org/10.22616/rrd.24.2018.057

Simpkins SB, Bocker T, Swisher EM et al (1999) MLH1 promoter methylation and gene silencing is the primary cause of microsatellite instability in sporadic endometrial cancers. Hum Mol Genet 8(4):661–666

Singh R, Mishra GP, Ahmed Z et al (2009) Effect of various greenhouse structures on yield and quality of different table tomato varieties under cold arid desert of trans-Himalayas. Indian J Agric Sci 79(4):243–247

Singh N, Aditika RS et al (2020) Vegetable microgreens farming in high-altitude region of trans-Himalayas to maintain nutritional diet of Indian troops. Proc Natl Acad Sci 90:743–752

Sujak A, Gabrielska J, Grudziński W et al (1999) Lutein and zeaxanthin as protectors of lipid membranes against oxidative damage: the structural aspects. Arch Biochem Biophys 371(2): 301–307

Sun J, Xiao Z, Lin LZ et al (2013) Profiling polyphenols in five *Brassica* species microgreens by UHPLC-PDA-ESI/HRMSn. J Agric Food Chem 61:10960–10970

Tak PP, Firestein GS (2001) NK-kappaB: a key role in inflammatory diseases. J Clin Investig 107(1):7–11

Tang D, Dong Y, Ren H et al (2014) A review of phytochemistry, metabolite changes, and medicinal uses of the common food mung bean and its sprouts (*Vigna radiata*). Chem Cent J 8:4

Treadwell D, Hochmuth R, Landrum L et al (2010) Microgreens: a new specialty crop (p. HS1164). University of Florida, Gainesville

Turner ER, Luo Y, Buchanan RL (2020) Microgreen nutrition, food safety, and shelf life: a review. J Food Sci 85(4):870–882. https://doi.org/10.1111/1750-3841.15049

USDA-ARS (2018a) Basic report: 11203, cress, garden, raw, National Nutrient Database for standard reference legacy release. https://ndb.nal.usda.gov/ndb/search/list?qlookup=11203

USDA-ARS (2018b) Full report (all nutrients): 11457, spinach, raw, National Nutrient Database for standard reference legacy release. https://ndb.nal.usda.gov/ndb/foods/show/3167?fgcd=&manu=&lfacet=&format=Full&count=&max=35&offset=&sort=&qlookup=11457. Accessed Apr 2018

Vaštakaitė V, Viršilė A (2015) Light emitting diodes (LEDs) for higher nutritional quality of Brassicaceae microgreens. In: Conference on 'research for rural development'. Held at Jelgava, Latvia, 11, pp 111–117

Vaštakaitė V, Virsile A, Brazaityte A et al (2015a) The effect of UV-A supplemental lighting on antioxidant properties of *Ocimum basilicum* L. microgreens in greenhouse. In: Proceedings of the 7th international scientific conference rural development, pp 1–7

Vaštakaitė V, Viršilė A, Brazaitytė A et al (2015b) The effect of blue light dosage on growth and antioxidant properties of microgreens. Sodininkystė ir Daržininkystė 34:25–35

Vaštakaitė V, Viršilė A, Brazaitytė A et al (2017) Pulsed light-emitting diodes for a higher phytochemical level in microgreens. J Agric Food Chem 65:6529–6534

Vaštakaitė V, Viršilė A, Brazaitytė A et al (2018) Pulsed light increases the phytochemical level of basil microgreens. Acta Hortic 1227:579–584

Vergari F, Tibuzzi A, Basile G (2010) An overview of the functional food market: from marketing issues and commercial players to future demand from life in space. In: Giardi MT, Rea G, Berra B (eds) Bio-farms for nutraceuticals. Springer, Boston, pp 308–321

Wagner AE, Terschluesen AM, Rimbach G (2013) Health promoting effects of Brassica-derived phytochemicals: from chemopreventive and anti-inflammatory activities to epigenetic regulation. Oxidative Med Cell Longev 2013:1–12

Walters RG (2005) Towards an understanding of photosynthetic acclimation. J Exp Bot 56:435–447. https://doi.org/10.1093/jxb/eri060

Wan XS, Ware JH, Zhou Z et al (2006) Protection against radiation induced oxidative stress in cultured human epithelial cells by treatment with antioxidant agents. Int J Rad Oncol Biol Phys 64:1475–1481. https://doi.org/10.1016/j.ijrobp.2005.11.024

Wang Q, Kniel KE (2016) Survival and transfer of murine norovirus within a hydroponic system during kale and mustard microgreen harvesting. Appl Environ Microbiol 82:705–713. https://doi.org/10.1128/aem.02990-15

Wang L, Luo Y, Nou X (2015) Proliferation of *Listeria monocytogenes* during microgreen production. In: Presented at poster session, international association for food protection annual meeting, Portland, OR, USA. https://iafp.confex.com/iafp/2015/webprogram/Paper9430.html

Warriner K, Ibrahim F, Dickinson M et al (2003) Internalization of human pathogens within growing salad vegetables. Biotechnol Genet Eng Rev 20:117–136. https://doi.org/10.1080/02648725.2003.10648040

Waterland NL, Moon Y, Tou JC et al (2017) Mineral content differs among microgreen, baby leaf, and adult stages in three cultivars of kale. HortScience 52(4):566–571

Weber CF (2017) Broccoli microgreens: a mineral-rich crop that can diversify food systems. Front Nutr 4:7. https://doi.org/10.3389/fnut.2017.00007

Wright KM, Holden NJ (2018) Quantification and colonisation dynamics of *Escherichia coli* O157:H7 inoculation of microgreen species and plant growth substrates. Int J Food Microbiol 273:1–10. https://doi.org/10.1016/j.ijfoodmicro.2018.02.025

Wu M, Hou C, Jiang C et al (2007) A novel approach of LED light radiation improves the antioxidant activity of pea seedlings. Food Chem 101:1753–1758

Xiao Z, Lester GE, Luo Y et al (2012) Assessment of vitamin and carotenoid concentrations of emerging food products: edible microgreens. J Agric Food Chem 60:7644–7651. https://doi.org/10.1021/jf300459b

Xiao Z, Nou X, Luo Y et al (2014) Comparison of the growth of *Escherichia coli* O157:H7 and O104:H4 during sprouting and microgreen production from contaminated radish seeds. Food Microbiol 44:60–63. https://doi.org/10.1016/j.fm.2014.05.015

Xiao Z, Lester GE, Park E et al (2015a) Evaluation and correlation of sensory attributes and chemical compositions of emerging fresh produce: microgreens. Postharvest Biol Technol 110:140–148

Xiao Z, Bauchan G, Nichols-Russell L et al (2015b) Proliferation of *Escherichia coli* O157:H7 in soil-substitute and hydroponic microgreen production systems. J Food Prot 78:1785–1790. https://doi.org/10.4315/0362-028x.jfp-15-063

Xonti A, Hunter E, Kulu N et al (2020) Diversification of health-promoting phytochemicals in radish (*Raphanus raphanistrum*) and kale (*Brassica oleracea*) micro-greens using high light bio-fortification. Funct Foods Health Dis 10(2):65–81

Ying Q, Kong Y, Zheng Y (2020) Applying blue light alone, or in combination with far-red light, during night time increases elongation without compromising yield and quality of indoor-grown microgreens. HortScience 55(6):876–881. https://doi.org/10.21273/HORTSCI14899-20

Yu S, Khor TO, Cheung KL et al (2010) *Nrf2* expression is regulated by epigenetic mechanisms in prostate cancer of TRAMP mice. PLoS One 5(1):e8579

Chapter 8
Antinutritional Factors: Nutrient Bioavailability and Health Beneficial Effects

Komal Soni, Mrinal Samtiya, Veda Krishnan, and Tejpal Dhewa

Abstract Antinutrients are naturally occurring substances in plants, well known to block the absorption of beneficial or essential organic nutrients and inorganic minerals. Major antinutrients such as enzymes (lipase, amylase, and protease), trypsin inhibitors, phytate, polyphenols, lectins, glucosinolates, oxalates, and saponins have been characterized in different plant species. In general, these antinutrients are reported to have bitter taste and are unpalatable with bad odor and have a role in plant defenses. Antinutrients, which are known to bind the nutrients, severely affect the latter's bio-accessibility and ultimately bioavailability. The current chapter briefly summarizes the various kinds of antinutrients and their role in limiting bioavailability of nutrients. Eventually, these antinutrients cause mineral deficiency and micronutrient malnutrition in humans. Hence, it is indispensable to reduce their contents in foods to a safe level for human consumption. Further, various strategies and concepts to tackle the deleterious effects of antinutrients are discussed. Many processing methods namely decortication, roasting, boiling, microwave heating, soaking, germination, autoclaving, fermentation, and extrusion technique are reported to decrease the antinutrient content in food crops. Further, the current understanding of the antinutrient's health promoting effects such as reduction of blood glucose, cholesterol levels, prevention of cardiovascular diseases and cancer are also discussed.

Keywords Antinutrients · Mineral malnutrition · Nutrient bioavailability · Plant based-micronutrients

K. Soni · M. Samtiya · T. Dhewa (✉)
Department of Nutrition Biology, Central University of Haryana, Mahendragarh, Haryana, India

V. Krishnan
Division of Biochemistry, ICAR-Indian Agricultural Research Institute, New Delhi, India

R. S. V., S. Praveen (eds.), *Conceptualizing Plant-Based Nutrition*,
https://doi.org/10.1007/978-981-19-4590-8_8

8.1 Introduction

A World Health Organization (WHO) report reveals that more than two billion people are encountering the problem of micronutrient deficiency due to improper nutrition leading to mass malnutrition. This condition is more specifically encountered in developing countries. Vitamin A, zinc, and iron are the most essential micronutrients whose deficiencies cause serious health concerns (Gupta et al. 2015). Though nutrients and antinutrients both are naturally present in plants, former has positive effects and latter pose deleterious effect on human body (Popova and Mihaylova 2019). In order to improve the proper mineral intake, several countries have endorsed dietary intake guidelines toward consumption of the whole grains, as these plant foods are exceptional sources of almost all the essential nutrients. However, the presence of several antinutritional factors (ANF) (for example phytic acids) could severely hinder the immense nutritional benefits of plant-based foods (Samtiya et al. 2021). Antinutrients are phytochemicals acquired or developed during the process of plant evolution for their own defense with limited biological functions. Upon consumption, antinutrients reduce the optimal utilization of food nutrients especially proteins, vitamins, and minerals thereby decreasing the overall nutritional value of foods (Ijeoma and Adeyemi 2020). Various antinutrients present in plant foods are depicted in Fig. 8.1. ANFs inhibit the proper utilization of nutrients by forming complexes with these compounds which eventually reduce their absorption in the gastrointestinal (GI) tract (Nikmaram et al. 2017). ANFs are found in appreciable concentration in legumes, grains, beans, and nuts. However, they are also known to occur in fruits, leaves, and roots of certain types of plants. The antinutrients in plant foods are enzyme inhibitors, phytates, tannins, oxalates, saponins, lectins, etc. (Popova and Mihaylova 2019). ANFs considerably affect the nutritional values of foods; hence, reduction or elimination of these factors from plant foods is now a major goal to improve human nutrition. There are several processing methods such as dehulling, milling, soaking, germination, and fermentation that can be employed to reduce these ANFs (Samtiya et al. 2020). This chapter aims to present updated information about antinutrients, their positive and negative effects, and existing strategies to reduce ANFs. Figure 8.2 depicts a brief overview of possible health beneficial properties of antinutrients.

8.2 Types of Antinutritional Factors

8.2.1 Lipase Inhibitors

On the basis of chemical structures, plant lipase inhibitors can be grouped into the following categories: phenols, saponins, alkaloids, terpenes, glycosides, carotenoids, and polysaccharides (Singh et al. 2015). Lipase inhibitors reduce the biochemical functioning of enzyme lipases, which hydrolyze the triglyceride to monoglycerides, glycerol esters, fatty acids, and glycerol. Lipase inhibitors primarily affect fat

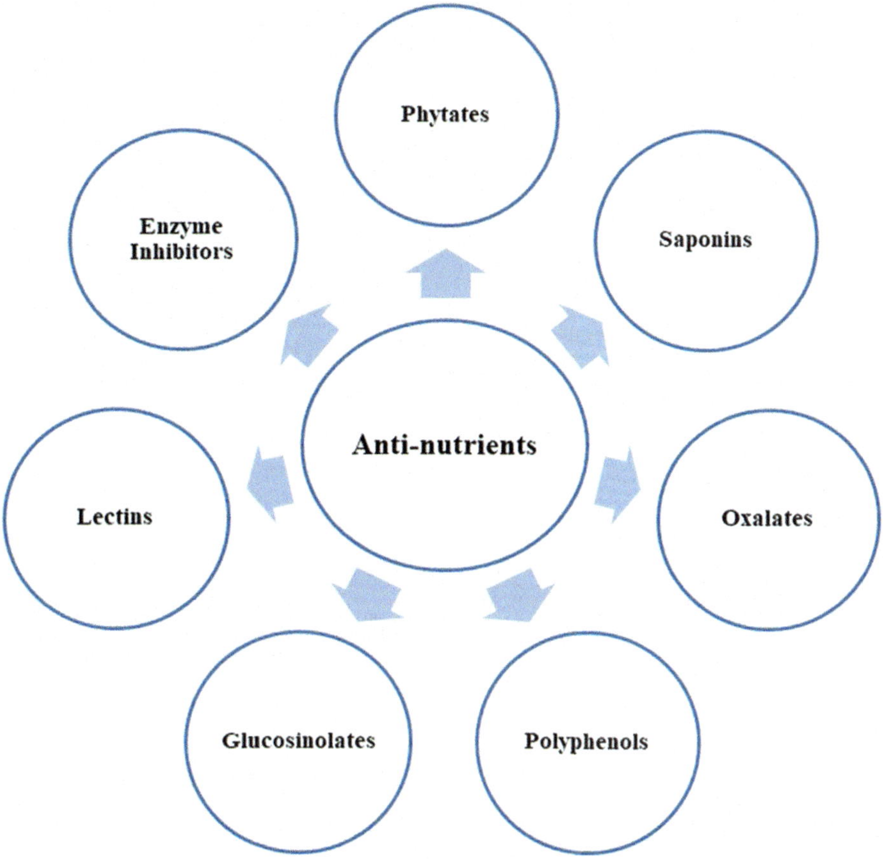

Fig. 8.1 Antinutrients present in plant food

metabolism, which inhibits lipid hydrolysis by macromolecules, reducing the absorption of small fat molecules and fat accumulation ultimately causing deficiency of fat-soluble vitamins (Liu et al. 2020; Yun 2010).

8.2.2 Amylase Inhibitors

Amylase inhibitors are the phytocompounds which bind to enzyme α-amylase and make them inactive. There are two main biological roles of α-amylase inhibitors in plants: protect the seeds against pests and microorganisms and inhibit mammalian α-amylases, insect α-amylases, and endogenous α-amylases (Popova and Mihaylova 2019; Wisessing and Choowongkomon 2012). Mammalian amylase enzyme is secreted by the pancreas into the small intestine, whereas α-glucosidase enzymes

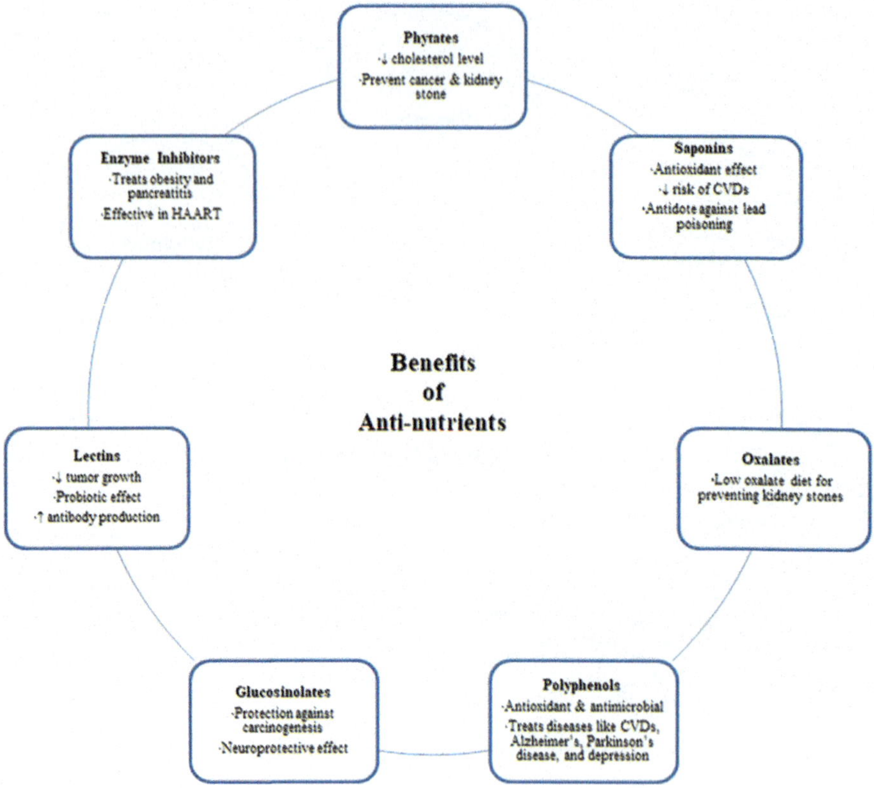

Fig. 8.2 Presents brief overview of possible health beneficial properties of antinutrients

are located in the brush border of the small intestines. Further, amylases convert the carbohydrates into oligosaccharides (Barrett and Udani 2011), and α-glucosidase acts on starch to convert them into glucose molecules (Brás et al. 2018). Amylase inhibitors impair the activity of salivary and pancreatic amylase and affect the growth and metabolism of animals at appreciably high levels are ingested (Grant et al. 2003). However, their ability to inhibit the action of α-amylase enzymes resulting in reduction of starch hydrolysis shows positive effects on glycemic index control in diabetics (Bhat et al. 2011). *Phaseolus* species (kidney beans) have relatively high content of amylase inhibitors of about 4.3 g per kg (Grant et al. 2003).

8.2.3 Protease Inhibitors

Proteases are important class of enzymes found in all cells and tissues that regulate multiple cellular processes (Popova and Mihaylova 2019). Protease inhibitors are relatively small proteins commonly found in raw cereals, legumes, specifically soybeans, tubers, and also in aerial parts of some plants. The metabolic functioning of protease, i.e., breaking down of hydrolytic cleavage of peptide bonds in proteins is restricted by these inhibitors (Popova and Mihaylova 2019; Habib and Fazili 2007). Protease inhibition occurs due to the formation of an enzyme–inhibitory molecule complex thereby restricting the availability of enzyme to perform substrate hydrolysis (Paiva et al. 2013). This comprehension has led to the development of drugs; for example, protease inhibitors play an effective role in treating AIDS in the strategy of HAART, i.e., highly active antiretroviral therapy (Wang et al. 2015).

8.2.4 *Trypsin Inhibitors*

These are found in a variety of foods such as potato, eggplant, millet, barley, wheat, mung beans, soybeans, red kidney beans, chickpeas, and adzuki beans belonging to diverse families *Solanaceae, Gramineae,* and *Leguminosae.* It inhibits the activity of digestive enzymes (trypsin and chymotrypsin) by forming complexes and prevents the absorption of nutrients and digestion of protein (Tibe and Amarteifio 2010; Vanga et al. 2020). For example, their presence in human food causes improper growth and impairs protein digestion, pancreatic hyperplasia and disturbance of sulfur and amino acid utilization (Nikmaram et al. 2017). Peas, lentils, and soybean contain Bowman–Birk-like trypsin inhibitors which have a low molecular weight, *i.e.,* 8–10 kDa and are double-headed to inhibit two enzyme molecules at a time (Grant et al. 2003).

8.2.5 *Phytates*

Phytates are the salts of phytic acid, chemically known as myo-inositol hexaphosphate and its general molecular formula is $C_6H_{18}O_{24}P_6$ (Diouf et al. 2019). Phytate chelates micronutrients (calcium, zinc, iron, copper, and magnesium) and makes them less bioavailable to monogastric animals, including poultry and humans, due to absence or low activity of phytase enzyme in their digestive tract (Gupta et al. 2015). Based on the type of cation, the minerals may bind with one or more phosphate groups of a phytate or may bridge with two or more phytate molecules (Nikmaram et al. 2017). Phytates are also known as demineralizing agents because they form insoluble salts with divalent and trivalent cationic metal ions. Phytates also interact with protein residues to form phytate–protein and phytate–mineral–protein complexes which inhibit many reactions of digestive enzymatic (Betancur-Ancona et al. 2012). Plants synthesize phytate to store phosphorus and phytate may represent approx. 50–85% of total phosphorous in some plants. It occupies 1–5% weight in legumes, cereals, nuts, and oil seeds (Vats and Banerjee

2004; Reddy et al. 1982). Decortication, soaking, germination, and fermentation are some of the traditional methods followed to reduce the antinutrients (Eltayeb et al. 2007).

8.2.6 Polyphenols

Polyphenols are a group of secondary metabolites which abundantly occur in vegetables, fruits, herbs, spices, tea, wine, chocolate, other cocoa products, and extra virgin olive oil. Phenolics are classified into simple phenolics which include phenolic acids, flavones, isoflavones, etc., and complex phenolics which include catechins, tannins, lignans, etc. Dietary polyphenols show many beneficial effects, such as protection against oxidative stress, and degenerative diseases like diabetes, cancer, cardiovascular diseases (Han et al. 2007). Different classes of phenolic compounds include tannins, flavonoids, phenolic acids, lignans, and stilbenes (Shahidi et al. 2019). Tannins are the polyphenols known to form reversible or irreversible complexes with proteins, reducing latter's digestibility and amino acid bioavailability (Lampart-Szczapa et al. 2003). Hydrolysable tannins mainly consist of phenolic acids or their derivatives attached to central unit of pentagalloylglucose with ester linkage. Gallotannins and ellagitanins are the two main classes of hydrolysable tannins, which consist of gallic acid and ellagic acid, respectively (Singh and Kumar 2019; Diouf et al. 2019). Condensed tannins are produced by the condensation of two or more flavanols units and have structure similar to flavonoids and they do not constitute sugar molecules (Hussain et al. 2019; Diouf et al. 2019). Dietary polyphenols show beneficial effects in reducing cancer, CVDs, diabetes, neurodegenerative diseases, and osteoporosis (Mattila et al. 2018; Vauzour et al. 2010). Polyphenolics are attributed with regulation of lipoprotein plasma concentrations and insulin resistance in a clinical trial involving men who have high risk of developing CVD (Chiva-Blanch et al. 2013).

8.2.7 Lectins

Lectins, known as phytohemagglutinins, are a glycoprotein compound that binds simple carbohydrates especially oligosaccharides and also agglutinates red blood cells (RBCs) in vitro (Klupšaitė and Juodeikienė 2015; Santos et al. 2014). Alternatively, lectins are known as carbohydrate-binding proteins found in plant foods like cereal grains and legumes (Van Buul and Brouns 2014). Lectins are synthesized at the time of seed development and are utilized by the plants as an amino acid source during germination as well as act as defensive compound against insects, fungi, and nematodes attack (Betancur-Ancona et al. 2012). Lectins are highly resistant to in vivo proteolytic degradation and survive while passing through the GI tract. Only if appropriate carbohydrate receptors present on epithelial cells of intestine, lectins can bind to them and are absorbed systematically. Thus, lectins can alter and modify many aspects of intestinal and systemic metabolism. The quantum of lectins in lentil and peas are comparable to that of soybean (2–4 g/kg) relatively low than what is reported in kidney bean (15–30 g/kg) (Grant et al. 2003).

8.2.8 Glucosinolates

Chemically, glucosinolates are S-β-thioglucoside N-hydroxysulfates which are found abundantly in cruciferous (*Brassicaceae*) plants but are also reported in other species like moringa, papaya, and capers. More than 120 different types of glucosinolates have been found in plants (Dinkova-Kostova 2012). Glucosinolates are water-soluble, nitrogen-containing compounds, having a glucopyranose moiety bound with sulfur in its molecular structure (Lopez-Rodriguez et al. 2020). Glucosinolates are the major secondary metabolites produced by plants, having crucial role in the physiology and defense of plants against various environmental stresses. Glucosinolates are enzymatically broken down by myrosinase (a thioglucosidase) whenever a plant tissue is damaged, to form glucose, sulfate, nitriles, indolic alcohols, isothiocyanates, thiocyanate, oxazolidinethions, amines, and epithionitriles. Glucosinolates along with their catabolized products play a vital role in plant defense (Międkus et al. 2020).

8.2.9 Oxalates

Oxalic acid forms potassium, sodium (soluble) or iron, calcium, magnesium (insoluble) salts, or esters called oxalates (Popova and Mihaylova 2019). By forming esters with these minerals, oxalates make them less available (Savage and Klunklin 2018). Compared to other ANFs, oxalates are found in less quantum in plants such as wheat, rye, millet, and barley (Siener et al. 2006). Foods rich in oxalate usually form a minor component of the human diet, but in some regions of the world, oxalates form an important ingredient of the seasonal diet. Calcium oxalate is responsible for the formation of kidney stones. People suffering from enteric and primary hyperoxaluria are advised to decrease the intake of oxalates because in the former more oxalates are absorbed and excreted via urine resulting in increased risk of kidney stone formation. In the latter condition, either liver does not produce adequate amount of enzymes to prevent the overproduction of oxalate or enzymes do not function properly (Popova and Mihaylova 2019; Bhasin et al. 2015).

8.2.10 Saponins

Saponins are a diverse group of chemicals and are called so because of their ability to form soap-like foams in aqueous solutions (Hill 2003). The structure of saponins contains a steroidal or triterpenoid aglycone, and one or more oligosaccharide moieties (Yildirım and Kutlu 2015). Saponins are found in broad beans, kidney beans, and lentils imparting bitter taste to food if present in high concentration hence low saponins foods are preferred (Shi et al. 2004). Saponins exhibit both the hypoglycemic and hypocholesteremic effects (Ikewuchi 2012; Barky et al. 2017).

8.2.11 Exorphins

The prolamins, *i.e.,* alcohol-soluble proteins found in dairy products and cereal grains which are known as gliadins, can be degraded into opioid-like polypeptides in GI tract which are called as exorphins (Tatham and Shewry 2008; Pruimboom and de Punder 2015). Recent studies indicated that the epigenetic effects of opiate peptides derived from milk protein alpha-casein may contribute to GI dysfunction and inflammation in susceptible people (Trivedi et al. 2015). The bioactivity of food-derived exorphins can affect behavioral characteristics i.e. memory, spontaneity, and pain perception (Lister et al. 2015). On the basis of origin, opioid peptides are of two types: endogenous and exogenous. Endogenous peptides are synthesized by the organism which may function as hormones and neuromodulators (Garg et al. 2016) whereas exogenous peptides are formed when plant or animal precursor proteins are hydrolyzed in the digestive tract (Janecka et al. 2004; Nyberg and Hallberg 2013).

8.2.12 Contextual Antinutrients

Some food or food additives can also act as antinutrients depending on the context. For example, foods rich in calcium can stop the absorption of iron. Also a mutual antagonism exist between copper and zinc during the absorption process which occurs in the intestinal epithelium (Van Campen 1969). Scientific literature states that phospholipids and phytosterols can hinder cholesterol absorption when added to low-fat or non-fat foods (Ostlund 2002; Cohn et al. 2010). It has been also noticed that some foods can interfere with the absorption of medications (Genser 2008). Food–drug interaction is also very common. For example, if a drug is taken along with grapefruit, the latter inactivates the enzyme of drug metabolism as it contains bergamottin-a natural furanocoumarin. Studies have also demonstrated that the polyphenol compound resveratrol present in peanuts and red wine inhibits platelet aggregation, thus when taken with anticoagulant drugs, it can increase the risk of bleeding (Jin and Han 2010). Similarly, foods that contain tyramine (beer, wine, chocolate, and avocados) are inhibitors of monoamine oxidase inhibitors (MAOIs). Hence, the activity of MAOI drugs such as anti-depressant drugs is affected when consumed with foods rich in tyramine (Vaquero et al. 2010). Likewise, foods rich in coumadin and vitamin K such as broccoli and spinach exhibit antagonism with anticoagulant drugs.

8.3 Health Beneficial Properties of Antinutritional Factors

Various health and beneficial properties of antinutritional factors derived from plant-based food are presented in Table 8.1. The health and beneficial effects of ANFs are known especially in the treatment of obesity, diabetes, antiviral treatment, neuroprotective effects, reduction in blood cholesterol levels, and inhibition of cancer.

8.4 Adverse Effects of Antinutritional Factors Relevance to Health

As stated below, the adverse effects of ANFs include reduced intestinal absorption of diet-derived nutrients, impaired digestion and growth, mal-absorption of mineral nutrients among others (Table 8.2).

8.5 Strategies for Reduction of Antinutrients in Plant Foods

Multiple studies have proven that antinutrients have negative effects on nutritional quality of food which eventually affect health. Several strategies are available to reduce antinutritional factors to great extent so as to improve food quality. Elimination of the antinutrients would be essential for effective utilization of nutrients like carbohydrates, proteins, and minerals in human nutrition (Ohiokpehai 2003; Tibe and Amarteifio 2010). Many traditional and modern techniques which include decortications, heating, soaking, germination, fermentation, and extrusion are available to reduce the concentration of antinutritional factors in food crops.

Table 8.1 Health and beneficial properties of antinutritional factors

Antinutrients	Health beneficial effects	Mode of action	References
Lipase inhibitors	• In the treatment of obesity	Prevents the absorption of fat in the body	Sridhar et al. (2019)
Amylase inhibitors	• In the treatment of diabetes mellitus II • Obesity treatment	Reduces starch hydrolysis which controls glycemic index	Bhat et al. (2011), Grant et al. (2003)
Protease inhibitors	• Effective role in HAART (highly active antiretroviral therapy), *i.e.,* treatment method for AIDS • Effective in treating hepatitis, thrombosis, cancer, and cirrhosis	Alters the protease configuration present in proteolytic events linked with the diseases	Wang et al. (2015), Adhikari et al. (2020)
Trypsin inhibitors	• In the treatment of pancreatitis	Inhibits trypsin production leads to no further cell damage in pancreas	Brandl et al. (2016), Ning et al. (2013)
Phytates	• Reduces cholesterol levels • Prevents coronary disease • Prevents kidney stone • Prevents cancer • Potential in the treatment of Alzheimer's disease, Parkinson's disease, and multiple sclerosis	Binds to cholesterol and calcium and makes them unavailable	Coulibaly et al. (2011), Vats and Banerjee (2004), Nikmaram et al. (2017), Oghbaei and Prakash (2016)
Polyphenols	• Antioxidant and antimicrobial property • Prevent cardiovascular diseases • In the treatment of Alzheimer's disease, Parkinson's disease, and neuropsychiatric disorders like depression • Flavonoids protect against heart diseases and stroke	By reversing extracellular amyloid beta deposition and intracellular tau hyperphosphorylation	Zhang et al. (2017), Grant et al. (2003), Hussain et al. (2019), Tungmunnithum et al. (2018), Hassan et al. (2020), Malar and Devi (2014)
Lectins	• Inhibits tumor growth • Probiotic • Also increases antibody production	Binds to membrane of cancer cell or their receptors, causing apoptosis, cytotoxicity, and inhibition of tumor growth	Betancur-Ancona et al. (2012), De Majia et al. (2005)
Glucosinolates	• Provides protection against carcinogenesis • Neuroprotective	• Hydrolyzed product of glucosinolates phenethyl isothiocyanate (PEITC), benzyl isothiocyanate	Dinkova-Kostova (2012), Tanito et al. (2005), Possenti et al. (2016), Soundararajan

(continued)

Table 8.1 (continued)

Antinutrients	Health beneficial effects	Mode of action	References
		(BITC) and sulforaphane (SFN) help in preventing cancer • Activates the Nrf2/ARE pathway, which enhances the functioning of neuronal natural phase 2 enzyme and acts as a powerful indirect antioxidant	and Kim (2018), Angeloni et al. (2017)
Saponins	• Reduces blood cholesterol levels • Antioxidant • Cancer inhibition • Antidote against lead poisoning	• Forms large micelles with bile acids and cholesterol • Act as potent Ca^{2+}-activated K^{+}channel opener, helpful for treating cardiovascular, urological, respiratory, neurological, and other disorders	Hill (2003), Shi et al. (2004), Gemede and Ratta (2014), Mohan et al. (2016)

8.5.1 Decortication

Decortication or dehulling involves the removal of outer covering (pericarp) of grains. In the pre-mechanization era, dehulling was done using mortar and pestle but currently automatic rice huller/rice milling machines are available for efficient processing (Kulkarni et al. 2018). Decortication significantly reduces many antinutrient components present in bran and also lowers the concentration of condensed tannins (Lestienne et al. 2007; Pal et al. 2015). Pal et al. (2016) observed that around 52–56% reduction of phytic acid content in lentils is achieved by following the decortication process. In different varieties of lentils, the combination of decortication and germination techniques have shown appreciable reduction in antinutritional factors including tannins, phytate, trypsin inhibitors, total polyphenols, etc. (Pal et al. 2015). Ghavidel and Prakash (2007) found a reduction of 43–52% and 47–52% in tannin and phytic acid contents, respectively, in various legume seeds such as green gram, cowpea, lentil, and chickpea. Himanshu et al. (2018) reported that this method decreases phytic phosphorus content by 39% in little millet, 23% in barnyard millet, 25% in kodo millet, and 12% in common millet. The activity of antinutritional factors i.e. trypsin inhibitor, phytic acid, and tannins was reported to be reduced by 7.59%, 20.7%, and 33.3%, respectively, after dehulling of mung bean seed (Oghbaei and Prakash 2016).

Table. 8.2 Adverse effects of antinutritional factors

Antinutrients	Adverse effects	References
Lipase inhibitors	• Reduced absorption of fats and lipids • Cause deficiency of fat-soluble vitamins • Other effects include high blood pressure, headache, dryness of mouth, insomnia, and constipation	Lunagariya et al. (2014), Yun (2010)
Amylase inhibitors	• Impairs growth and metabolism • Prevents starch digestion	Grant et al. (2003), Barrett et al. (2011)
Protease inhibitors	• Inhibits growth • Poor utilization of food • Pancreatic hypertrophy • Interferes in blood clotting and cellular apoptosis	Popova and Mihaylova (2019), Paiva et al. (2013)
Trypsin inhibitors	• Inhibit protein digestion • Pancreatic hyperplasia • Interference in sulfur and amino acid utilization	Nikmaram et al. (2017)
Phytates	• Cause mineral deficiency (Zn, Fe, Ca, Mg)	Nikmaram et al. (2017)
Polyphenols	• High concentration of tannin could be a reason for throat and esophageal cancer	Hussain et al. (2019)
Lectins	• Joint pain and migraine • Acne and inflammation • Agglutinate red blood cells (RBCs)	Popova and Mihaylova (2019), Van Buul and Brouns (2014)
Glucosinolates	• Enlargement of thyroid • Reduce reproductive performance • Damage GI tract	Prieto et al. (2019), Bischoff (2016)
Oxalates	• Prevent calcium absorption, i.e., hypocalcemia • Kidney stone formation • Urinary calculi	Savage and Klunklin (2018), Nikmaram et al. (2017)
Saponins	• Hinder absorption of vitamin A, E, and lipids • Effect epithelial lining of intestine	Samtiya et al. (2020)
Exorphins	• Dizziness • Physical tolerance • Nausea and vomiting	Garg et al. (2016)

8.5.2 Milling

Milling is a processing method which removes the outer layer, i.e., pericarp of the grain (Kulkarni et al. 2018). It is commonly employed to reduce phytic acid levels from grains but it also has some demerits as it removes dietary fibers and minerals from grains (Gupta et al. 2015). The process of milling can be of two types: (1) The whole grain is ground into flour without separating any parts or, (2) Differential milling to separate the grain into different parts (Oghbaei and Prakash 2016). Former results into grain flour whereas latter provides many products such as germ, bran, semolina, and refined wheat flour. Milled wheat flour is used to make *chapattis* which on heating decrease the phytic acid and polyphenol content and improve protein and starch digestion (Chowdhury and Punia 1997).

8.5.3 Heating

Heat from different sources is applied as processing method in roasting, cooking, boiling, and microwave heating. Adeyemo and Onilude (2013) found appreciable reduction in tannin (74.6%), phytate (28.4%), trypsin inhibitor (98.3%), and protease inhibitor (97.5%) after roasting soybean in comparison with cooking which eliminated tannin (42%), phytate (75.8%), trypsin inhibitor (95.8%), and protease inhibitor (95.8%). Microwave processing degrades the bioavailability of glucosinolates and significantly reduces the polyphenolic content in millets (Miękus et al. 2020; Hithamani and Srinivasan 2014). Vanga et al. (2020) reported that microwave heating can eliminate 70% of trypsin inhibitors in soy milk. Barba et al. (2016) reported that boiling decreases glucosinolates level more significantly than steaming. Ertop and Bektas (2018) stated that pressure cooking of black gram eliminates tannins and increases its protein digestibility. A comparative analysis of the effect of boiling and baking of taro leaves was conducted by Savage and Mårtensson (2010) which showed that boiling taro leaves for 40 min reduced 47% oxalate content whereas no such significant reduction of oxalate was obtained after baking. Many studies have demonstrated that autoclaving is best suited method to reduce levels of various antinutritional factors like tannin, phytic acid, and free phenolics compared to other processing treatments (Samtiya et al. 2020; Vijayakumari et al. 1996). The findings of Kadam et al. (1987) concluded that the methods like boiling and autoclaving improved the protein quality of winged beans by eliminating antinutrients.

8.5.4 Soaking

Soaking is a widely used process which generally precedes other treatments like germination, cooking, and fermentation. It is one of the easiest ways to reduce antinutrients (Kumari et al. 2014). Soaking is effective to eliminate tannins, phytic acid, total phenols, and trypsin inhibitor activity of many cereals, legumes, and millets (Oghbaei and Prakash 2016). It is also effective in reducing saponins on domestic as well as on industrial levels (Shi et al. 2004). Soaking for 12–18 h was very effective for the reduction of phytic acid and enzyme inhibitors in legumes (Handa et al. 2017). Phytate being water-soluble compound can be easily eliminated by soaking and discarding the soaked water (Greiner and Konietzy 2006). Soaking at room temperature for 24 h eliminated 16–21% of phytic acid levels in sorghum flour (Mahgoub and Elhag 1998). The combination of dehulling and soaking reduced

25% and 57% amylase inhibitors in *Lathyrus sativa* and *Lathyrus* beans, respectively (Srivastava 1994). Rehman and Shah (2001) found that soaking of black gram at 30 °C removed 18.45% of the tannins in 3 h; whereas 22.14% of the tannins were removed on soaking at 100 °C for 45 min.

8.5.5 Germination

Germination is suitable for minimizing the antinutrient components present in plant-based foods (Nkhata et al. 2018). During the process of germination, an increase in phytate-degrading enzyme activity was observed by Greiner and Konietzy (2006). About 40% of phytate content can be reduced by employing this technique (Masud et al. 2007) and 40.00–59.38% reduction in phytic acid contents was observed in lentils (Pal et al. 2016). Trypsin inhibitor content was eliminated to the range of 19.2–88.2% in different types of beans by germination (Avilés-Gaxiola et al. 2017). Gupta et al. (2015) observed that longer duration of germination has caused greater elimination of antinutrients. For instance, mungbean and kidney bean following germination revealed continuous decrease of phytic acid for 6 days (Rasha Mohamed et al. 2011).

8.5.6 Fermentation

Fermentation is a process where microorganisms effect some desirable biochemical changes in food material with the aid of their enzymes (Admassie 2018). It increases protein digestibility, reduces antinutritional factors, and enhances texture (Adewumi and Odunfa 2009). During the process of fermentation, metabolic activities of microorganisms modify the concentration of bioactive compounds present in the food crops. The cell wall of cereal grain ruptures as a result of fermentation which leads to production of several bioactive compounds. Some enzymes like amylases, proteases, and xylanases derived from cereals along with microorganisms modify the grain nutritional content (Đorđević et al. 2010). This process is really helpful in reduction of phytic acid and trypsin inhibitor activity in legumes (Oghbaei and Prakash 2016). Coulibaly et al. (2011) reported that 12- and 24-h fermentation of millet grains eliminates significant amount of tannins, phytates, and protease inhibitors. Villacrés et al. (2020) concluded that fermentation utilizing *Rhizopus oligosporus* significantly reduces the content of antinutrients such as phytic acid (70.06%), tannins (82.10%), and trypsin inhibitors (76.76%). Mohapatra et al. (2019) observed that fermentation eliminated 30% tannin from grain sorghum whereas Dlamini et al. (2007) reported even more (49–68%) reduction. Fermentation reduces antinutrients like oxalates and phytate content to a very large extent (Ijeoma and Adeyemi 2020). Mohapatra et al. (2019) concluded that during fermentation of whole-grain sorghum, the total phenolic content decreases by 28% and tannin content decreases by 30–39%.

8.5.7 *Extrusion Cooking Technique*

It is a food processing technique that combines different steps including mixing, kneading, cooking, shearing, shaping, and forming (Bordoloi and Ganguly 2014). It is one of the most widely used technique and modern food unit operation that converts plant-based foods, usually in a granular or powdered form, into partially cooked, low moisture, and highly shelf-stable food products. It results in enhanced functional properties of food (Ciudad-Mulero et al. 2020). Extrusion cooking technique is a high-temperature short-time (HTST) process that inactivates inherent enzymes and mitigates microbial contamination (Bordoloi and Ganguly 2014). This processing treatment shows significant reduction in antinutritional factors; for example, about 30% phytates are eliminated through extrusion (Chai and Liebman 2005; Harland et al. 2004). This technique completely inactivates lectin and trypsin inhibitors in peas and lentils (Grant et al. 2003).

8.5.8 *Biotechnological Interventions*

Several biotechnological approaches have been used to down-regulate or even eliminate the genes engaged in the metabolic pathways for reducing the production, aggregation, and/or inactivation of antinutrients. Low phytate rice and soybean with about 40–50% reduction in phytate without detrimental effects on their nutrient quality have been developed (Kumar et al. 2019; Punjabi et al. 2018; Larson et al. 2000). Single nucleotide substitution in rice Khira caused mutation in *SPDT* gene coding sequence which inhibited the accumulation of phytic acid in plant (Kumar et al. 2021). *lpa* mutants of rice have 45–95% less phytic acid content than wild-type seeds (Perera et al. 2018). To reduce phytic acid levels in rapeseed, *ITPK* gene encoding an enzyme that stimulates the last step of phytate synthesis was blocked using CRISPR/Cas9 (Liu et al. 2021). Shukla et al. (2009) utilized zinc-finger nucleases to mutate the *IPK1*, one of the phytic acid biosynthesis gene in *Zea mays*. Further, work has also been performed to reduce cyanogenic glycosides in cassava through expression of hydroxynitrile lyase enzyme in cassava roots (Siritunga et al. 2004). Likewise, the solanine content of potato has been reduced significantly using an antisense RNA approach, and efforts are ongoing to reduce the level of the other major potato glycoalkaloid and chaconine (McCue et al. 2003). In oilseed rape, Shashidhar et al. (2020) reported 35% reduction phytic acid by knocking out three essential *BnITPK* genes with an enhanced amount of phosphorus.

8.6 Current Trends in Antinutritional Factors

In the current scenario, our comprehension of dietary requirements of human body and associated complications has improved to great extent. Also, awareness regarding ANF in pulses and cereals has grown. Even though these ANFs cannot be detoxified by the human body, it can be diminished to an extent by adopting various processing methods. On the other hand, phenolic compounds especially flavonoids are added into beverages which make them more valuable to prevent early-stage diseases (i.e., hypertension and diabetes). It has been found that tannin can be used as therapeutic agent due to its laxative effect which helps in treating constipation (Youn Hwang 2019). In recent researches, tannins are introduced into cellulose nanofibrils to make a packaging material which has been proved to be sustainable, eco-friendly, non-toxic packaging material for pharmaceuticals as well as food. In addition, tannins showed antibacterial and antioxidant properties and are used as preservatives in food industries (Singh and Kumar 2019). Total pomegranate tannin (TPT) extract from *Punica granatum* L. when evaluated for anti-proliferative activity in vitro on human oral (KB, CAL27), prostate (RWPE-1, 22Rv1), and colon (HT-29, HCT116, SW480, SW620) tumor cells, and apoptotic effects suggest that it induces apoptosis and decreases the viable cell number of human oral, prostate, and colon tumor cells (Yildirım and Kutlu 2015). Flavonoids are associated with large number of health-promoting effects and are essential components in pharmaceutical, medicinal, nutraceutical, and cosmetic applications. Flavonoids have been shown to possess anti-cholinesterase activity which reduces the level of acetylcholinesterase (AChE) enzyme in the CNS and inhibition of it results in elevated levels of neural acetylcholine levels which is one of the therapeutic strategies to combat Alzheimer's disease (Panche et al. 2016). Glucosinolates present in moringa leaves are extracted and used for decreasing the risk of developing non-communicable diseases (Lopez-Rodriguez et al. 2020). Also, glucosinolates have been experimented in the prevention of fungal and bacterial spoilage of food products by using advanced atmospheric packaging technology (MAP) that improves the shelf-life of these products (Melrose 2019).

8.7 Conclusions

Plant contains both nutrients and antinutrients. Antinutrients are a major area of concern for those whose diet predominantly comprises unprocessed plant-based foods. Plant foods especially cereals and grains can be processed to diversify their uses, and to enhance their nutritional value and consumer acceptability. Antinutritional factors can be easily removed by using traditional and advanced processing techniques. Traditional methods include soaking, boiling, germination, and fermentation whereas modern technique includes autoclaving, microwave heating, and extrusion technique. These techniques have been proved to reduce a great amount of antinutrients like phytates, oxalates, saponins, enzyme inhibitors, etc. Some antinutrients bind to different minerals and make them less bioavailable, some inhibit digestive enzymes, and some can cause health problems. Exorphins and contextual antinutrients are also present in foods. The former category of ANF is present in milk and cereals whereas the latter category interacts with other food and drugs resulting in its poor absorption in the digestive system which results in poor functioning of medicines. Therefore, they have to be eliminated from plant-based foods before consumption. Biotechnological interventions in plants by suppressing the gene responsible for the antinutrient production form an integral component of alternative strategies to reduce ANFs.

References

Adewumi GA, Odunfa SA (2009) Effect of lactic fermentation on anti-nutritional factors in Nigerian Local Beans *(Vigna unguiculata)* varieties. Nigerian Food J 27(2):73–77

Adeyemo SM, Onilude AA (2013) Enzymatic reduction of anti-nutritional factors in fermenting soybeans by *Lactobacillus plantarum* isolates from fermenting cereals. Nigerian Food J 31(2): 84–90

Adhikari B, Marasini BP, Rayamajhee B, Bhattarai BR, Lamichhane G, Khadayat K, Adhikari A, Khanal S, Parajuli N (2020) Potential roles of medicinal plants for the treatment of viral diseases focusing on COVID-19: a review. Phytother Res. https://doi.org/10.1002/ptr.6893

Admassie M (2018) A review on food fermentation and the biotechnology of lactic acid bacteria. World J Food Sci Technol 2(1):19. https://doi.org/10.11648/j.wjfst.20180201.13

Angeloni C, Hrelia S, Malaguti M (2017) Neuroprotective effects of glucosinolates. In: Mérillon JM, Ramawat K (eds) Glucosinolates. Reference series in phytochemistry. Springer, Cham. https://doi.org/10.1007/978-3-319-25462-3_20

Avilés-Gaxiola S, Chuck-Hernández C, Serna Saldívar SO (2017) Inactivation methods of trypsin inhibitor in legumes: a review. J Food Sci 83(1):17–29. https://doi.org/10.1111/1750-3841.13985

Barba FJ, Nikmaram N, Roohinejad S, Khelfa A, Zhu Z, Koubaa M (2016) Bioavailability of glucosinolates and their breakdown products: impact of processing. Front Nutr 3. https://doi.org/10.3389/fnut.2016.00024

Barky AR, Hussein SA, Alm-Eldeen A, Hafiz YA, Mohamed TM (2017) Saponins and their potential role in diabetes mellitus. Diab Manage 7(1):148–158

Barrett ML, Udani JK (2011) A proprietary alpha-amylase inhibitor from white bean (*Phaseolus vulgaris*): a review of clinical studies on weight loss and glycemic control. Nutr J 10(1). https://doi.org/10.1186/1475-2891-10-24

Betancur-Ancona D, Segura-Campos M, Rosado-Rubio JG, Franco LS, Chel-Guerrero L (2012) Chemical composition and anti-nutritional factors in five tropical legume seeds. Nutr Consum Health, Beans:117–141

Bhasin B, Ureki HM, Atta MG (2015) Primary secondary hyperoxaluria: understanding the enigma. World J Nephrol 4(2):235–244. https://doi.org/10.5527/wjn.v4.i2.235

Bhat M, Zinjarde SS, Bhargava SY, Kumar AR, Joshi BN (2011) Antidiabetic Indian plants: a good source of potent amylase inhibitors. Evid Based Complement Alternat Med 1–6. https://doi.org/10.1093/ecam/nen040

Bischoff KL (2016) Glucosinolates. Forum Nutr 551–554. https://doi.org/10.1016/b978-0-12-802147-7.00040-1

Bordoloi R, Ganguly S (2014) Extrusion technique in food processing and a review on its various technological parameters. Indian J Scientific Res Technol 2(1):1–3

Brandl T, Simic O, Skaanderup PR, Namoto K, Berst F, Ehrhardt C, Schiering N, Mueller I, Woelcke J (2016) Trypsin inhibitors for the treatment of pancreatitis. Bioorg Med Chem Lett 26(17):4340–4344. https://doi.org/10.1016/j.bmcl.2016.07.029

Brás NF, Santos-Martins D, Fernandes PA, Ramos MJ (2018) Mechanistic pathway on human α-glucosidase maltase-glucoamylase unveiled by QM/MM calculations. J Phys Chem B 122(14):3889–3899. https://doi.org/10.1021/acs.jpcb.8b01321

Chai W, Liebman M (2005) Oxalate content of legumes, nuts, and grain-based flours. J Food Compos Anal 18(7):723–729. https://doi.org/10.1016/j.jfca.2004.07.001

Chiva-Blanch G, Urpi-Sarda M, Ros E, Valderas-Martinez P, Casas R, Arranz S, Guillén M, Lamuela-Raventós RM, Llorach R, Andres-Lacueva C, Estruch R (2013) Effects of red wine polyphenols and alcohol on glucose metabolism and the lipid profile: a randomized clinical trial. Clin Nutr 32(2):200–206

Chowdhury S, Punia D (1997) Nutrient and anti-nutrient composition of pearl millet grains as affected by milling and baking. Food Nahrung 41(2):105–107

Ciudad-Mulero M, Fernández-Ruiz V, Cuadrado C, Arribas C, Pedrosa MM, Berrios JD, Pan J, Morales P (2020) Novel gluten-free formulations from lentil flours and nutritional yeast: evaluation of extrusion effect on phytochemicals and non-nutritional factors. Food Chem 315: 126175. https://doi.org/10.1016/j.foodchem.2020.126175

Cohn JS, Kamili A, Wat E, Chung RW, Tandy S (2010) Dietary phospholipids and intestinal cholesterol absorption. Nutrients 2(2):116–127. https://doi.org/10.3390/nu2020116

Coulibaly A, Kouakou B, Chen J (2011) Phytic acid in cereal grains: structure, healthy or harmful ways to reduce phytic acid in cereal grains and their effects on nutritional quality. Am J Plant Nutr Fertil Technol 1(1):1–22. https://doi.org/10.3923/ajpnft.2011.1.22

De Mejía EG, Prisecaru VI (2005) Lectins as bioactive plant proteins: a potential in cancer treatment. Crit Rev Food Sci Nutr 45(6):425–445. https://doi.org/10.1080/10408390591034445

Dinkova-Kostova AT (2012) Chemoprotection against cancer by isothiocyanates: a focus on the animal models and the protective mechanisms. Top Curr Chem 329:179–201. https://doi.org/10.1007/128_2012_337

Diouf A, Sarr F, Sene B, Ndiaye C, Fall SM, Ayessou NC (2019) Pathways for reducing anti-nutritional factors: prospects for *Vigna unguiculata*. J Nutr Health Food Sci 7(2):1–10. https://doi.org/10.15226/jnhfs.2019.001157

Dlamini NR, Taylor JR, Rooney LW (2007) The effect of sorghum type and processing on the antioxidant properties of African sorghum-based foods. Food Chem 105(4):1412–1419. https://doi.org/10.1016/j.foodchem.2007.05.017

Đorđević TM, Šiler-Marinković SS, Dimitrijević-Branković SI (2010) Effect of fermentation on antioxidant properties of some cereals and pseudo cereals. Food Chem 119(3):957–963. https://doi.org/10.1016/j.foodchem.2009.07.049

Eltayeb MM, Babiker HA, Sulieman MA, Babiker EE (2007) Effect of processing followed by fermentation on antinutritional factors content of pearl millet (*Pennisetum glaucum L.*) cultivars. Pak J Nutr 6(5):463–467

Ertop MH, Bektas M (2018) Enhancement of bioavailable micronutrients and reduction of anti-nutrients in foods with some processes. Food Health 4(3):159–165. https://doi.org/10.3153/FH18016

Garg S, Nurgali K, Mishra VK (2016) Food proteins as source of opioid peptides: a review. Curr Med Chem 23(9):893–910

Gemede HF, Ratta N (2014) Antinutritional factors in plant foods: potential health benefits and adverse effects. Int J Nutr Food Sci 3(4):284–289. https://doi.org/10.11648/j.ijnfs.20140304.18

Genser D (2008) Food and drug interaction: consequences for the nutrition/health status. Ann Nutr Metab 52(Suppl. 1):29–32. https://doi.org/10.1159/000115345

Ghavidel RA, Prakash J (2007) The impact of germination and dehulling on nutrients, antinutrients, in vitro iron and calcium bioavailability and in vitro starch and protein digestibility of some legume seeds. LWT- Food Sci Technol 40(7):1292–1299. https://doi.org/10.1016/j.lwt.2006.08.002

Grant G, Duncan M, Alonso R, Marzo F (2003) Peas and lentils. Encycl Food Sci Nutr:4433–4440. https://doi.org/10.1016/b0-12-227055-x/00899-3

Greiner R, Konietzny U (2006) Phytase for food application. Food Technol Biotechnol 44(2): 125–140

Gupta RK, Gangoliya SS, Singh NK (2015) Reduction of phytic acid and enhancement of bioavailable micronutrients in food grains. J Food Sci Technol 52(2):676–684. https://doi.org/10.1007/s13197-013-0978-y

Habib H, Fazili KM (2007) Plant protease inhibitors: a defense strategy in plants. Biotechnol Mol Biol Rev 2(3):068–085

Han X, Shen T, Lou H (2007) Dietary polyphenols and their biological significance. Int J Mol Sci 8(9):950–988. https://doi.org/10.3390/i8090950

Handa V, Kumar V, Panghal A, Suri S, Kaur J (2017) Effect of soaking and germination on physicochemical and functional attributes of horsegram flour. J Food Sci Technol 54(13): 4229–4239. https://doi.org/10.1007/s13197-017-2892-1

Harland BF, Smikle-Williams S, Oberleas D (2004) High performance liquid chromatography analysis of phytate (IP6) in selected foods. J Food Compos Anal 17(2):227–233. https://doi.org/10.1016/j.jfca.2003.08.005

Hassan S, Faiza N, Farooq MA, Egbuna C, Habib-ur-Rehman, Olatunde A (2020) Role of nutraceuticals in maternal nutrition. In: Functional foods and nutraceuticals. Springer, Cham, pp 527–541. https://doi.org/10.1007/978-3-030-42319-3_24

Hill GD (2003) Plant antinutritional factors | characteristics. In: Encyclopedia of food sciences and nutrition. Elsevier, pp 4578–4587. https://doi.org/10.1016/b0-12-227055-x/01318-3

Himanshu CM, Sonawane SK, Arya SS (2018) Nutritional and nutraceutical properties of millets: a review. Clin J Nutr Diet 1(1):1–10

Hithamani G, Srinivasan K (2014) Effect of domestic processing on the polyphenol content and bioaccessibility in finger millet (Eleusine coracana) and pearl millet (Pennisetum glaucum). Food Chem 164:55–62. https://doi.org/10.1016/j.foodchem.2014.04.107

Hussain G, Huang J, Rasul A, Anwar H, Imran A, Maqbool J, Razzaq A, Aziz N, Konuk M, Sun T (2019) Putative roles of plant-derived tannins in neurodegenerative and neuropsychiatry disorders: an updated review. Molecules 24(12):2213. https://doi.org/10.3390/molecules24122213

Ijeoma O, Adeyemi OO (2020) Effect of fermentation on some minerals and antinutrient content of *Telfaira Occidentalis* and *Gnetum Africanum* leaves. Int J Adv Sci Res Eng 6(2):6. https://doi.org/10.31695/IJASRE.2020.33703

Ikewuchi CC (2012) Hypocholesterolemic effect of an aqueous extract of the leaves of *Sansevieria senegambica* Baker on plasma lipid profile and atherogenic indices of rats fed egg yolk supplemented diet. Exp Clin Sci J (EXCLI J) 11:346–356

Janecka A, Fichna J, Janecki T (2004) Opioid receptors and their ligands. Curr Top Med Chem 4(1): 1–17. https://doi.org/10.2174/1568026043451618

Jin MJ, Han HK (2010) Effect of piperine, a major component of black pepper, on the intestinal absorption of fexofenadine and its implication on food-drug interaction. J Food Sci 75(3):H93–H96. https://doi.org/10.1111/j.1750-3841.2010.01542.x

Kadam SS, Smithard RR, Eyre MD, & Armstrong DG (1987) Effects of heat treatments of antinutritional factors and quality of proteins in winged bean. J Sci Food Agric 39(3): 267–275doi: https://doi.org/10.1002/jsfa.2740390310

Klupšaitė D, Juodeikienė G (2015) Legume: composition, protein extraction and functional properties. A review. Chem Technol 1(66). https://doi.org/10.5755/j01.ct.66.1.12355

Kulkarni DB, Sakhale BK, Giri NA (2018) A potential review on millet grain processing. Int J Nutr Sci 3(1)

Kumar A, Kumar V, Krishnan V, Hada A, Marathe A, Jolly M, Sachdev A (2019) Seed targeted RNAi-mediated silencing of GmMIPS1 limits phytate accumulation and improves mineral bioavailability in soybean. Sci Rep 9(1):7744. https://doi.org/10.1038/s41598-019-44255-7

Kumar A, Nayak S, Ngangkham U, Sah RP, Lal MK, Tp A, Behera S, Swain P, Behera L, Sharma S (2021) A single nucleotide substitution in the *SPDT* transporter gene reduced phytic acid and increased mineral bioavailability from Rice grain (*Oryza sativa* L.). J Food Biochem 45(7): e13822. https://doi.org/10.1111/jfbc.13822

Kumari S, Sachdeva A, Krishnan V (2014) Impact of soaking and germination durations on antioxidants and antinutrients of black and yellow soybean (*Glycine max.* L) varieties. J Plant Biochem Biotechnol 24(3):355–358. https://doi.org/10.1007/s13562-014-0282-6

Lampart-Szczapa E, Siger A, Trojanowska K, Nogala-Kalucka M, Malecka M, cholek B. (2003) Chemical composition and antibacterial activities of lupin seeds extracts. Nahrung/Food 47(5): 286–290

Larson SR, Rutger N, Young KA, Raboy V (2000) Isolation and genetic mapping of a non-lethal rice (*Oryza sativa* L.) low phytic acid 1 mutation. Crop Sci J 40:1397–1405. https://doi.org/10.2135/cropsci2000.4051397x

Lestienne I, Buisson M, Lullien-Pellerin V, Picq C, Trèche S (2007) Losses of nutrients and anti-nutritional factors during abrasive decortication of two pearl millet cultivars (*Pennisetum glaucum*). Food Chem 100(4):1316–1323. https://doi.org/10.1016/j.foodchem.2005.11.027

Lister J, Fletcher PJ, Nobrega JN, Remington G (2015) Behavioral effects of food-derived opioid-like peptides in rodents: implications for schizophrenia? Pharmacol Biochem Behav 134:70–78. https://doi.org/10.1016/j.pbb.2015.01.020

Liu T-T, Liu X-T, Chen Q-X, Shi Y (2020) Lipase inhibitors for obesity: a review. Biomed Pharmacother 128. https://doi.org/10.1016/j.biopha.2020.110314

Liu Q, Yang F, Zhang J, Liu H, Rahman S, Islam S, Ma W, She M (2021) Application of CRISPR/Cas9 in crop quality improvement. Int J Mol Sci 22(8):4206. https://doi.org/10.3390/ijms22084206

Lopez-Rodriguez NA, Gaytán-Martínez M, de la Luz R-VM, Loarca-Piña G (2020) Glucosinolates and isothiocyanates from *Moringa oleifera*: chemical and biological approaches. Plant Foods Hum Nutr. https://doi.org/10.1007/s11130-020-00851-x

Lunagariya NA, Patel NK, Jagtap S, Bhutani KK (2014) Inhibitors of pancreatic lipase: state of the art and clinical perspectives. Exp Clin Sci J (EXCLI J) 13:897–921. https://doi.org/10.17877/DE290R-6941

Mahgoub SE, Elhag SA (1998) Effect of milling, soaking, malting, heat-treatment and fermentation on phytate level of four Sudanese sorghum cultivars. Food Chem 61(1–2):77–80. https://doi.org/10.1016/s0308-8146(97)00109-x

Malar DS, Devi KP (2014) Dietary polyphenols for treatment of Alzheimer's disease--future research and development. Curr Pharm Biotechnol 15(4):330–342. https://doi.org/10.2174/1389201015666140813122703

Masud T, Mahmood T, Latif A, Sammi S, Hameed T (2007) Influence of processing and cooking methodologies for reduction of phytic acid content in wheat (*Triticum aestivum*) varieties. J Food Process Preserv 31:583–594

Mattila PH, Pihlava JM, Hellström J, Nurmi M, Eurola M, Mäkinen S, Jalava T, Pihlanto A (2018) Contents of phytochemicals and antinutritional factors in commercial protein-rich plant products. Food Qual Safety 2(4):213–219. https://doi.org/10.1093/fqsafe/fyy021

McCue KF, Allen PV, Rockhold DR, Maccree MM, Belknap WR, Shephard LV, Davies H, Joyce PE, Corsini DL, Moehs CP (2003) Reduction of total steroidal glycoalkaloids in potato tubers using antisense constructs of a gene encoding a solanidine glucosyl transferase. Acta Horticulturae 619:77–86. https://doi.org/10.17660/ActaHortic.2003.619.9

Melrose (2019) The glucosinolates: a sulphur glucoside family of mustard anti-tumour and antimicrobial phytochemicals of potential therapeutic application. Biomedicine 7(3):62. https://doi.org/10.3390/biomedicines7030062

Miękus N, Marszałek K, Podlacha M, Iqbal A, Puchalski C, Świergiel AH (2020) Health benefits of plant-derived sulfur compounds, glucosinolates, and organosulfur compounds. Molecules 25(17):3804. https://doi.org/10.3390/molecules25173804

Mohan VR, Tresina PS, Daffodil ED (2016) Antinutritional factors in legume seeds: characteristics and determination. Encycl Food Health:211–220. https://doi.org/10.1016/B978-0-12-384947-2.00036-2

Mohapatra D, Patel AS, Kar A, Deshpande SS, Tripathi MK (2019) Effect of different processing conditions on proximate composition, anti-oxidants, anti-nutrients and amino acid profile of grain sorghum. Food Chem 271:129–135. https://doi.org/10.1016/j.foodchem.2018.07.196

Nikmaram N, Leong SY, Koubaa M, Zhu Z, Barba FJ, Greiner R, Oey I, Roohinejad S (2017) Effect of extrusion on the anti-nutritional factors of food products: an overview. Food Control 79:62–73. https://doi.org/10.1016/j.foodcont.2017.03.027

Ning W, Wang Y, Zhang F, Wang H, Wang F, Wang X, Tang H, Liang S, Shi X, Liu Z (2013) Beneficial effects of trypsin inhibitors derived from a spider venom peptide in l-arginine-induced severe acute pancreatitis in mice. PLoS One 8(4):e61049. https://doi.org/10.1371/journal.pone.0061049

Nkhata SG, Ayua E, Kamau EH, Shingiro JB (2018) Fermentation and germination improve nutritional value of cereals and legumes through activation of endogenous enzymes. Food Sci Nutr 6(8):2446–2458

Nyberg FAC, Hallberg M (2013) Casomorphins/hemorphins. In: Kastin A (ed) Handbook of biologically active peptides. USA, Academic Press, pp 1550–1555

Oghbaei M, Prakash J (2016) Effect of primary processing of cereals and legumes on its nutritional quality: a comprehensive review. Cogent Food Agric 2(1). https://doi.org/10.1080/23311932.2015.1136015

Ohiokpehai O (2003) Promoting the nutritional goodness of traditional food products. Pak J Nutr 2(4):267–270

Ostlund RE Jr (2002) Phytosterols in human nutrition. Annu Rev Nutr 22:533–549. https://doi.org/10.1146/annurev.nutr.22.020702.075220

Paiva PMG, Pontual E, Coelho L, Napoleão TH (2013) Protease inhibitors from plants: biotechnological insights with emphasis on their effects on microbial pathogens. In: Microbial pathogens and strategies for combating them: science, technology and education, vol 1, pp 641–649

Pal RS, Bhartiya A, ArunKumar R, Kant L, Aditya JP, Bisht JK (2015) Impact of dehulling and germination on nutrients, antinutrients, and antioxidant properties in horsegram. J Food Sci Technol 53(1):337–347. https://doi.org/10.1007/s13197-015-2037-3

Pal RS, Bhartiya A, Yadav P, Kant L, Mishra KK, Aditya JP, Pattanayak A (2016). Effect of dehulling, germination and cooking on nutrients, anti-nutrients, fatty acid composition and antioxidant properties in lentil (*Lens culinaris*). J Food Sci Technol 54(4):909–920. doi: https://doi.org/10.1007/s13197-016-23

Panche AN, Diwan AD, Chandra SR (2016) Flavonoids: an overview. J Nutr Sci 5. https://doi.org/10.1017/jns.2016.41

Perera I, Seneweera S, Hirotsu N (2018) Manipulating the phytic acid content of rice grain toward improving micronutrient bioavailability. Rice 11(1):4. https://doi.org/10.1186/s12284-018-0200-y

Popova A, Mihaylova D (2019) Antinutrients in plant-based foods: a review. Open Biotechnol J 13: 68–76. https://doi.org/10.2174/1874070701913010068

Possenti M, Baima S, Raffo A, Durazzo A, Giusti AM, Natella F (2016) Glucosinolates in food. In: Glucosinolates. Springer, Cham, pp 1–46. https://doi.org/10.1007/978-3-319-26479-0_4-1

Prieto MA, López CJ, Simal-Gandara J (2019) Glucosinolates: molecular structure, breakdown, genetic, bioavailability, properties and healthy and adverse effects. Adv Food Nutr Res. https://doi.org/10.1016/bs.afnr.2019.02.008

Pruimboom L, de Punder K (2015) The opioid effects of gluten exorphins: asymptomatic celiac disease. J Health Popul Nutr 33(24). https://doi.org/10.1186/s41043-015-0032-y

Punjabi M, Bharadvaja N, Jolly M, Dahuja A, Sachdev A (2018) Development and evaluation of low Phytic acid soybean by siRNA triggered seed specific silencing of inositol polyphosphate 6-/3-/5-kinase gene. Front Plant Sci 9:804. https://doi.org/10.3389/fpls.2018.00804

Rasha Mohamed K, Abou-Arab EA, Gibriel AY, Rasmy NM, Abu-Salem FM (2011) Effect of legume processing treatments individually or in combination on their phytic acid content. Afr J Food Sci Technol 2(2):036–046

Reddy NR, Sathe SK, Salunkhe DK (1982) Phytates in legumes and cereals. Adv Food Res 28:1–92. https://doi.org/10.1016/s0065-2628(08)60110-x

Rehman Z, Shah WH (2001) Tannin contents and protein digestibility of black grams (*Vigna mungo*) after soaking and cooking. Plant Foods Hum Nutr 56:265–273

Samtiya M, Aluko RE, Dhewa T (2020) Plant food anti-nutritional factors and their reduction strategies: an overview. Food Prod Process Nut 2(6). https://doi.org/10.1186/s43014-020-0020-5

Samtiya M, Aluko RE, Puniya AK, Dhewa T (2021) Enhancing micronutrients bioavailability through fermentation of plant-based foods: a concise review. Fermentation 7(2):63. https://doi.org/10.3390/fermentation7020063

Santos AFS, da Silva MDC, Napoleão TH, Paiva PMG, Correia MTS, Coelho LCBB (2014) Lectins: function, structure, biological properties and potential applications. Curr Top Peptide Protein Res 15:41–62

Sashidhar N, Harloff HJ, Potgieter L, Jung C (2020) Gene editing of three *BnITPK* genes in tetraploid oilseed rape leads to significant reduction of phytic acid in seeds. Plant Biotechnol J 18(11):2241–2250. https://doi.org/10.1111/pbi.13380

Savage G, Klunklin W (2018) Oxalates are found in many different European and Asian foods—effects of cooking and processing. J Food Res 7(3):76. https://doi.org/10.5539/jfr.v7n3p76

Savage GP, Mårtensson L (2010) Comparison of the estimates of the oxalate content of taro leaves and corms and a selection of Indian vegetables following hot water, hot acid and in vitro extraction methods. J Food Compos Anal 23(1):113–117. https://doi.org/10.1016/j.jfca.2009.07.001

Shahidi F, Ramakrishnan VV, Oh WYJ (2019) Bioavailability and metabolism of food bioactives and their health effects: a review. J Food Bioactives 8:6–41. https://doi.org/10.31665/JFB.2019.8204

Shi J, Arunasalam K, Yeung D, Kakuda Y, Mittal G, Jiang Y (2004) Saponins from edible legumes: chemistry, processing, and health benefits. J Med Food 7(1):67–78. https://doi.org/10.1089/109662004322984734

Shukla VK, Doyon Y, Miller JC, DeKelver RC, Moehle EA, Worden SE, Mitchell JC, Arnold NL, Gopalan S, Meng X, Choi VM (2009) Precise genome modification in the crop species *Zea mays* using zinc-finger nucleases. Nature 459(7245):437–441. https://doi.org/10.1038/nature07992

Siener R, Hönow R, Voss S, Seidler A, Hesse A (2006) Oxalate content of cereals and cereal products. J Agric Food Chem 54(8):3008–3011. https://doi.org/10.1021/jf052776v

Singh AP, Kumar S (2019) Applications of tannins in industry. In: Tannins-structural properties, biological properties and current knowledge. https://doi.org/10.5772/intechopen.85984

Singh G, Suresh S, Bayineni VK, Kadeppagari RK (2015) Lipase inhibitors from plants and their medical applications. Int J Pharmacy Pharm Sci 7:1–5

Siritunga D, Arias-Garzon D, White W, Sayre RT (2004) Over-expression of hydroxynitrile lyase in cassava roots accelerates cyanogenesis and detoxification. Plant Biotechnol J 2(1):37–43. https://doi.org/10.1046/j.1467-7652.2003.00047.x

Soundararajan P, Kim J (2018) Anti-carcinogenic glucosinolates in cruciferous vegetables and their antagonistic effects on prevention of cancers. Molecules 23(11):2983. https://doi.org/10.3390/molecules23112983

Sridhar SNC, George G, Verma A, Paul AT (2019) Natural products-based pancreatic lipase inhibitors for obesity treatment. In: Natural bio-active compounds. Springer, Singapore, pp 149–191. https://doi.org/10.1007/978-981-13-7154-7_6

Srivastava S (1994). Study on the effects of processing on nutrient and non-nutrient composition of Lathyrus sativus. M.Sc. Thesis, CCS Haryana Agricultural University, Hisar, India.

Tanito M, Masutani H, Kim Y-C, Nishikawa M, Ohira A, Yodoi J (2005) Sulforaphane induces thioredoxin through the antioxidant-responsive element and attenuates retinal light damage in mice. Invest Ophthalmol Vis Sci 46:979–987

Tatham AS, Shewry PR (2008) Allergens to wheat and related cereals. Clin Exp Allergy 38(11): 1712–1726. https://doi.org/10.1111/j.13652222.2008.03101.x

Tibe O, Amarteifio J (2010) Trypsin inhibitor activity and condensed tannin content in Bambara Groundnut (*Vigna Subterranea* (L.) Verdc) Grown in Southern Africa. J Appl Sci Environ Manag 11(2). https://doi.org/10.4314/jasem.v11i2.55021

Trivedi MS, Hodgson NW, Walker SJ, Trooskens G, Nair V, Deth RC (2015) Epigenetic effects of casein-derived opioid peptides in SH-SY5Y human neuroblastoma cells. Nutr Metab 12:54. https://doi.org/10.1186/s12986-015-0050-1

Tungmunnithum D, Thongboonyou A, Pholboon A, Yangsabai A (2018) Flavonoids and other phenolic compounds from medicinal plants for pharmaceutical and medical aspects: an overview. Medicines 5(3):93

Van Buul VJ, Brouns FJPH (2014) Health effects of wheat lectins: a review. J Cereal Sci 59(2): 112–117. https://doi.org/10.1016/j.jcs.2014.01.010

Van Campen DR (1969) Copper interference with the intestinal absorption of zinc-65 by rats. J Nutr 97(1):104–108. https://doi.org/10.1093/jn/97.1.104

Vanga SK, Wang J, Raghavan V (2020) Effect of ultrasound and microwave processing on the structure, in-vitro digestibility and trypsin inhibitor activity of soymilk proteins. LWT 131: 109708. https://doi.org/10.1016/j.lwt.2020.109708

Vaquero MP, Muniz FS, Redondo SJ, Oliván PP, Higueras FJ, Bastida S (2010) Major diet-drug interactions affecting the kinetic characteristics and hypolipidaemic properties of statins. Nutr Hosp 25(2):193–206

Vats P, Banerjee UC (2004) Production studies and catalytic properties of phytases (myo-inositol-hexakis-phosphate phosphohydrolases): an overview. Enzyme Microb Technol 35:3–14. https://doi.org/10.1016/s0141-0229(04)00087-0

Vauzour D, Rodriguez-Mateos A, Corona G, Oruna-Concha MJ, Spencer JP (2010) Polyphenols and human health: prevention of disease and mechanisms of action. Nutrients 2(11):1106–1131. https://doi.org/10.3390/nu2111106

Vijayakumari K, Siddhuraju P, Janardhanan K (1996) Effect of different post-harvest treatments on antinutritional factors in seeds of the tribal pulse, *Mucuna pruriens* (L.) DC. Int J Food Sci Nutr 47(3):263–272. https://doi.org/10.3109/09637489609012587

Villacrés E, Quelal MB, Fernández E, Garcìa G, Cueva G, Rosell CM (2020) Impact of debittering and fermentation processes on the antinutritional and antioxidant compounds in *Lupinus mutabilis* sweet. LWT 131:109745. https://doi.org/10.1016/j.lwt.2020.109745

Wang Y, Lv Z, Chu Y (2015) HIV protease inhibitors: a review of molecular selectivity and toxicity. HIV/AIDS: Res Palliative Care 7:95. https://doi.org/10.2147/hiv.s79956

Wisessing A, Choowongkomon K (2012) Amylase inhibitors in plants: structures, functions and application. Funct Plant Sci Biotechnol 6(1):31–41

Yildirım I, Kutlu T (2015) Anticancer agents: saponin and tannin. Int J Biol Chem 9:332–340. https://doi.org/10.3923/ijbc.2015.332.340

Youn Hwang D (2019) Therapeutic role of natural products containing tannin for treatment of constipation. Constipation. https://doi.org/10.5772/intechopen.81837

Yun JW (2010) Possible anti-obesity therapeutics from nature—a review. Phytochemistry 71(14-15):1625–1641. https://doi.org/10.1016/j.phytochem.2010.07.011

Zhang L, Li J, Han F, Ding Z, Fan L (2017) Effects of different processing methods on the antioxidant activity of 6 cultivars of foxtail millet. J Food Qual:1–9.: Article ID 8372854. https://doi.org/10.1155/2017/8372854

Chapter 9
Metabolic Fate of Food and Its Bioavailability

R. Sivaranjani, Ramesh S. V., and Shelly Praveen

Abstract Food bioactive components have garnered greater attention due to their effect in the prevention and therapeutic value against diseases. In this context, bioavailability of food bioactives refers to their prevalence in body fluids and accessibility for the tissues so that beneficial effects are harnessed. Hence, the metabolic processes that a food undergoes inside human system have greater implications for its bioavailability. The ultimate aim of the research is to identify factors responsible for improving the bioavailability of food so as to enhance the utility of food-derived components in according multiple health benefits. This chapter deliberates upon the metabolic processes of food-derived bioactive components, and factors affecting their bioavailability. Also, the role of gut microbiome in the process of food metabolism, the concept of food-derived modulations in host epigenetics, disease progression, and wellness are discussed. Finally, the effect of food on host epigenetic-based gene regulation, referred to as nutrigenomics, is also discussed.

Keywords Bioaccessibility · Food metabolism · Epigenetics · Gut microbiome · Nutrigenomics

R. Sivaranjani
ICAR-Indian Institute of Spices Research, Kozhikode, Kerala, India

R. S. V. (✉)
Physiology, Biochemistry and Post-Harvest Technology Division, ICAR-Central Plantation Crops Research Institute, Kasaragod, Kerala, India
e-mail: ramesh.sv@icar.gov.in

S. Praveen
Division of Biochemistry, ICAR-Indian Agricultural Research Institute, New Delhi, Delhi, India
e-mail: shellyparveen@icar.gov.in

R. S. V., S. Praveen (eds.), *Conceptualizing Plant-Based Nutrition*,
https://doi.org/10.1007/978-981-19-4590-8_9

9.1 Introduction

The nutrients derived from the food can be classified into primary metabolites comprising carbohydrates, proteins, fats, and secondary metabolites namely phenolics, flavonoids, tannins, saponins, lignin, alkaloids, etc. Each category of nutrients has definite mode of metabolic processing due to the involvement of numerous hydrolytic enzymes of human digestive system starting from mouth to large intestines (Fig. 9.1). The digested nutrients are absorbed in small and large intestines and are used in the biochemical processes of energy production or stored in liver, adipose, and peripheral tissues for future energy needs or utilized in structural process or exert functional role by having specific bioactivity like antioxidants, anti-carcinogenic, and anti-inflammatory.

The digestive potential of nutrients present in each food constituent is assessed based on their bioaccessibility and bioavailability. Bioaccessibility is defined as the fraction or quantity of nutrients in the food which is accessible for the digestive enzymes in the gastrointestinal (GI) tract and becomes available for absorption through the intestinal cells (Hayes 2018). Bioaccessibility of a nutrient is decided by many factors like food matrix, processing methods employed, presence of antinutritional factors, etc. Likewise, the term bioavailability can be defined as the fraction or quantity of the digested nutrients getting assimilated and utilized by cells/tissues. The process includes digestion, absorption, metabolism, and bioactivities of the nutrient. Bioavailability is a key term for functional foods containing health beneficial bioactive metabolites. It addresses several phases of food metabolism such as absorption, distribution, metabolism, and elimination (ADME). Evaluation of

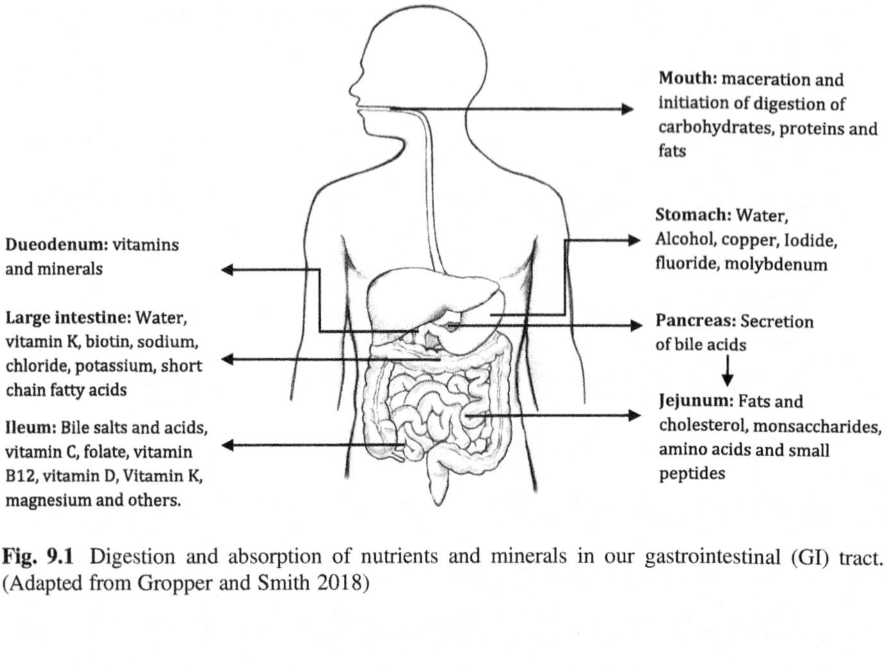

Fig. 9.1 Digestion and absorption of nutrients and minerals in our gastrointestinal (GI) tract. (Adapted from Gropper and Smith 2018)

ADME properties of individual nutrients throws light on its bioavailability and several in vitro models are available to find out the bioaccessibility and bioavailability of a particular nutrient from foods (Ting et al. 2015). Apart from them, several in vivo models, utilizing laboratory animals, are also available to ascertain ADME of foods.

This chapter discusses the metabolic fate of major and minor nutrients from food namely carbohydrates, proteins and peptides, fats (including sterols), vitamins, and bioactive secondary metabolites from plants. It also deliberates about the role of microbiota in food metabolism, their effect on host epigenetics, progression of diseases, and human wellness.

9.2 Carbohydrates

Carbohydrates, comprising sugars and starches, contribute around 40–70% of total energy requirements of human. The sources of sugar in our diet include fruits (fructose), milk (lactose), table sugar (sucrose), and other foods containing five carbon sugars (xylulose, arabinose, ribose, and ribulose). The process of digestion of these sugars is initiated by the salivary enzyme amylase, which breaks down the complex carbohydrates like starches into constituent sugars. Later enzymes like lactase, sucrase, and maltase secreted by the epithelial cells of small intestine degrade these complex sugars into its monomers namely glucose, galactose, or fructose. These monomers are then absorbed by the epithelial cells by both active and passive transport mechanisms in the circulatory system. Once inside the target cells, these sugars are converted into glucose and are used in different metabolic pathways for (i) energy production *via* glycolytic and electron transport chain, (ii) synthesis of glycogen in the liver and skeletal muscle, and (iii) synthesis of triglycerides and stored in the adipose tissue (Dashty 2013).

The starch derived from foods (grains, tubers, fruits, and vegetables) can be classified into rapidly digestible starch (RDS), slowly digestible starch (SDS), and resistant starch (RS) based on their ability to release free sugars during the process of digestion. Starch is a homo-polysaccharide consisting of repeating unit of D-glucose linked to one another via α-glycosidic linkages. The two types of polysaccharides namely amylose and amylopectin constitute 98–99% of dry weight of starch. Some classifications categorize starch-containing foods as 'waxy' (<15% amylose), 'normal' (20–35%), and 'high' amylose (≥40%) based on their content of amylose.

9.2.1 *Metabolic Fate of Starch*

The digestion of starch begins in the mouth where secretion of salivary amylases (α-amylase) breaks them down into short-chain maltose (maltotriose and maltotetraose), dextrins, and soluble sugars. The partially digested starch then passes

Table 9.1 Classification of resistant starch (Birt et al. 2013; Yang et al. 2017)

Type of RS	Structural features	Food source(s)
Resistant starch I	Physically remain inaccessible by entrapment in non-digestible matrix	Coarsely ground or whole-kernel grains
Resistant starch II	Ungelatinized granular starch with the B or C polymorph	High-amylose maize starch, raw potato, raw banana starch
Resistant starch III	Retrograded starch	Cooked and cooled starchy foods
Resistant starch IV	Chemically modified starched	Cross-linked starch and octenyl succinate starch
Resistant starch V	Amylose–lipid complex	Stearic acid complexed high-amylose starch

on to small intestine, where the pancreatic α-amylase and α-glucosidase hydrolyze them to release sugars in the intestinal cavity where it gets absorbed by gut epithelium and transported to different tissues and organs through circulatory system. Small intestine is the place where more than 60% of starch hydrolysis happens. The glucose produced in the process is metabolized in the same way as sugars as mentioned above.

Rapidly digestible starch (RDS) is the fraction of starch which is digested very quickly (within 20 min) and they are commonly present in white rice, potato (freshly cooked), and white bread. Upon consumption, RDS causes sudden increase in blood glucose level. Slowly digestible starch (SDS) is the fraction of starch which is digested slowly (120 min) and complete digestion happens in the small intestine. They are common in whole-grain bread, pasta, potato (cooked and cooled), coarse cereals like sorghum, maize, and legumes. Resistant starch (RS) is the portion of starch that cannot be digested by amylases in the small intestine and is fermented by the microbiota present in the large intestine. They do not release sugars within 120 min of ingestion. The common foods that contain resistant starches are beans, unripened banana, and high-amylose maize. Not much structural differences were noticed among the above-mentioned classification of starches. The difference in their digestion depends on the physical accessibility of starch-degrading enzymes into the polymers. The RS is further classified into five groups based on their structures and interaction with other food components (Tables 9.1).

9.2.2 *Dietary Fiber*

American Association of Cereal Chemists (AACC) has defined dietary fiber as 'the edible parts of plant or analogous carbohydrates that are resistant to digestion and absorption in the human small intestine with complete or partial fermentation in the large intestine'. The dietary component of fiber includes polysaccharides like cellulose, hemicellulose, pectins, chitin, gums, mucilages, and non-polysaccharides like lignin and associated plant substances. Dietary fiber is classified into soluble and insoluble fibers: wheat bran, cellulose, hemicellulose, and lignin are not soluble in water whereas pectins, gums, and mucilages are soluble and become swollen in water.

Owing to its structural complexity and unavailability of digestive enzymes to break down the β-glycosidic linkages prevalent in these components, most of the dietary fibers pass on from small intestine to large intestine where some of them are disintegrated by the microbes residing there. The assimilation of insoluble fiber in the colon is sparse and they provide bulking to the stool. On the other hand, soluble fiber is fermented in the colon to release physiologically active by-products such as short-chain fatty acids which get absorbed by the colonic epithelial cells. The dietary fibers increase the volume of food passage through the GI tract to colon which provides satiety and reduce the appetite. The sugars accessible for digestive enzymes from soluble fiber are released in the intestine and are processed in a manner similar to that of sugars released from starch.

Consumption of dietary fiber is reported to reduce the α-amylase activity and thereby arrests the sugar release from starch which in turn reduces the postprandial glucose level. Moreover, the dietary fibers interact with other nutrients in the GI tract and slow down the rate of their absorption by altering the viscosity and increasing the solute diffusion coefficient. Regular intake of dietary fiber especially soluble fibers like pectin has been reported to reduce the absorption of cholesterol present in the food and also induces the synthesis of bile acids from cholesterol in liver thereby reducing the risk of cardiovascular diseases. Small-chain fatty acids released from the bacterial actions on dietary fiber in the colon are found to have profound health benefits (Al-Lahham et al. 2010).

9.3 Proteins

Proteins are ubiquitous macromolecule in a cell/tissue/organ involved in various biological activities. Proteins differ in their structures and functions based on the sequence and composition of 20 amino acids. They are essential nutritional requirement to maintain body functions as structural, regulatory, enzymatic activities, signaling protein, and transport proteins (Elango et al. 2009).

Optimal dietary protein intake will provide all the 20 amino acids including essential, non-essential, and conditionally essential amino acids in appropriate proportions. Human body can synthesize non-essential and some conditionally essential amino acids, and dietary proteins are the only source of essential amino acids. Quality of the proteins obtained from the diet is determined by its amino acid composition especially its essential amino acid content and the digestibility of the protein (Tome 2012).

The active digestion of proteins starts in the proximal end of small intestine by the action of several proteolytic enzymes such as trypsin, chymotrypsin, and elastase, and carboxypeptidases A and B. The resultant amino acids are absorbed by the brush border epithelial cells which ultimately feed them to circulatory network for different tissues. Amino acid composition and physiochemical properties of the protein decide their kinetics of digestion and uptake. Proteins obtained from several sources were compared, and it was found that whey protein digestion causes short but drastic increase in amino acid concentration in plasma and is considered as 'fast protein' whereas casein digestion produced prolonged release of amino acids and was designated as 'slow protein' (Bendtsen et al. 2013).

The digestion of protein in the small intestines releases amino acids and peptides in the lumen. Most of the peptides are also absorbed by the various transport proteins located in the intestinal wall epithelium (Fernández-Tomé et al. 2017). Studies suggest that bioactive peptides obtained from diet have diverse role as antimicrobial, anti-diabetic, DNA stimulating, and antioxidants. These protective effects might act on intestinal cells and microbiota and positively influence the proper development of the gut (González-Montoya et al. 2018).

Amino acids derived from food are utilized in multiple catabolic and anabolic pathways, and the resultant products include polyamines, long-chain and short-chain fatty acids, urea, uric acid, nitric oxide, hydrogen sulfide, and non-amino acid bioactive metabolites like gamma-aminobutyric acid (GABA), taurine, ornithine, agmatine, etc. The catabolic products are also involved in the synthesis of various nitrogen-containing compounds in the cellular pathways.

Like other classes of nutrients, the food processing methods like fermentation, soaking, germination, milling, and protease treatments determine the digestibility and amino acid availability in many protein-containing foods (Ketnawa and Ogawa 2021). Normally, protein is not utilized as the energy source but when the primary calorie-rich food is not available and fat stored in the body is fully utilized, which is the case in extreme fasting, proteins are taken up for energy production by synthesizing glucose *via* glucogenic amino acids namely isoleucine, valine, threonine, and methionine *via* gluconeogenesis pathway.

9.4 Fats and Oils

Around 35–40% of dietary energy requirements of human are met by fats and oils, which are collectively termed as lipids. Their calorific value is higher than that of carbohydrates and proteins. Apart from meeting out the energy requirements, lipids play an important role in growth and development of brain and nervous system.

Fats and oils are obtained in the form of triacylglycerol from plants and animal sources. In general, fats obtained from animal sources contain more saturated fatty acids and are solid in room temperature whereas the oil obtained from plant sources is rich in unsaturated fatty acid and is liquid in room temperature (Lichtenstein 2013). The digestion of fats starts in the mouth with the help of salivary lipase and release fatty acids which are absorbed in the stomach. But, most of the digestion process happens in the small intestine where fats form micelles with bile acids secreted by the liver which are then digested to release free fatty acids and monoacylglycerol by the action of pancreatic lipase. The released fatty acids are carried in micelles and absorbed by the intestinal epithelium. In intestinal mucosal cells, fatty acids are conjugated with monoacylglycerol to from triacylglycerol, packed into lipoprotein complexes named chylomicron. They are transported via lymphatic system which feeds them to circulatory system. These lipoprotein complexes reach adipose tissues for storage and to muscles where they are again degraded to fatty acids and monoacylglycerol for energy production through the process of oxidation.

Humans are capable of synthesizing variety of fatty acids from simple precursors obtained from dietary nutrients and they are called non-essential fatty acids. On the other hand, essential fatty acids must be obtained from dietary sources. They fall into two categories: omega-3 (linolenic acid and docosahexaenoic acid) and omega-6 (linoleic and oleic) fatty acids. They are precursors for the synthesis of eicosanoid hormones that control important body functions in nervous and immune systems. The appropriate ratio of omega-3 and omega-6 fatty acids is a prerequisite for maintaining good health.

9.4.1 Metabolic Fate of Cholesterol

Cholesterol falls in the major nutrient category of sterols. Sterol is classified into phytosterol and cholesterol; the former is present in plants and latter is derived from animal products. Normally, humans do not need sterols in our diet for nutrition purpose which means they are not essential because human body can synthesize an average 11 mg/kg body weight of cholesterol per day without an intake of external cholesterol-containing food. The synthesis of cholesterol happens in liver and to some extent in intestine too. Though cholesterol is non-essential, it has numerous biological functions in our body. It is the precursor for the synthesis of bile acids, which are secreted into small intestines and help in the digestion and absorption of fats in our diet. It is also the precursor of the synthesis of hormones like estrogen and progesterone. Another main function of the cholesterol is maintaining the fluidity of the plasma membrane owing to its structural peculiarity of having both hydrophobic and hydrophilic group and cyclic structures which helps the fatty acid present in the plasma membrane to interact with and reduce the compactness of the plasma membrane.

The cholesterol esters obtained from the diet are processed more like fats by the enzyme esterase secreted by the pancreas. The de-esterified cholesterol is packed into lipoprotein complexes namely chylomicron, very low-density lipoprotein (VLDL), low-density lipoprotein (LDL), and high-density lipoprotein (HDL) in the small intestine and enters into circulatory network. Among them, VLDL and LDL carry substantial portion of cholesterol in the blood. Through various apolipoprotein receptors, these circulating phospholipids enter liver, muscles, and adipose tissues where lipid components are degraded and released inside the cell.

Phytosterols are structurally very similar to cholesterol except the substitution at the C24 position on the sterol side chain. Phytosterols are reported to reduce the dietary cholesterol absorption mainly by displacing cholesterol in the micelles and LDLs (Lin et al. 2010) thereby found to reduce the cardiovascular disease risk. Though poorly absorbed from the intestine, some phytosterols are metabolized in the liver into bile acids. They are also reported to have anti-tumor properties especially reduction in colon cancer development.

9.5 Phenolics and Flavonoids

Growing epidemiological evidences state that consumption of phenolics and flavonoid-rich foods decreases the risk of developing certain lifestyle diseases such as diabetes, obesity, coronary heart diseases, and even certain cancers (Hodgson and Kroft 2006; Scalbert et al. 2005). Plants synthesize variety of secondary metabolites which impart evolutionary advantage to withstand biotic and/or abiotic stresses prevailing in their ecosystem. The secondary metabolite pool of plant kingdom is enormously diverse and used in traditional medicinal preparations since time immemorial. They do not participate in energy production but exert multiple health benefits.

The bioaccessibility and bioavailability of many secondary metabolites from unprocessed food products are restricted due to the digestive barrier posed by the plant cell wall where most of these metabolites reside. Bioavailability of these metabolites is functions of many factors like their structure, solubility, interactions with other dietary nutrients, molecular transformations, cellular transportation, interaction with gut microbiota, etc. (Fernandez-Garcia et al. 2012). Nevertheless, Cassidy et al. (2006) and Mateo-Anson et al. (2011) proved that processing of food products like fermentation and milling increased the bioavailability of flavonoids and phenolics in soy and wheat products, respectively. After bypassing the challenge of being released from the food matrix and becoming bioaccessible, bioactive food compounds are processed in the GI tract.

9.5.1 Metabolic Fate of Bioactive Metabolites

In contrast to metabolic fate of carbohydrates, proteins, and fats, the metabolism of plant secondary metabolites is complicated. They are processed like that of xenobiotics in our system. Most of the digestion process happen in colon and very little, mainly of aglycone metabolites, are being absorbed in the small intestine and transported to liver for biotransformation. Even though studies provide evidence that simple glycosylation of some of the metabolites happens in the oral cavity by the glycosidase enzymes secreted by the oral microorganisms (Velderrain-Rodríguez et al. 2014), most of the glycosylated compounds and other conjugated metabolites reach colon with little or no absorption in the small intestine. In colon, these compounds are subjected to hydrolysis or fermentation by the enzymes secreted by the gut microbiota. Some amount of enzymatic hydrolysis of conjugated polyphenols takes place at the brush border epithelial cells of small intestine. The released aglycones then enter into liver where they are biotransformed.

The metabolism of these compounds is divided into two phases of biotransformation: Phase I biotransformation reactions consist mainly of oxidation, reduction, and hydrolysis. This phase is intended to change the structure of the exogenous compounds by adding hydroxyl, carboxyl, and amino groups, etc., with the help of enzymes like cytochrome P450-dependent mixed-function oxidases (CYPs) and catechol-O-methyltransferase. This addition changes the polarity of these compounds facilitating their absorption or excretion. These changes can also increase or decrease the bioactivity of these compounds. Though liver is the main site of transformation, fraction of phase I transformation also happens in small and large intestine (Fig. 9.2).

Phase II biotransformation involves the incorporation of methyl, glucuronic acid, and sulfate groups to phenolics/flavonoids by the action of methyl transferase, uridine 5′-diphosphate glucuronide transferase, and sulfonate transferase in the small intestine, liver, and kidney and enters into systemic circulation or excretion. Many studies have proved that the health benefits obtained from the consumption of phenolic-rich foods are in fact due to the metabolically transformed compounds. The structure, position of hydroxyl group, and type of conjugation reaction during biotransformation reactions severely influence the biological activities of these biotransformed compounds (Cosme et al. 2020).

For instance, retention properties of strawberry anthocyanins revealed that the biochemicals are detected in plasma of the human subjects at both 45 and 90 days of assessment period. Further, many metabolic processes like changes in gut microbiome, upregulation of enzymes involved in phase I and phase II biotransformation, changes in the activities of efflux transporters to maintain equilibrium, among others could contribute to production of different metabolites derived from the anthocyanins. Remarkable inter-individual variability in the concentration of urolithin metabolites was also detected in the plasma (Sandhu et al. 2018).

Metabolomic approach was utilized to analyze the phenolic metabolites of polyphenol-rich bur-erh tea and biotransformed metabolites excreted in the urine. Such metabonomic approach could unravel the complex interactions between multi-component nutraceuticals and the human metabolic system which could be utilized in nutritional intervention (Xie et al. 2012). Table 9.2 lists out some of the major food crop derived phenolics/flavonoids/carotenoids and their biotransformed metabolites.

The importance of food matrix on the absorption and bioavailability of isoflavones from soy-rich foods was reported. The pharmacokinetic profile of these compounds is influenced by the food matrix as liquid matrix (soy milk) has showed higher rate of absorption of isoflavone than solid matrix whereas the fermented foods like tempeh which is rich in aglycones due to partial hydrolysis of glycosides present are rapidly absorbed. The influence of gender on the absorption profile of isoflavones was reported; however, age showed no influence on the absorption profile (Cassidy et al. 2006) implying the multi-factorial nature of food absorption.

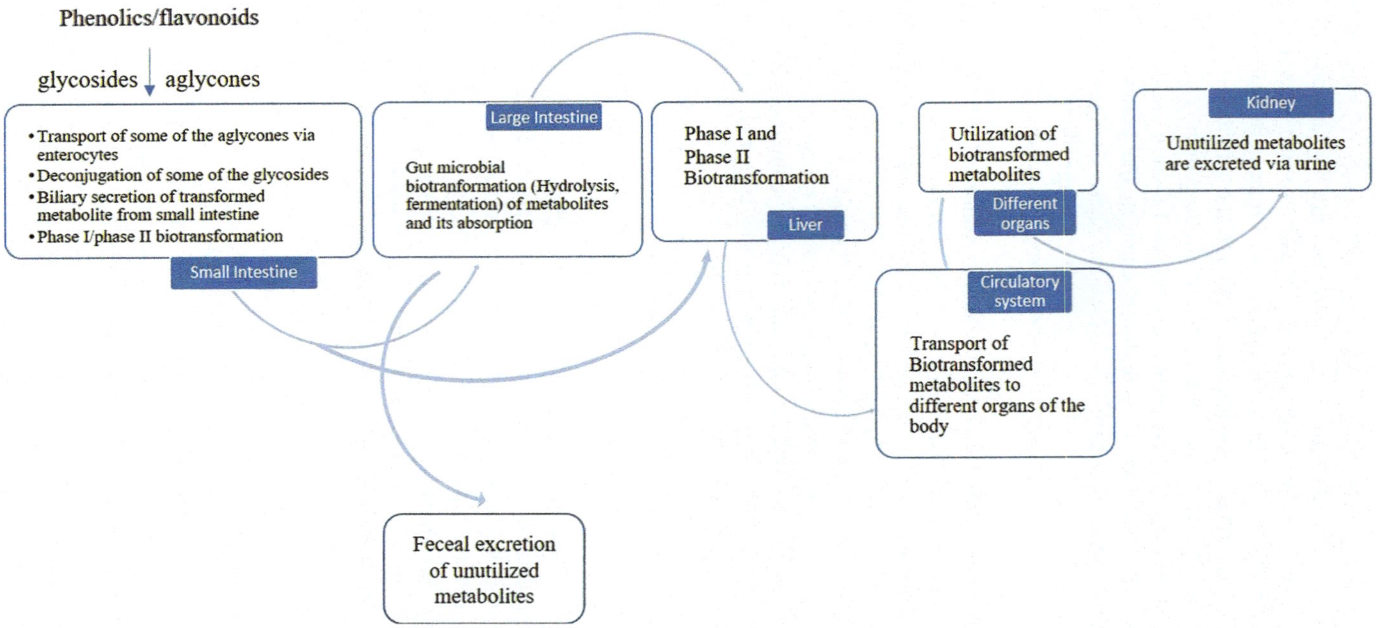

Fig. 9.2 Overview of phenolics/flavonoid metabolism in human gut

Table 9.2 Food sources with bioactive plant secondary metabolites

Crop	Polyphenols/flavonoids/ carotenoids	Biotransformed bioactive metabolite	References
Tea	Phenolics (theophylline, 1, 3 dimethyluric acid, theobromine, caffeine, nicotinic acid, epigallocatechin, 4-aminobutanoic acid, 3,5 dihydrobenzoic acid)	1, methyluric acid, 1,7 methyl uric acid, 2-hydroxybenzoic acid, paraxanthine, theophylline, hippuric acid, 1-methylxanthine, 2-hydroxyphenylacetic acid	Xie et al. (2012)
Strawberry	Phenolics (ellagitannins, pelargonidin-3-*O*-glucoside, pelargonidin glucuronide, pelargonidin-3-*O*-rutinoside, urolithin A glucuronide, isourolithin A glucuronide, and urolithin B glucuronide)	3, 4-Dihydroxybenzaldehyde, hippuric acid, 4-hydroxybenzaldehyde, *p*-coumaric acid and 3-hydroxybenzoic acid, *p*-coumaric acid and cinnamic acid, vanillic acid glucuronide	Sandhu et al. (2018)
Pomegranate	Phenolics (Ellagitannins)	Urolithin A glucuronide, urolithin B glucuronide, dimethyl ellagic acid	González-Sarrías et al. (2010)
Soybean	Isoflavones (daidzein, glycitein, and genistein)	Equol, *O*-desmethylangolensin	Cassidy et al. (2006), Setchell et al. (2001)
Olive oil	Phenolics (tyrosol, hydroxytyrosol, elenolic acid, deacetoxy-ligstroside aglycon, oleuropein aglycone)	Conjugated hydroxytyrosol, oleuropein, homovanillic acid, homovanillic alcohol	de Bock et al. (2013), Visioli et al. (2008)
Fruits and vegetables	Carotenoids (lycopene, β-carotene, α-carotene, β-cryptoxanthin, lutein, zeaxanthin)	Astaxanthin, capsanthin, violaxanthin, neoxanthin, fucoxanthin	Nagao (2011)

The compounds, which are not absorbed in the small intestines, reach colon where they are catabolized into smaller phenolic acids by the action of microbiome which may increase the bioavailability and getting absorbed by intestinal epithelia to systemic circulation.

9.6 Carotenoids

Carotenoids are polyene hydrocarbon metabolites obtained from fruits and vegetables rich in yellow, orange, and red pigments, egg yolk, and some marine products. The most common carotenoids are carotenes (α-carotene and β-carotene) and xanthophylls (β-cryptoxanthin, lutein, zeaxanthin, and lycopene). Among them, carotenes and cryptoxanthin are called pro-vitamin A carotenoids as they serve as the precursor for the synthesis of retinol, retinal, and retinaldehyde in human body. Though not directly involved in the synthesis of vitamin A, carotenoids like lutein and zeaxanthin have important role in filtering the blue light and protect eyes from light induced oxidative damage. Since dietary intervention is the only source to obtain these nutrients, their metabolism and bioavailability are the major determinants to avoid age-related macular degeneration and related diseases such as certain cancers, skin and bone diseases, and cardiovascular diseases (Meléndez-Martínez et al. 2021).

9.6.1 *Metabolic Fate of Carotenoids*

Carotenoids like α-carotene, β-carotene, and lycopene are highly hydrophobic compounds and their absorption is inefficient in humans. Upon ingestion, when released from the food matrix, they get mixed with phospholipids, free fatty acids, and bile acids and are solubilized into mixed micelles. This composition of the micelles is a major determining factor for their uptake by the intestinal epithelia by simple diffusion as well as for its bioavailability. The uptake mechanism of carotenes and xanthophylls varies due to their structural differences and hydrophilicity. The metabolism and bioavailability of more polar epoxyxanthophyll compounds such as neoxanthin and fucoxanthin in healthy human participants revealed that their plasma concentration was very low even after one week intervention period compared to less polar carotenoids such as luetin and β-carotene (Asai et al. 2008). It suggests that the polar carotenoids have low bioavailability due to poor intestinal absorption from micelles or rapid metabolism in the body.

The carotenoids absorbed through micelles into epithelial are packed into chylomicron for circulation and reach liver for biotransformation. Cytosolic β-carotene oxygenase 1 (BCO1) and mitochondrial β-carotene oxygenase 2 (BCO2) are the two carotenoid cleaving enzymes found in human. BCO1 catalyzes the formation of two retinal molecules by cleaving on 15, 15′ double bond site of one carotene molecule, whereas BCO2 cleaves at the 9, 10 and/or 9′, 10′ double bonds of almost all carotenes to yield various apocarotenoid products in the inner membrane of mitochondria (Amengual et al. 2013). The kinetics of β-carotene conversion to retinol in healthy adults divulged that of total bioconversion, 82%, 17%, and 0.83% occurs in the intestine, liver, and other tissues, respectively (Green et al. 2021).

In humans, the metabolism, genes, and enzymes involved in the biotransformation of carotene-derived compounds are very well understood; however, the process of understanding the xanthophyll biotransformation and the biological activity of the resultant metabolites in humans are gaining momentum and are yet to be deciphered fully.

9.7 Interaction of Major Nutrients and Bioavailability of Secondary Metabolites

Food we consume often contains many nutrients in different proportions, thereby influencing the process of digestion and bioavailability. Studying the biological activity of the nutrients and their interaction with other nutrients provides valuable information about the positive and negative health effects associated with those nutrients which would help nutritionists take informed choices about the healthy dietary meals. Here, we give few examples of interactions between different biomolecules and their nutritional importance.

Dietary polyphenols obtained from fruits, vegetables, and spices are often associated with dietary fiber. Fiber-polyphenol complexes may be present as soluble polymers or insoluble macromolecular assemblies or as swollen, hydrated networks. Polyphenols from soluble polymer complex are readily available in the GI tract whereas non-extractable polyphenol fractions, mainly tannins and proanthocyanidins, are not readily available in the prevailing conditions of GI tract. However, added dietary fiber can also negatively affect the absorption of nutrients because of gel formation, increased viscosity, or binding and entrapment. Other compounds, present in fruits and vegetables, like antinutritional factors such as phytic acid, oxalates, protease inhibitors, lectins, and tannins also limit the bioavailability of nutrients present in the food (Bohn 2014). The fats and proteins present in the foods have positive effect on the bioavailability of bioactive metabolites. The bioavailability of isoflavonoids from foods rich in fat and protein is more than that of extracted isoflavonoid supplements without these nutrients (Walsh et al. 2003). Likewise, the carotenoid absorption and bioavailability are higher when consumed along with fat (Brown et al. 2004) and bioavailability is reduced when co-ingested with soluble dietary fibers and phytosterols. The interaction between different bioactive metabolites also affects their bioavailability as increased bioavailability of curcumin was observed if ingested along with piperine (Shoba et al. 1998).

9.8 Role of Gut Microbiome in Metabolism and Bioavailability

The human gut microbiota comprises a complex and diverse set of microorganisms and not less than 1000 bacterial species were identified where most of them were unculturable. Bacteria constitute one of the largest groups of microbiota that occupies >99% of human gut along with archaea and viruses. In general, the gut microbiome interacts with host resulting in diverse beneficial effects such as digestion of dietary substrates, production of nutrients, and regulation of host immune system and arresting the growth of harmful microorganisms. The colonic or gut microbial organisms of human contribute extensively to the process of food metabolism by secreting enzymes that complement the repertoire of human digestive enzymes (Rajilić-Stojanović and de Vos 2014). Microbe-derived enzymes in metabolism cover the catabolism of polysaccharides, polyphenols, and biosynthesis of vitamins among others. Furthermore, the combined genetic repertoire of microbiota would account for about three million genes way more than the genetic coding potential of human genome (Zhang et al. 2010). Numerous studies have provided evidence for the role of microbiota in metabolism of food components and its impact on the health of an individual after analyzing human–microbiota association and in vitro investigations. Additionally, alterations in the composition of gut microbiome have been implicated in the development of diseases as diverse as inflammatory bowel disease (IBD), irritable bowel syndrome (IBS), colon cancer, and antibiotic-associated diarrhea and in the etiology of diseases like diabetes and obesity (Marchesi et al. 2016).

Dietary carbohydrates are acted upon by the gut microorganisms to produce bacterial fermentation products, short-chain fatty acids (SCFAs) namely acetic acid, propionic acid butyric acid, and gases (Rowland et al. 2018). These three SCFAs are present in the molar ratio of 3:1:1–10:2:1. Butyric acid has anticancer properties besides being the energy supplier of colonocytes. The anticancer properties of butyrate are due to its capacity to induce programmed cell death of colon cancer cells and gene expressional changes due to its inhibitory activities on histone deacetylases (De Vadder et al. 2014). Propionic acid, besides serving as an energy source, is involved in the gluconeogenesis process in liver. Additionally, it acts as satiety signaling molecule by binding to the intestinal G-protein-coupled receptors, thereby promoting intestinal gluconeogenesis (Tazoe et al. 2008). Acetate acts as co-factor that induces growth of other bacteria and plays a significant role in lipogenesis and appetite regulation (Frost et al. 2014). This comprehension has led to the devising of a diet low in fermentable oligo-saccharides, disaccharides, monosaccharides, and polyols (FODMAP) to ensure the reduced bacterial fermentation as a viable treatment of IBS (Halmos et al. 2015).

Microorganisms of the colon exert tremendous proteolytic activities to convert the dietary proteins, endogenous enzymes into short peptides, amino acids and their derivatives, short-chain or branched-chain fatty acids, and gases such as hydrogen, carbon dioxide, and hydrogen sulfide. The aromatic amino acids are converted into phenylpropanoid metabolites, phenylacetic acid, etc. (Russell et al. 2013). Further, it was also deduced that formation of polypeptides from free amino acids due to the activity of microorganisms greatly influences the amino acid metabolism and bioavailability in mammalian gut (Dai et al. 2013).

Gut microbiota are involved in the biosynthesis of vitamins including vitamin K and vitamin B. It was estimated that gut microbiota could contribute a little over one fourth of recommended dietary intake for some of the vitamins namely cobalamin, folate, niacin, and pyridoxine (Magnúsdóttir et al. 2015). Also, the human colon epithelial cells are adept at absorbing B vitamins (Said 2013).

Bile acids (cholic acid and chenodeoxycholic acid) biosynthesized from cholesterol by the human liver cells are secreted into the small intestine to facilitate digestion and absorption of lipids. The residual bile acids that escape the enterohepatic circulation and reach colon are acted upon by the microbes residing there to produce potent variants deoxycholic acid and ursodeoxycholic acid. These variant bile acids have greater implications for gut microbial diversity, digestive function of humans including absorption of dietary lipids, fat-soluble vitamins, etc. These interactions, however, underscore the importance of bile acids in serving as a mediator molecule that influences the gut microbiome and metabolic status of host.

Polyphenols derived from fruits and vegetables are intensively researched owing to their supposed health benefits and bioactive potential. The inherent structural diversity, conjugated nature (remain as glycosides—e.g., flavonoids), and high molecular weight polymeric nature (proanthocyanidins, ellagitannins, etc.) severely affect their digestion and bioavailability. Hydrolytic activity of colon microbes (e.g., *Bacteroides distasonis* and *Eubacterium cellulosolvens*) ensures that the undigested dietary polyphenols are converted into aglycones or monomers so that polyphenols are converted into simpler counterparts for absorption (Marín et al. 2015). Further, the inter-individual variations in the ability to metabolize certain dietary polyphenol have been linked to the gut microbial diversity. For instance, to harvest the potential health benefits of consumption of soy isoflavone daidzein or ellagitannins, conversion of these compounds into bioactive superior derivatives such as equols or urolithins, respectively, by the activity of microbial community is of paramount importance (Landete et al. 2015; Tomas-Barberan et al. 2016).

It is apparent that gut microbiota-derived products are subsumed into the human metabolic pathways consequently influencing the metabolic phenotype of an individual. Conversely, host metabolites also serve as substrates for the gut microbial activity. Collectively, it can be concluded that the metabolic cross talk between the host and gut microbial community determines the metabolic phenotype of the host.

9.9 Nutrigenomics: Link of Nutrients and Epigenetics for Well-Being

Dietary components have been shown to markedly influence the epigenetic-based gene regulation in human and thereby modulate the gene expression patterns especially when the immunity of an individual is compromised. Even though the specific mechanisms by which diet-derived components alter the epigenetics of humans remain unclear, their potential in regulating the human health is evident. Molecular interaction of dietary components and gene is recognized to play a direct and indirect role in the well-being of humans. The advent of genomics-based revolution in human medicine, especially the advancements made in the field of human genome sequencing project, has greatly aided in unraveling the nexus of food, genes and disease. Hence, nutrition research has encompassed the effects of food on our genes or the response of an individual gene for a food in the field called nutrigenomics (Nicastro et al. 2012). Food greatly influences the metabolic response and gene expression pattern thereby affecting the health of an individual. Thus, the branch of food science and nutrigenomics depends on two facets of food (a) effects of food-derived nutrients on the gene expression (b) differential metabolism of food components depending upon the genotype of an individual causing difference in the health conditions (Nasir et al. 2020).

The host enzymes namely DNA methyltransferases, histone acetyltransferases, DNA hydroxylases, histone deacetylases, and histone demethylases are known to be involved in these epigenetic changes as metabolites derived from dietary components regulate these changes. For example, sirtuin deacetylases are controlled by NAD^+/NADH ratio, acetyl-CoA, O-acetyl-ADP-ribose, and nicotinamide (Ringel et al. 2018).

Secondary plant metabolites such as polyphenols have potential beneficial effects against diseases like cancer, GI disorders, and neurodegenerative diseases owing to their inherent antioxidant potential. Research evidences have proven that the beneficial effects of polyphenols are mediated through modulation of expression of NF-κB, alteration of the activities of histone deacetylases, and DNA methyltransferases consequently reversing the phenomenon of abnormal gene expression patterns. Dietary components such as curcumin, epigallocatechin gallate, genistein, resveratrol have been known to effect chromatin remodeling through various epigenetic mechanisms (Remely et al. 2015). Daily administration of soybean-derived genistein (a phytoestrogen) in premenopausal women increased DNA demethylation and reversed the silencing effects of methylated genes, *RARβ2* and *CCND*2 (Qin et al. 2009). Similarly, coffee and tea polyphenols inhibited the DNA methylation in human breast cancer cell lines (Lee and Zhu 2006). Curcumin has been known to decrease DNA methylation, inhibit the activity of acetyl transferase, and block histone hyperacetylation and also regulates miRNA expression in the alleviation of effects of leukemia, prostate, and pancreatic cancers, respectively (Remely et al. 2015). Curcumin from turmeric inactivates the active site of human dinucleotide methylase transferase, and its epigenomic effect causes hypomethylation of leukemia cells. Nutrition derived from the food serves as substrates for the DNA methylation process and thus the precursors of one-carbon metabolite (S-adenosylmethionine) namely folic acid, choline, vitamins B2, B12, and B6, etc., have a significant influence on the DNA methylation phenomenon and hence their role in epigenetic control is further emphasized (Anderson et al. 2012).

Various diet-derived plant bioactives with potential and proven epigenetic effects in human are depicted in Table 9.3. Food-derived bioactives have anticancerous properties owing to their epigenetic effects such as causing DNA demethylation, DNA repair, inhibition of dinucleotide methylase transferase, inhibiting the activity of histone deacetylases and activation of silenced tumor suppressor genes (Table 9.3). Dietary polyphenols such as coumaric acid, cinnamic acid in cinnamon; resveratrol from grapes, epigallocatechin from green tea; curcumin from turmeric have capability to inhibit DNA methyltransferases and to modify the histone proteins. Notably, green tea-derived epigallocatechin has been shown to reactivate the silenced genes by interacting with dinucleotide methylase transferase. Apigenin—a plant-derived flavone prevalent in parsley, celery, etc., has dinucleotide

Table 9.3 Food components and their epigenetic effects (Adapted from Nasir et al. 2020)

Sl. No	Dietary bioactives	Source plants	Epigenetic effects
1	Phloretin	Apple	Demethylation, inhibition of histone deacetylases (HDAC), and activation of tumor suppressor gene (TSG)
2	Isothiocyantes	Broccoli	Chromatin remodeling and activation of TSG, p21
3	Anacardic acid	Cashew nut	Involved in DNA repair and inhibits histone acetyltransferase
4	Hesperidin	Citrus	Inhibits dinucleotide methylase transferase (DMTs)
5	Coumaric acid	Cinnamon	Inhibits dinucleotide methylase transferase
6	Caffeic acid	Coffee	Inhibits dinucleotide methylase transferase
7	Allyl mercaptan	Garlic	Inhibition of histone deacetylases, promotes histone acetylation
8	Resveratrol	Grapes	Inhibits dinucleotide methylase transferase
9	Genistein	Soybean	Inhibits dinucleotide methylase transferase
10	Epigallocatechin gallate	Tea	Inhibits dinucleotide methylase transferase
11	Lycopene	Tomato	–
12	Curcumin	Turmeric	Inhibits dinucleotide methylase transferase
13	Phytosterols, phenolics	Peanut, extra virgin olive oil	Enhanced methylation of *cg01081346*
14	β-glucan	Rye, barley, oats	Substrate for bacteroidetes producing propionate which in turn acts as inhibitor of histone deacetylases
15	Anthocyanins, quercetin, resveratrol, flavonoids	Wine, beer	Inhibitor of DNA methyltransferase
16	Flavanols (epicatechin, catechin, procyanidins), flavonols (quercetin)	Cocoa	Attenuates DNA methyltransferase and promotes hypomethylation

methyltransferase and histone deacetylase inhibitory activities. Besides the plant bioactives, minerals and vitamins such as zinc and folate have proven effect in DNA repair activities. Food-derived plant bioactives may also affect the epigenetic mechanism through various other processes. For instance, folate, B vitamins, etc., that act as methyl donor in 1-carbon metabolism could affect the processes of DNA methylation and histone methylation (Montgomery and Srinivasan 2019).

9.10 Food–Gut Microbiome and Epigenetic Linkage

Evidences from the epidemiological investigations have highlighted the significance of exposure to microbes, especially the composition of gut microbes, in determining the epigenetic response of human which in turn, albeit partly, explains the occurrence or disease progression in many instances. As stated above, microbial community inhabiting human gut produces several low molecular weight bioactive molecules including SCFAs, neurotransmitters (serotonin, etc.), and gases (H_2S, NO, NH_3, etc.). These biomolecules not only function as signaling molecules of digestion, neurotransmission, or inflammation but also as mediator of epigenetic regulation (BerniCanani et al. 2012). Further, the influence of gut microbiota on defining the metabolic disorders and phenotype (obese or lean) has led to consideration of microbiota-based therapeutics to manage these health complications. The variations in the gut microbiota and its link with obesity and other disorders have been interconnected with the signature methylome patterns suggesting the potential microbe–methylome–phenome linkage (Kumar et al. 2014). Though the molecular mechanism of involvement of microbes in epigenetic changes remains subtle, the role of microbial composition in effecting differential methylation of free fatty acid receptors in obese and type 2 diabetic individuals had been proven (Remly et al. 2014). Butyric acid, a main product of gut *Firmicutes*, is known to inhibit human histone deacetylases thereby offering protection against low-grade inflammation (BerniCanani et al. 2012). It is certain that dysbiosis of human microbiota potentially alters the levels of s-adenosyl methionine (SAM) and consequently affects the methylation status of DNA and histone complexes. Also, it is worth exploring if dysregulation of α-ketoglutarate and succinate levels could alter the epigenetic profile of peripheral host tissues. Another epigenetic activity that is potentially linked to microbial action is phosphorylation of histone protein mediated through AMP-activated protein kinase (AMPK) in response to energy status of cells since modulations in the activities of AMPK are observed during the physiological conditions of type 2 diabetes, metabolic syndrome, cardiovascular disease, and obese phenotype individuals. In summary, dysregulation of microbial community potentially depletes the food-derived metabolites which act as regulators of histone or DNA modification leading to aberrant phenotypes (Miro-Blanch and Yanes 2019).

Alterations in the composition of gut microbiota have been linked to the development of many diseases in human. For instance, the composition of *Firmicutes* to *Bacteroidetes* increases to cause irritable bowel syndrome whereas reduced ratio of *Bacteroidetes* to *Firmicutes* causes obesity; abundance of Fusobacteria is associated with colorectal cancer; production of trimethylamine-N-oxide from phospholipids leads to atherosclerosis; and excess ammonia production by gut microbiota causes Alzheimer's disease (Paul et al. 2015). Evidences have started emerging from our improved understanding of gut microbiota-dietary metabolism-host epigenetic axis about various diseases such as cancer, diabetes, arthritis, irritable bowel syndrome and the alteration in microbiota associated epigenetic changes in the disease development (Table 9.4)

Table 9.4 Gut microbiome and their epigenetic effects in human diseases

Disease/ physiological disorder	Alterations in gut microbiome/ changes in metabolites due to microbiota	Epigenetic modulations	References
Colon cancer	High TNF-α expression	Suppression of butyric acid-induced differentiation and potentiated cell death	Erdman et al. (2009)
Estrogen-dependent cancers	Bacterial-derived β-glucuronidases and β-glucuronides involved in estrogen modulations	Hepatic conjugation reactions of methylation and glucuronidation	Mageroy et al. (2012)
Gastric cancer	128-kDa protein derived from *H. pylori*	Acetylates promoter of p21 gene	Ding et al. (2010)
Liver cancer	Lipopolysaccharides from gut bacteria	Epigenetic modification of TLR4 gene expression in intestinal epithelial cells	Dapito et al. (2012)
Lung cancer	Short-chain fatty acids generated by gut bacteria modulate GPCR43 thereby affecting inflammatory responses	SCFAs inhibit histone deacetylases	Maslowski et al. (2009)
Diabetes mellitus 2	Increased number of *Bacteroides* and *Clostridium* and particularly increased *Firmicutes/Bacteroidetes* ratio	Increases the intestinal permeability causing low-grade inflammation and epigenetic modulation of Toll-like receptors Epigenetic regulation of free fatty acid receptors; decreased methylation in promoters of genes	Remely et al. (2014)
Schizophrenia	–	Gut microflora produced low molecular weight molecules (namely folate, butyrate, biotin, and acetate) interferes with epigenetic processes	Zhuo et al. (2019)
Depression	–	Gut microflora-derived butyrate, β-hydroxybutyrate, and GABA epigenetically modulate factors such as receptors or mediators	Zalar et al. (2018)
Obesity	Increased proportion of *Firmicutes* to *Bacteroidetes*	Aberrant methylation pattern of metabolism, obesity-related genes	Kumar et al. (2014)

9.11 Brain Health: Bioavailability Linkage

Though the link between GI comorbidities and brain disorders is known since time immemorial, the biochemical basis involving the interaction of neural, immune, endocrine, and metabolic pathways has started emerging. The human central nervous system (CNS), of which brain is an important constituent, is immunologically privileged due to blood–brain barrier (BBB). This selective permeability due to BBB leads to poor bioavailability of dietary nutrients warranting pharmacological interventions to improve the bioavailability of biomolecules. Dietary polyphenols derived from varied sources, such as tea, *Gingko Biloba*, cocoa, and blueberries, have exerted beneficial effects on the memory and learning capabilities of humans by suppressing neuroinflammation and protecting against neurotoxicity, etc. (Zhang et al. 2021). Further, several dietary interventions have reiterated the role of polyphenols in providing improved cognitive performance. Despite the potential therapeutic and cognition enhancer roles of dietary polyphenols, their bioavailability in brain tissues is a major concern. Bioavailability of important polyphenols, *viz.*, resveratrol and curcumin or their metabolites, is found to be in traces in liver and blood suggesting the need for research in identifying various factors associated in this process (Garcea et al. 2004; Walle et al. 2004). Dietary folates and vitamin B12 are indispensable for one-carbon metabolism, and folate deficiency has been shown to cause neural tube defects during fetal development. Hence, enhancing the bioavailability of folates in expectant mothers during the early stages of pregnancy is a major concern (Saini et al. 2016).

The term 'brain-gut axis' has been coined to denote the interactions that occur between the gut living microbes and the central nervous system and their implications for human wellness. The gut microbiota exerts significant influence on the multiple brain processes such as activation of the stress responsiveness, neurotransmission, neurogenesis, and neuroinflammation. Biochemicals produced by the gut microbiota along with the metabolic products of host influence the gut–immune–brain axis. The microbial products such as lipopolysaccharides trigger immune responses and alter the levels of neurotransmitters thereby known to control several neuropsychiatric disorders. Serotonin is a neurotransmitter or signal hormone with profound influence on human metabolism. The relative proportion of neuron serotonin and mucosa-derived serotonin has been implicated in the development of diabetes mellitus as former is an inflammatory shield whereas the latter functions as pro-inflammatory molecule.

9.12 Conclusions and Way Forward

The science of food bioavailability is even more challenging since the process depends on number of factors and also the bioactive potential of a food-derived biochemical component greatly relies on the process of bioavailability. Hence, there are several major gaps in our comprehension of bioavailability ranging from the effects of food processing, dynamics of food digestion, cellular components involved in the influx or efflux of bioactives in the GI tract, colonic fermentation-induced changes in biochemical composition, and their metabolism following the process of absorption to highlight a few. Prior to this stage, our knowledge regarding food matrix and its influence on the bioavailability or fate of food products are limited due to deprived understanding of various facets including effect of interplay of complex mixtures, effect of stabilization or protective effect from other food components, process of micellarization, or its effects on the process of digestion, etc. The diverse structural features of various food bioactive components and the resultant absorption mechanism warrant novel tools to study their interaction effect and tools to detect multiple bioactive forms (such as circulating forms) to portray the complete picture.

The science of nutrigenomics has thrown light upon the field of metabolic fate of food, especially in the arena of interaction of food and its components in modifying the host gene expression, influence of diet on the intestinal microbiota composition. The molecular basis of epigenetic modifications in the process of disease progression such as the missing links between the production of serotonin enterochromaffin cells and its plausible role in the alleviation (or otherwise) of diabetes mellitus warrants thorough investigation utilizing modern genomic tools. It would lead to development of therapeutic models to treat human disorders. Further, the idea that nutritional factors could effectively reverse the age-related epigenetic markers warrants in-depth studies so that the underlying mechanisms of food-linked physiological changes in aging process could be decoded.

References

Al–Lahham SH, Peppelenbosch MP, Roelofsen H, Vonk RJ, Venema K (2010) Biological effects of propionic acid in humans; metabolism, potential applications and underlying mechanisms. Biochim Biophys Acta 1801:1175–1183

Amengual J, Widjaja-Adhi MA, Rodriguez-Santiago S, Hessel S, Golczak M, Palczewski K, Von Lintig J (2013) Two carotenoid oxygenases contribute to mammalian provitamin A metabolism. J Biol Chem 288(47):34081–34096. https://doi.org/10.1074/jbc.M113.501049

Anderson OS, Sant KE, Dolinoy DC (2012) Nutrition and epigenetics: an interplay of dietary methyl donors, one-carbon metabolism and DNA methylation. J Nutr Biochem 23:853–859

Asai A, Yonekura L, Nagao A (2008) Low bioavailability of dietary epoxyxanthophylls in humans. Br J Nutr 100:273–277

Bendtsen LQ, Lorenzen JK, Bendsen NT, Rasmussen C, Astrup A (2013) Effect of dairy proteins on appetite, energy expenditure, body weight, and composition: a review of the evidence from controlled clinical trials. Adv Nutr 4(4):418–438. https://doi.org/10.3945/an.113.003723

BerniCanani R, Di Costanzo M, Leone L (2012) The epigenetic effects of butyrate: potential therapeutic implications for clinical practice. Clin Epigenetics 4:4

Birt DF, Boylston T, Hendrich S, Jane JL, Hollis J, Li L, McClelland J, Moore S, Phillips GJ, Rowling M, Schalinske K (2013) Resistant starch: promise for improving human health. Adv Nutr 4(6):587–601. https://doi.org/10.3945/an.113.004325

Bohn T (2014) Dietary factors affecting polyphenol bioavailability. Nutr Rev 72:429–452. https://doi.org/10.1111/nure.12114

Brown MJ, Ferruzzi MG, Nguyen ML, Cooper DA, Eldridge AL, Schwartz SJ, White WS (2004) Carotenoid bioavailability is higher from salads ingested with full–fat than with fat-reduced salad dressings as measured with electrochemical detection. Am J Clin Nutr 80(2):396–403. https://doi.org/10.1093/ajcn/80.2.396

Cassidy A, Brown JE, Hawdon A, Faughnan MS, King LJ, Millward J, Zimmer-Nechemias L, Wolfe B, Setchell KD (2006) Factors affecting the bioavailability of soy isoflavones in humans after ingestion of physiologically relevant levels from different soy foods. J Nutr 136(1):45–51. https://doi.org/10.1093/jn/136.1.45

Cosme P, Rodríguez AB, Espino J, Garrido M (2020) Plant phenolics: bioavailability as a key determinant of their potential health-promoting applications. Antioxidants 9:1263. https://doi.org/10.3390/antiox9121263

Dai ZL, Li XL, Xi PB, Zhang J, Wu G, Zhu WY (2013) L-Glutamine regulates amino acid utilization by intestinal bacteria. Amino Acids 45:501–512

Dapito DH, Mencin A, Gwak GY, Pradere JP, Jang MK, Mederacke I, Caviglia JM, Khiabanian H, Adeyemi A, Bataller R, Lefkowitch JH (2012) Promotion of hepatocellular carcinoma by the intestinal microbiota and TLR4. Cancer Cell 21(4):504–516

Dashty M (2013) A quick look at biochemistry: carbohydrate metabolism. Clin Biochem 46:1339–1352. https://doi.org/10.1016/j.clinbiochem.2013.04.027

De Bock M, Thorstensen EB, Derraik JG, Henderson HV, Hofman PL, Cutfield WS (2013) Human absorption and metabolism of oleuropein and hydroxytyrosol ingested as olive (*Olea europaea* L.) leaf extract. Mol Nutr Food Res 57(11):2079–2085. https://doi.org/10.1002/mnfr.201200795

De Vadder F, Kovatcheva-Datchary P, Goncalves D, Vinera J, Zitoun C, Duchampt A, Bäckhed F, Mithieux G (2014) Microbiota-generated metabolites promote metabolic benefits via gut-brain neural circuits. Cell 156:84–96

Ding S-Z, Goldberg JB, Hatakeyama M (2010) Helicobacter pylori infection, oncogenic pathways and epigenetic mechanisms in gastric carcinogenesis. Future Oncol 6(5):851–862

Elango R, Ball RO and Pencharz PB (2009) Amino acid requirements in humans: with a special emphasis on the metabolic availability of amino acids. Amino Acids 37(1):19–27. doi:10.1007/s00726–009–0234–y

Erdman SE, Rao VP, Poutahidis T, Rogers AB, Taylor CL, Jackson EA, Ge Z, Lee CW, Schauer DB, Wogan GN, Tannenbaum SR (2009) Nitric oxide and TNF-a trigger colonic inflammation and carcinogenesis in *Helicobacter hepaticus*-infected, Rag2-deficient mice. Proc Natl Acad Sci 106(4):1027–1032

Fernández-García E, Carvajal-Lérida I, Jarén-Galán M, Garrido-Fernández J, Pérez-Gálvez A, Hornero-Méndez D (2012) Carotenoids bioavailability from foods: from plant pigments to efficient biological activities. Food Res Int 46:438–450

Fernández-Tomé S, Sanchón J, Recio I, Hernández-Ledesma B (2017) Transepithelial transport of lunasin and derived peptides: inhibitory effects on the gastrointestinal cancer cells viability. J Food Compos Anal 68:101–110. https://doi.org/10.1016/j.jfca.2017.01.011

Frost G, Sleeth ML, Sahuri-Arisoylu M, Lizarbe B, Cerdan S, Brody L, Anastasovska J, Ghourab S, Hankir M, Zhang S, Carling D (2014) The short-chain fatty acid acetate reduces appetite via a central homeostatic mechanism. Nat Commun 5:3611

Garcea G, Jones DJ, Singh R, Dennison AR, Farmer PB, Sharma RA, Steward WP, Gescher AJ, Berry DP (2004) Detection of curcumin and its metabolites in hepatic tissue and portal blood of patients following oral administration. Br J Cancer 5:1011–1015. https://doi.org/10.1038/sj.bjc.6601623

González-Montoya M, Hernández-Ledesma B, Mora-Escobedo R, Martínez-Villaluenga C (2018) Bioactive peptides from germinated soybean with anti-diabetic potential by inhibition of dipeptidyl peptidase-IV, α-amylase, and α-glucosidase enzymes. Int J Mol Sci 19:E2883. https://doi.org/10.3390/ijms19102883

González-Sarrías A, Giménez-Bastida JA, García-Conesa MT, Gómez-Sánchez MB, García-Talavera NV, Gil-Izquierdo A, Sánchez-Álvarez C, Fontana-Compiano LO, Morga-Egea JP, Pastor-Quirante FA, Martínez-Díaz F (2010) Occurrence of urolithins, gut microbiota ellagic acid metabolites and proliferation markers expression response in the human prostate gland upon consumption of walnuts and pomegranate juice. Mol Nutr Food Res 54(3):311–322. https://doi.org/10.1002/mnfr.200900152

Green MH, Ford JL, Green JB (2021) A compartmental model describing the kinetics of β-carotene and β-carotene-derived retinol in healthy older adults. J Nutr 151(2):434–444. https://doi.org/10.1093/jn/nxaa306

Gropper SAS, Smith JL, Carr TP (2018) Advanced nutrition and human metabolism. Cengage Learning, Boston, MA

Halmos EP, Christophersen CT, Bird AR, Shepherd SJ, Gibson PR, Muir JG (2015) Diets that differ in their FODMAP content alter the colonic luminal microenvironment. Gut 64:93–100

Hayes M (2018) Bioavailability, bioaccessibility, and nutritional measurement of proteins. In: Hayes M (ed) Novel proteins for food pharmaceuticals and agriculture, John Wiley & Sons, Ltd., pp 183–195. https://doi.org/10.1002/9781119385332.ch9

Hodgson J, Kroft KD (2006) Dietary flavonoids: Effects on endothelial function and blood pressure. J Sci Food Agric 86:2492–2498

Ketnawa S, Ogawa Y (2021) In vitro protein digestibility and biochemical characteristics of soaked, boiled and fermented soybeans. Sci Rep 11:14257

Kumar H, Lund R, Laiho A, Lundelin K, Ley RE, Isolauri E, Salminen S (2014) Gut Microbiota as an epigenetic regulator: pilot study based on whole-genome methylation analysis. mBio 5: e02113–e02114

Landete JM, Arqués J, Medina M, Gaya P, de Las RB, Muñoz R (2015) Bioactivation of phytoestrogens: intestinal bacteria and health. Crit Rev Food Sci Nutr 56:1826–1843

Lee WJ, Zhu BT (2006) Inhibition of DNA methylation by caffeic acid and chlorogenic acid, two common catechol-containing coffee polyphenols. Carcinogenesis 2:269–277

Lichtenstein AH (2013) Fats and Oils. In: Caballero B (ed) Encyclopedia of human nutrition, 3rd edn. Academic Press, pp 201–208. https://doi.org/10.1016/b978-0-12-375083-9.00097-0

Lin X, Racette SB, Lefevre M, Spearie CA, Most M, Ma L, Ostlund RE (2010) The effects of phytosterols present in natural food matrices on cholesterol metabolism and LDL–cholesterol: a controlled feeding trial. Eur J Clin Nutr 64:1481–1487

Mageroy MH, Tieman DM, Floystad A, Taylor MG, Klee HJ (2012) A *Solanum lycopersicum* catechol-O-methyltransferase involved in synthesis of the flavor molecule guaiacol. Plant J 69(6):1043–1051

Magnúsdóttir S, Ravcheev D, de Crécy-Lagard V, Thiele I (2015) Systematic genome assessment of B-vitamin biosynthesis suggests co-operation among gut microbes. Front Genet 6:148

Marchesi JR, Adams DH, Fava F, Hermes GD, Hirschfield GM, Hold G, Quraishi MN, Kinross J, Smidt H, Tuohy KM, Thomas LV (2016) The gut microbiota and host health: a new clinical frontier. Gut 65:330–339

Marín L, Miguélez EM, Villar CJ, Lombó F (2015) Bioavailability of dietary polyphenols and gut microbiota metabolism: antimicrobial properties. Biomed Res Int 2015:905215

Maslowski KM, Vieira AT, Ng A, Kranich J, Sierro F, Yu D, Schilter HC, Rolph MS, Mackay F, Artis D, Xavier RJ (2009) Regulation of inflammatory responses by gut microbiota and chemoattractant receptor GPR43. Nature 461(7268):1282–1286

Mateo-Anson N, Aura AM, Selinheimo E, Mattila I, Poutanen K, Van Den Berg R, Havenaar R, Bast A, Haenen GR (2011) Bioprocessing of wheat bran in whole wheat bread increases the bioavailability of phenolic acids in men and exerts anti-inflammatory effects ex vivo. J Nutr 141: 137–143

Meléndez-Martínez AJ, Böhm V, Borge GI, Cano MP, Fikselová M, Gruskiene R, Lavelli V, Loizzo MR, Mandić AI, Brahm PM, Mišan AČ (2021) Carotenoids: Considerations for their use in functional foods, nutraceuticals, nutricosmetics, supplements, botanicals, and novel foods in the context of sustainability, circular economy, and climate change. Annu Rev Food Sci Technol 12:433–460

Miro-Blanch J, Yanes O (2019) Epigenetic regulation at the interplay between gut microbiota and host metabolism. Front Genet 10:638

Montgomery M, Srinivasan A (2019) Epigenetic gene regulation by dietary compounds in cancer prevention. Adv Nutr 10(6):1012–1028. https://doi.org/10.1093/advances/nmz046

Nagao A (2011) Absorption and metabolism of dietary carotenoids. Biofactors 37(2):83–87. https://doi.org/10.1002/biof.151

Nasir A, Bullo MM, Ahmed Z, Imtiaz A, Yaqoob E, Jadoon M, Ahmed H, Afreen A, Yaqoob S (2020) Nutrigenomics: epigenetics and cancer prevention: a comprehensive review. Crit Rev Food Sci Nutr 60(8):1375–1387. https://doi.org/10.1080/10408398.2019.1571480

Nicastro HL, Trujillo EB, Milner JA (2012) Nutrigenomics and cancer prevention. Curr Nutr Rep 1(1):37–43. https://doi.org/10.1007/s13668-011-0007-6

Paul B, Barnes S, Demark-Wahnefried W, Morrow C, Salvador C, Skibola C, Tollefsbol TO (2015) Influences of diet and the gut microbiome on epigenetic modulation in cancer and other diseases. Clin Epigenetics 7(1):1–11

Qin W, Zhu W, Shi H, Hewett JE, Ruhlen RL, MacDonald RS, Rottinghaus GE, Chen YC, Sauter ER (2009) Soy isoflavones have an antiestrogenic effect and alter mammary promoter hypermethylation in healthy premenopausal women. Nutr Cancer 2:238–244

Rajilić-Stojanović M, de Vos WM (2014) The first 1000 cultured species of the human gastrointestinal microbiota. FEMS Microbiol Rev 38:996–1047

Remely M, Aumueller E, Merold C, Dworzak S, Hippe B, Zanner J, Pointner A, Brath H, Haslberger AG (2014) Effects of short chain fatty acid producing bacteria on epigenetic regulation of FFAR3 in type 2 diabetes and obesity. Gene 537:85–92

Remely M, Lovrecic L, De La Garza AL, Migliore L, Peterlin B, Milagro FI, Martinez AJ, Haslberger AG (2015) Therapeutic perspectives of epigenetically active nutrients. Br J Pharm 172:2756–2768

Ringel AE, Tucker SA, Haigis MC (2018) Chemical and physiological features of mitochondrial acylation. Mol Cell 72:610–624. https://doi.org/10.1016/j.molcel.2018.10.023

Rowland I, Gibson G, Heinken A, Scott K, Swann J, Thiele I, Tuohy K (2018) Gut microbiota functions: metabolism of nutrients and other food components. Eur J Nutr 57(1):1–24. https://doi.org/10.1007/s00394-017-1445-8

Russell WR, Duncan SH, Scobbie L, Duncan G, Cantlay L, Calder AG, Anderson SE, Flint HJ (2013) Major phenylpropanoid derived metabolites in the human gut can arise from microbial fermentation of protein. Mol Nutr Food Res 57:523–535

Said HM (2013) Recent advances in transport of water-soluble vitamins in organs of the digestive system: a focus on the colon and the pancreas. Am J Physiol Gastrointest Liver Physiol 305: G601–G610

Saini RK, Nile SH, Keum YS (2016) Folates: chemistry, analysis, occurrence, biofortification and bioavailability. Food Res Int 89:1–13. https://doi.org/10.1016/j.foodres.2016.07.013

Sandhu AK, Miller MG, Thangthaeng N, Scott TM, Shukitt-Hale B, Edirisinghe I, Burton-Freeman B (2018) Metabolic fate of strawberry polyphenols after chronic intake in healthy older adults. Food Funct 9(1):96–106. https://doi.org/10.1039/c7fo01843f

Scalbert A, Manach C, Morand C, Rémésy C, Jiménez L (2005) Dietary polyphenols and the prevention of diseases. Crit Rev Food Sci Nutr 45:287–306

Setchell KD, Brown NM, Desai P, Zimmer-Nechemias L, Wolfe BE, Brashear WT, Kirschner AS, Cassidy A, Heubi JE (2001) Bioavailability of pure isoflavones in healthy humans and analysis of commercial soy isoflavone supplements. J Nutr 131(Suppl. 4):1262S–1375S. https://doi.org/10.1093/jn/131.4.1362S

Shoba G, Joy D, Joseph T, Majeed M, Rajendran R, Srinivas PS (1998) Influence of piperine on the pharmacokinetics of curcumin in animals and human volunteers. Planta Med 64:353–356

Tazoe H, Otomo Y, Kaji I, Tanaka R, Karaki SI, Kuwahara A (2008) Roles of short-chain fatty acids receptors, GPR41 and GPR43 on colonic functions. J Physiol Pharmacol 59(Suppl 2): 251–262

Ting Y, Zhao Q, Xia C, Huang Q (2015) Using *in vitro* and *in vivo* models to evaluate the oral bioavailability of nutraceuticals. J Agric Food Chem 63:1332–1338

Tomás-Barberán FA, González-Sarrías A, García-Villalba R, Núñez-Sánchez MA, Selma MV, García-Conesa MT, Espín JC (2016) Urolithins, the rescue of 'old' metabolites to understand a 'new' concept: metabotypes as a nexus between phenolic metabolism, microbiota dysbiosis and host health status. Mol Nutr Food Res 61:1500901

Tome D (2012) Criteria and markers for protein quality assessment—a review. Br J Nutr 108:S222–S229

Velderrain-Rodríguez GR, Palafox-Carlos H, Wall-Medrano A, Ayala-Zavala JF, Chen CO, Robles-Sánchez M, Astiazaran-García H, Alvarez-Parrilla E, González-Aguilar GA (2014) Phenolic compounds: their journey after intake. Food Funct 5(2):189–197

Visioli F, Ieri F, Mulinacci N, Vincieri FF, Romani A (2008) Olive-oil phenolics and health: potential biological properties. Nat Prod Commun 3(12):2085–2088

Walle T, Hsieh F, DeLegge MH, Oatis JE, Walle UK (2004) High absorption but very low bioavailability of oral resveratrol in humans. Drug Metab Dispos 12:1377–1382. https://doi.org/10.1124/dmd.104.000885

Walsh KR, Zhang YC, Vodovotz Y, Schwartz SJ, Failla ML (2003) Stability and bioaccessibility of isoflavones from soy bread during in vitro digestion. J Agric Food Chem 51:4603–4609

Xie G, Zhao A, Zhao L, Chen T, Chen H, Qi X, Zheng X, Ni Y, Cheng Y, Lan K, Yao C (2012) Metabolic fate of tea polyphenols in humans. J Proteome Res 11:3449–3457. https://doi.org/10.1021/pr300318m

Yang X, Darko KO, Huang Y, He C, Yang H, He S, Li J, Li J, Hocher B, Yin Y (2017) Resistant starch regulates gut microbiota: structure, biochemistry and cell signalling. Cell Physiol Biochem 42:306–318. https://doi.org/10.1159/000477386

Zalar B, Haslberger A, Peterlin B (2018) The role of microbiota in depression—a brief review. Psychiatr Danub 30(2):136–141

Zhang Q, Raoof M, Chen Y, Sumi Y, Sursal T, Junger W, Brohi K, Itagaki K, Hauser CJ (2010) Circulating mitochondrial DAMPs cause inflammatory responses to injury. Nature 464:104–107

Zhang Y, Lv C, Zhao G (2021) Ways to enhance the bioavailability of polyphenols in the brain: a journey through the blood-brain barrier. Food Rev Int:1–17. https://doi.org/10.1080/87559129.2021.1888973

Zhuo C, Yao Y, Xu Y, Liu C, Chen M, Ji F, Li J, Tian H, Jiang D, Lin C, Chen C (2019) Schizophrenia and gut-flora related epigenetic factors. Prog Neuro-Psychopharmacol Biol Psychiatry 90:49–54

Chapter 10
Nutrigenomics: Insights and Implications for Genome-Based Nutrition

S. Rajesh, S. Varanavasiappan, and Ramesh S. V.

Abstract Nutrigenomics encompasses crosstalk among nutrients, diet, and gene expression. Recent advances in 'Omics' technologies have opened up platforms for comprehensive analysis of how the intake of certain nutrients in diet would categorically influence the gene expression consequently affecting the metabolic health of an individual. Several genes that are linked to metabolic disorders are being characterized which could pave way for designing therapeutic system on a case-by-case basis of treating an individual and to have informed decision of administering personalized nutrition. Nutrigenomics, amid offering several benefits in nutritional guidance for human disease management, has also been implicated in ethical and social issues associated with it. This chapter would briefly discuss the role of diet supplementation and its influence on regulation of energy metabolism in individual, nutrient-regulated gene expression, and its impact on metabolic disorders and suggestions for genome-based nutritional guidance for better health.

Keywords Nutrients · Diet · Metabolic disorders · Gene expression · Omics

10.1 Introduction

Nutrigenomics is a rapidly emerging research field that studies the diet-induced changes on the genome, and thus considers the intersection of three topics, namely, health, diet, and genomics. Nutrigenomics can be mainly conducted through various 'Omics' techniques, which (among others) include microarrays or RNA-Seq analysis (transcriptomics) for the measurement of changes in mRNAs expression; proteomics that identify changes in polypeptides expression or in post-translational

S. Rajesh (✉) · S. Varanavasiappan
Department of Plant Biotechnology, Centre for Plant Molecular Biology and Biotechnology, Tamil Nadu Agricultural University, Coimbatore, Tamil Nadu, India
e-mail: rajesh.s@tnau.ac.in

R. S. V.
Physiology, Biochemistry and Post-Harvest Technology Division, ICAR-Central Plantation Crops Research Institute, Kasaragod, Kerala, India

R. S. V., S. Praveen (eds.), *Conceptualizing Plant-Based Nutrition*,
https://doi.org/10.1007/978-981-19-4590-8_10

modifications; metabolomics that mainly focus on the study of metabolites; and also epigenomics that measure the epigenetic changes in the genetic material.

Unhealthy diet and resulting malnutrition are linked to several non-communicable diseases (NCDs), including obesity, elevated blood pressure, high cholesterol, diabetes, cardiovascular disease, stroke, cancers, and resistance to the action of insulin. NCDs cause major deaths globally over the past two decades. Thus, NCDs are a considerable burden on limited health budgets, particularly in emerging economies. With the success of the human genome project and the advances in molecular biology, nutrigenomics could unfold the molecular basis underlying nutrition–gene interactions and may provide the strategies for developing safe and effective nutri-therapies for individuals such as those who are under siege of chronic diseases (Lau et al. 2008). Thus, the concept of nutrigenomics offers promises for both developed and developing countries (Neeha and Kinth 2013). The broad scope of nutrigenomics involves studying the effect of nutrition or dietary components on the structure, integrity, and function of the genome. It is an offshoot of the science of genomics and is being shaped by evolving and powerful genomic technologies. In this chapter, the basics and applications of nutrigenomics, diet supplementation, and genome-based nutrient guidance are discussed.

10.2 Nutrigenomics and Diet Supplementation

As stated above, nutrigenomics is defined as the effect of food on the gene expression. Consumption of unbalanced diet and adoption of unhealthy lifestyle lead to the development of chronic illness such as heart diseases, cancer, and diabetes. Strong interactions of genetic and epigenetic factors play a key role in determining individual's response to these illnesses. In this context, precision nutrition takes a lead role in establishing nutritional guidelines and diet supplementation in prevention and management of major illness and chronic diseases. Recent advancements in genome sequencing and cohort studies enable us in understanding the interplay of multiple factors in chronic disorders which opens up a field of customized intervention strategies. Nutrigenomics helps us in identification of genetic variants associated with disease susceptibility through interaction with dietary factors and diet supplement plan.

The practice of plant-based medicine, in the form of diet supplementation, is in existence since ancient times. And this forms the basis of Ayurvedic medicine too. As a disease prevention strategy, many spices are added to our daily diet ever since unknown. In recent times, the molecular pathways of the medicinal compounds from these spices are studied extensively to prove their nutrigenomics effect of chronic illnesses. Several natural products in the form of extracts or pure compounds have been shown to lower the risk of chronic diseases, by modulating signaling pathways, in model organisms (Fig. 10.1; Ramos-Lopez et al. 2017). For instance, curcumin an active ingredient of turmeric, has shown to prevent or treat diabetic retinopathy (Mrudula et al. 2007). The expression of vascular endothelial growth

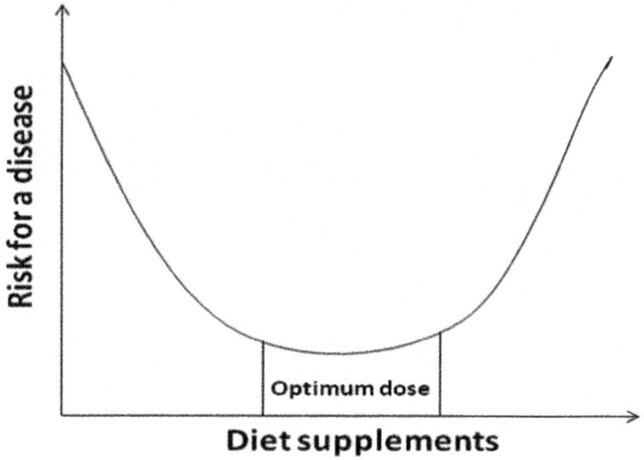

Fig. 10.1 Relationship between diet supplementation and disease risk levels. At optimal dietary dose of diet supplements (plant/microbes-based extracts or pure compounds) reduces the risk for chronic disease

factor (VEGF) is inhibited in the retina of streptozotocin-induced diabetic rat. In addition, turmeric has been proved to be a potent antioxidant, anti-inflammatory agent, and chemoprotective agent (Yue et al. 2014; Huang et al. 2018; Elifani et al. 2019). Low energy fruit and vegetable-enriched diet along with specific diet supplements are suggested for the management of obesity (Singh et al. 1994; He et al. 2004; Ello-Martin et al. 2007). A novel derivative from *Garcinia cambogia*, hydroxycitric acid (HCA), is clinically proven to be three times more effective for weight loss than diet and exercise alone. HCA-SX supplement is conditionally effective in weight management and lowered abdominal fat leptin expression in experimental animals and as well as in humans (Roy et al. 2003, 2007; Lau et al. 2008). In addition, it was reported that HCA and niacin bound chromium III (NBC) is safe and effective for weight loss and recommended as diet supplement. The use of novel bioactive foods and nutraceuticals in cardioprotection and management is growing (Alissa et al. 2012; Barreca et al. 2021). Foods rich in omega 3 fatty acids, antioxidant vitamins, and fibers are beneficial to cardiovascular health (Kris-Etherton et al. 2002; Psota et al. 2006). Fish oils and nutraceuticals in vegetable fat-free diet along with a healthy lifestyle enhance cardioprotection (Thompkinson et al. 2014). A dialyzed aqueous extract of fenugreek seeds stimulates insulin signaling pathways in adipocytes and liver cells and thereby possess hypoglycemic properties (Vijayakumar et al. 2005, 2008). A novel thermo-stable extract of fenugreek seeds has a potential application in the management of dyslipidemia and its associated metabolic disorders (Vijayakumar et al. 2010). Cumin is proved to modulate the alpha-crystallin chaperone activity and delays development of diabetic cataract in rat model system (Kumar et al. 2009).

Insect model systems are used to address the age-related disorders. Supplementation of rosemary extract, in a dose-dependent manner, increased the longevity (Wang et al. 2017). Ginger extract regulates the expression of superoxide dismutase (*Sod*) and catalase (*Cat*) genes in fruit flies (Zhou et al. 2018). This extract is found to alter the metabolism of amino acids, carbohydrates, and lipids and this indicates that anti-aging effect is achieved by protecting mitochondrial function, coordinating the oxidant-antioxidant balance, and ameliorating metabolic dysfunction. The extracts from *Rhodiola rosea*, *Curcuma longa* (rhizome), and *Emblica officinalis* (fruit) are reported to extend the lifespan (Evangelakou et al. 2019). Supplementation of resveratrol, a stress responsive polyphenol produced in plants, and epigallocatechin gallate from green tea also proved to extend the longevity by increasing the activity of SOD and CAT enzymes (Wang et al. 2013; Wagner et al. 2015). In addition to plant-based compounds, fungal and marine-derived products are also reported as diet supplements and regulate the immune system to inhibit tumor cell growth and various chronic disorders. Extract from *Ganoderma lucidum* increased lifespan of male flies by 42.32% and female flies by 29.24% by enhancing the antioxidant stress responses through modulating nutrient signaling pathways (Huang et al. 2011). The edible mushroom extracts aid in modifying nutrient signaling pathways through enhancement of responses to antioxidant stress and the dosage of these extracts will have positive impacts in promoting longevity and sex-dependent effects of Drosophila.

10.3 Nutritional Regulation of Gene Expression

Every living organisms exhibit varied responses depending on their ability to detect changes in nutrient levels. Adaptations of organisms to this variability in nutrient intake stipulate absolute regulation of metabolic pathways. Mammals display mechanisms that can reflect the abundance of nutrients such as sugars, lipids, amino acids and can provide an integrated response to these changes at the level of transcription to translation. Any alteration of these mechanisms may lead to the development of metabolic diseases. Understanding the 'cause' and 'effects' of nutrients on gene expression helps to enhance our knowledge of metabolic diseases and will provide ways for personalized nutrition based on individual genetic makeup.

Metabolic homeostasis can be achieved by modulation of the gene expression when energy sources such as carbohydrates, lipids, and amino acids are effectively used, thus maintaining the homeostatic energy balance (Fig. 10.2). For instance, sugars signal through the carbohydrate-responsive element binding protein (ChREBP). Peroxisome proliferator-activated receptors (PPARs) sense the fat, and the GCN2/activating transcription factor 4 (ATF4) and mTORC1 pathways regulate amino acid concentrations.

10.3.1 Regulation of Sugar Metabolism

Due to increased levels of glucose in the liver, the metabolic pathways associated with glucose homeostasis are regulated by key cellular enzymes involved in glycolysis and lipogenesis. Diets rich in carbohydrate induce transcription of the genes coding for enzymes of glycolysis (pyruvate kinase and glucokinase (GK)),

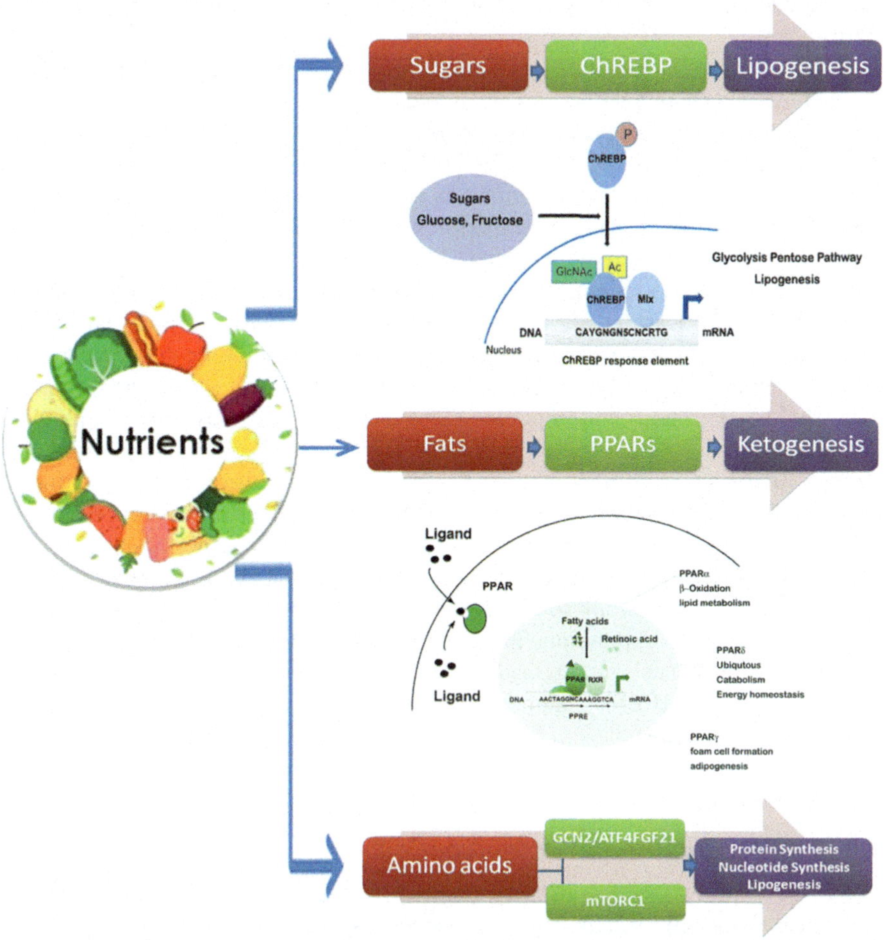

Fig. 10.2 Metabolic homeostasis in mammals through nutrient-regulated gene expression. Regulation of gene expression induced through various nutrients modulating the transcriptional activity in cells (Based on Haro et al. 2019)

lipogenesis (fatty acid synthase (FASN), acetyl CoA carboxylase, ATP citrate lyase, and stearoyl-CoA desaturase), and glucose 6-phosphate dehydrogenase involved in pentose pathway which in turn enhances the storage of sugars in the form of triglycerides (TGs).

The mechanism of regulation of sugar-induced lipogenesis was understood from the discovery of the carbohydrate-responsive element binding protein (ChREBP). ChREBP is structurally a basic helix–loop–helix (bHLH) leucine zipper transcription factor (TF); the gene encoding the factor is localized in the chromosome 7q11.23 and is absent in patients with Williams–Beuren syndrome. ChREBP forms a heterodimer with Mlx as a response to glucose and fructose which triggers the enzymes of the genes possessing carbohydrate response element (ChoRE) motifs.

ChREBP serves as glucose sensor and is reported to play key role in lipogenesis induced by fructose in the liver and small intestine. Loss of function of this regulator ChREBP causes drastic increase in the levels of FGF21 and absence of it causes liver disease (Lee and Cha 2018; Herman and Samuel 2016). ChREBP has two isoforms, ChREBP-α and ChREBP-β (Herman et al. 2012). Glucose-induced ChREBPα transcriptional activity triggers expression of ChREBPβ. In pancreatic islets, ChREBPα signaling is downregulated by ChREBPβ demonstrating the role of ChREBPβ in glucose-regulated gene expression (Jing et al. 2016; Ortego-Preito and Postic 2019; Katz et al. 2021). Glucose levels affect the post-translational modifications of the key regulator, ChREBP which modulate the subcellular localization, stability, and the transcriptional activity of ChREBP through the interaction with the 14-3-3 proteins and importins (Tsatsos et al. 2008; Kawaguch et al. 2001; Kawaguchi et al. 2002; Merla et al. 2004; Sakiyama et al. 2008; Kabashima et al. 2003). ChREBP recruits other partners like hepatic nuclear factor 4 (HNF-4), liver X receptor (LXR), farnesoid X receptor (FXR), or the thyroid hormone receptor (TR) for gene regulation. FXR represses ChoRE of glycolytic genes through interaction with ChREBP (Meng et al. 2016; Pupeau and Postic 2011; Caron et al. 2013). Also, there exists a cross-talk between ChREBP and PPAR for the glucose-mediated induction of FGF21 expression. In human beings, lower ChREBP activity along with de novo lipogenesis represents insulin resistance whereas in mice it is attributed to knockout of ChREBP in adipose tissues (Vijayakumar et al. 2017; Sanchez-Gurmaches et al. 2018).

10.3.2 Regulation of Fat Metabolism

Anomalies in the lipid metabolism increase the risk of cardiovascular issues, obesity, diabetes, and fatty liver problems. The discovery of pesticide-induced proliferation of peroxisomes in rat liver led to recognition of peroxisome proliferator-activated receptor (PPAR), a nuclear receptor that binds these pesticide molecules. It belongs to ligand-activated nuclear receptor and steroid receptor super family which specifically binds to the nuclear receptor responsive elements with a consensus of AGGTCA recognized by its DNA binding domain (Feige et al. 2006; Sever and Glass 2013).

Binding of the ligands (lipids) with PPAR triggers subsequent dimerization with retinoic acid receptor (RXR) followed by the binding to PPAR responsive element (PPRE) sequence that brings about change in chromatin structure and release of the histone H1 (Monsalve et al. 2013). PPARs are lipid sensors that are activated by the fatty acids and their derivatives and thus PPAR control lipid homeostasis. Three different isoforms of PPARs are reported, *viz.*, PPARα, PPARγ, and PPARδ. PPARα is involved in fatty acid oxidation and is majorly expressed in liver and lesser in heart, kidney, skeletal muscle, and brown adipose tissues (Hong et al.

Table 10.1 Role of PPARs in energy metabolism of organs

Organs	PPAR types		
	PPAR α	PPARγ	PPARβ/δ
Heart	Increased fatty acid oxidation[a]; Increased glucose uptake[a]		Increased glucose uptake[a]
Intestine	Higher levels of SCFA production[a]; fatty acid oxidation[a]; ketogenesis[a]	Improved gut microbiota composition[a]; Irritable bowel syndrome[a]	Higher levels of SCFA production[a]; fatty acid oxidation[a]; ketogenesis[a]; high level of glucose transport[a]
Pancreas	Increased fatty acid oxidation[a]	Increased glucose uptake[a]	High mitochondrial energy metabolism[a]; Elevated insulin secretion[a]
Skeletal muscle	Increased fatty acid oxidation[a]	Increased glucose uptake[a]	Increased fatty acid oxidation[a]; Increased glucose uptake[a]; Increased glucose utilization[a]
White adipose tissue	–	Reduced de novo lipogenesis[b]; Increased adipocyte differentiation[a]	Increased fatty acid oxidation[a]; Decreased lipogenesis[a]
Brown adipose tissue	Increased fatty acid oxidation[a]; Increased thermogenesis[a]	Increased de novo lipogenesis[a]; Increased adipocyte differentiation[a]	Increased thermogenesis[a]; Increased fatty acid oxidation[a]
Brain	–	Active glucose metabolism[a]	–
Liver	Increased fatty acid oxidation[a]; higher ketogenesis[a]; Decreased lipid storage[a]	Increased lipid storage[b] Gluconeogenesis[b]	Decreased lipogenesis[a]

[a]Represents beneficial effect
[b]Represents harmful effect (based on Hong et al. 2019)

2019). Role of PPARs in various organs influencing the energy metabolism is presented in Table 10.1. PPARγ is involved in adaptive response to fasting and has implications in the energy homeostasis (Desvergne et al. 2006; Napal et al. 2005; Rodriguez et al. 1994; Evans et al. 2004; Kersten et al. 1999) and is a master effector of adipogenesis. This molecule has been reported for its clinical significance in regulation of cardiovascular diseases, inflammation, and tumorogenesis (Kim et al. 2015). PPARδ is profoundly ubiquitous and is involved in fatty acid catabolism and energy homeostasis. It has effect on reducing the triglyceride levels and improving the cardiac contractility simultaneously increasing the HDL levels. In liver cells, it functions as ameliorator of glucose homeostasis (Barish et al. 2006).

Recently, a dual approach for strengthening the immune system using synthetic and nutritional PPAR-γ ligands to check the cytokine storm in the wake of COVID-

19 infection has been presented (Ciavarella et al. 2020). The anti-inflammatory drugs, thiazolidinediones (TZDs), like pioglitazone, agonist of PPAR-γ are reported to have ameliorating effects on severe viral pneumonia. Also, the nutritional ligands of PPAR-γ, like turmeric (*Curcuma longa*), lemongrass (*Cymbopogon sp.*), and pomegranate (*Punica granatum*), possess anti-inflammatory properties through PPAR-γ activation.

Angiopoietin-like 4 (ANGPTL4) is a potent regulator of triacylglycerol metabolism; however, the mechanisms underlying its transcription in response to fatty acids are limited. Molecular characterization of ANGPTL4 in large yellow croaker (*Larimichthys crocea*) demonstrated expression of *angptl4* is positively regulated by PPAR (α, β, and γ), and more particularly, the expression of *PPARγ* was found to be significantly increased in response to oleic and palmitic acids (Xiang et al. 2021).

10.3.3 Regulation of Protein Metabolism

Protein turnover ensures appropriate protein functionality. In the event of protein turnover imbalance, the transcriptome and metabolome are severely impaired causing more intakes of proteins and less synthesis affecting the amino acid pools. Cell senses the amino acid pool for maintenance of amino acid homeostasis (Chou et al. 2012).

The essential amino acids are obtained only through the dietary protein intake. The deficiency of the amino acid triggers amino acid response pathway. When essential amino acid level decreases below a threshold limit in the cells, deacetylation of corresponding tRNA takes place and these tRNAs can bind and activate general control non-depressible 2 kinase thus switching on the cascade of events in the amino acid response pathway (Qiu et al. 2001). Further, there is increase in the mRNA levels of activating transcription factor 4 (ATF4) (Kilberg et al. 2009; Vattem and Wek 2004), which subsequently triggers the specific target genes that can adapt to dietary stress caused by low amino acid levels (Shan et al. 2009).

Apart from this canonical pathway, methionine restricted diet activates a non-canonical pathway involving protein kinase R-like endoplasmic reticulum kinase (PERK)/nuclear factor like 2 axis (Wanders et al. 2016) which triggers increased energy expenditure and improved insulin sensitivity. Similar case is observed with low protein diets involving the signal transduction pathway.

The amino acid restricted or deprived diets have serious implications of the protein homeostasis and direct impact on lipid metabolism. Amino acid starvation inflicts metabolic response which are linked to FGF21, a fibroblast growth factor family, produced by liver, white and brown adipose tissues, skeletal muscles, etc. (Domouzoglou and Maratos-Flier 2011; Johnson et al. 2009). The expression of FGF21 is regulated, among other transcription factors (TFs), by ATF4 suggesting that GCN2/eIF2α/ATF4 as the major pathway that induces FGF21 expression under low-protein diets or leucine-deprived diet regimes (De Sousa-Coelho et al. 2012).

Another signaling pathway that is activated by amino acid intake is mTOR (mammalian target of rapamycin). mTOR is a serine/threonine kinase which is expressed ubiquitously. mTOR is a multiprotein complex of TORC1 and TORC2, of which TORC1 activation is by amino acids and some growth factors (Sancak et al. 2008, 2010). TORC1 complex controls cell growth and blocks catabolism and autophagy. Subsequent induction of glycolysis and the reduction in oxidative phosphorylation facilitate the incorporation of nutrients as biosynthetic precursors instead of energy suppliers. There are several amino acid sensors that activate this alternate pathway. Impairment of mTORC1 transduction pathway signals the development of cancer, obesity, and cardiovascular disease (Düvel et al. 2010; Festuccia 2021). Understanding the gene regulatory control of metabolism during nutrient intake helps to develop nutritional intervention-based new strategies to tackle metabolic pathologies.

10.4 Nutrients and Gene Expression in Metabolic Pathologies

Nutrients and dietary factors elicit health implications by regulating the gene expression at molecular level through modulation of transcriptional activity involving the TFs. Among various ill health effects, due to nutritional responses, obesity, diabetes, and cancer are the major ones. Nutritional intervention impacting the health by modulation of gene expression is presented in Table 10.2.

10.4.1 Obesity

Obesity is a lifestyle disorder and a chronic condition due to accumulation of excessive fat in the body because of lack of balance between energy consumption and expenditure. Obesity culminates as an interaction between various genetic, epigenetic, environmental, and behavioral factors profoundly associated with changes in dietary habit and sedentary life style.

Obesity is of majorly two types, monogenic obesity and common (or) polygenic obesity. Monogenic obesity is relatively rare form and is associated with malfunction in the endocrine glands. Mutation in genes that regulate and integrate signals in controlling food intake is considered as a main reason associated with this malady. Monogenic obesity is largely manifested as an altered phenotype. Common obesity is polygenic and often has multifactorial origins and is associated with the environmental and behavioral changes. Genome-wide association studies (GWAS) have

Table 10.2 Nutritional interventions and their effect on target genes impacting health

Nutritional intervention	Target genes	Gene expression changes	Potential health implications
High PUFA	*POMC, GALP*	Upregulated	Anti-obesity
	HCRT, MCH	Downregulated	Anti-obesity
Apple polyphenols	*LEP, SREBF1, PLIN, PPARGC1A, AQP7, AEBP1*	Downregulated	Anti-obesity
Energy-restricted diet with eicosapentaenoic acid and a-lipoic acid	Lipid catabolism genes	Upregulated	Antilipidemic
	Lipid storage genes	Downregulated	Antilipidemic
High MUFA	*APOBR*	Downregulated	Antilipidemic, antiatherogenic
Curcumin	*MMP9, MMP13, EMMPRIN*	Downregulated	Antiatherogenic
High protein	*PPARGC1A, PCK1, GSTA, CPT1A*	Upregulated	Antisteatotic
	FGF21, SCD1	Downregulated	Antisteatotic
Resveratrol	*FASN*	Downregulated	Antisteatotic

AEBP1, adipocyte enhancer binding protein 1; *APOBR*, apolipoprotein B receptor; *AQP7*, aquaporin 7; *CPT1A*, carnitine palmitoyltransferase 1A; *EMMPRIN*, extracellular matrix metalloproteinase inducer; *FASN*, fatty acid synthase; *FGF21*, fibroblast growth factor 21; *GALP*, galanin-like peptide; *GSTA*, glutathione S-transferase cluster; *HCRT*, hypocretin neuropeptide precursor; *LEP*, leptin; *MCH*, melanin-concentrating hormone; *MMP13*, matrix metallopeptidase 13; *MMP9*, matrix metallopeptidase 9; *PCK1*, phosphoenolpyruvate carboxykinase 1; *PLIN*, perilipin; *POMC*, proopiomelanocortin; *PPARGC1A*, peroxisome proliferative activated receptor g coactivator 1a; *SCD1*, stearoyl-coenzyme A desaturase 1; *SREBF1*, sterol regulatory element binding transcription factor 1. (Adapted based on Ramos-Lopez et al. 2017)

allowed identification of novel genetic loci that regulate changes in dietary intake, insulin signaling, inflammation, and muscle metabolism (Milagro et al. 2020).

Limited studies demonstrate the effect of diet on obesity as an influence of DNA sequence variants regulating nutrient altered gene expression. Approaches for understanding the nutrient-regulated gene expression influencing obesity can be performed by integrating GWAS with the gene expression profiles of specific tissues.

Adipose tissues play vital roles in the development of obesity. There are two types of adipose tissues, *viz.*, white adipose tissue (WAT) and brown adipose tissue (BAT) with contrasting functions of energy storage and energy dissipation, respectively. Adipocytes are key regulators maintaining the daily influx of fat whereas the WAT-derived factors exert auto, para, and endocrine signaling in the regulation of adipogenesis and energy metabolism thus playing a major role in obesity-related disorders. Acylation of histone causes changes in the chromatin structure and regulates gene expression. Histone deacetylase (HDAC) catalyzes the removal of acetyl groups in the histone proteins. Histone deacetylase inhibitors alter the expression of thermogenic gene encoding uncoupling protein 1, PPAR-γ, and also cause browning of WAT thus increasing the energy expenditure. Among various classes of

HDACs, Class I, Class II, and Class IV HDAC are Zn^+-dependent which increases the incidence of obesity due to binding on the Zn^+, whereas Class III HDAC, also called as SIRT, is NAD+-dependent which reduces the incidence of obesity (Sharma et al. 2021).

Omics approaches like transcriptome profiling of adipose tissue in a low-calorie diet regimen have identified predictors that would influence obesity in obese non-diabetic responders and non-responders. Also, it is reported that the expansion of adipose tissue during obesity is linked with altered expression of non-coding RNAs (ncRNAs). Long ncRNAs possibly affect the gene expression in adipose tissue and mediate changes in the adipocyte metabolism.

Presently, incidence of obesity and type 2 diabetes mellitus continues unabated and the physicians recommend making lifestyle changes as a panacea have little to do with the impact these metabolic disorder causes. More pertinent cause that challenges the life style changes as a recommendation is the continued access to the nutrient poor junk food without time limitations. Chrono-nutrition is recommended in such cases to overcome these metabolic pathologies which shall optimize metabolism that helps to improve insulin sensitivity and glycemic control yielding metabolic health (Hawley et al. 2020).

Exercise-induced genes, that regulates mitochondrial biogenesis, oxidative phosphorylation, antioxidant defense, and the amelioration of insulin resistance, are identified in the skeletal muscle transcriptomic analysis (Erlich et al. 2017; Vainshtein et al. 2015; Wang et al. 2016; Hu et al. 2019). These findings would suggest therapies for obesity-related disorders by linking the exercise benefits with gene expression and mapping the effect of the molecular pathways that are significantly impacted due to exercise. This could help achieve metabolic healthy individual and also have pharmacovigilance based on genetic profiling, which ultimately aids in developing an exercise pill mimicking exercise (Ghanemi et al. 2020).

10.4.2 Diabetes

Among chronic diseases, type 2 diabetes poses serious concern and the cause is attributed to the interaction between genetic and environmental factors. Unhealthy lifestyle of individual is the prime reason that is aggravated by poor nutritional intake and lack of physical activities in daily routine. Although environmental influence on the susceptibility to the development of this disease is highly variable, genetic susceptibility is high. Nutrigenomics may come handy through the personalized nutrition based on the knowledge of food components in daily dietary intake and how it modulates gene expression in an individual and the repercussions of the response to nutrients in the individual can be addressed.

In recent years, GWAS have detected some of the common variants of this type 2 diabetes; however, the limitation of identification of low frequency alleles particularly in specific target groups is less interesting and may have lesser clinical relevance (Fuchsberger et al. 2016).

Studies on the evaluation of the complex traits have often met with limited success. Exploration of the gene expression profile, gene × environment (GxE) interaction through expression quantitative trait loci (eQTL) analysis, has linked the genes of adipose tissue with the obesity and diabetes-related traits. GWAS has showed involvement of the genetic component on the expression profile of the adipose tissue (Emilsson et al. 2008). The pathogenesis of type 2 diabetes is directly regulated at the transcriptional level by the dietary nutrients through modulation of mechanisms, *viz.*, glucotoxicity, lipotoxicity, oxidative stresses, and inflammation. PPARs, most studied nutrient sensor, regulate metabolism and inflammation in variety of tissues (Gross et al. 2017). Regulatory role of PPARs has been described elsewhere in this chapter.

The pathway for de novo lipogenesis leading to fatty liver disease induced by the ChREBP in adipose tissue is often associated with better insulin sensitivity, hence could prevent the development of resistance to insulin and type 2 diabetes. In the type 2 diabetes, a group of essential amino acids, the branched-chain amino acids (BCAAs) serve as nutrient signals. Diets rich in BCCAs regulate body mass, muscle protein synthesis, glucose homeostasis thus improving the overall metabolic health of an individual (Bifari and Nisoli 2017). In metabolic processes, level of BCCAs changes since in catabolic condition, they can be play energy substrate role whereas under anabolic state, it can lead to induction of protein synthesis and effect cell growth. Impaired catabolism of BCCAs gene expression may have different role in increased risk of insulin resistance in humans. Insulin resistance has been reported to be regulated by the enhancement of the inflammatory pathway by saturated fatty acids mediated by Toll-like receptor (TLR) dependent and independent mechanisms (Glass and Olefsky 2012).

Calorie restriction has often been advised for the management of obesity and type 2 diabetes, which is presumed to improve the metabolic health of obese individuals. Omic approaches deployed for understanding the dietary intervention with low calorie diets and its implication in adipose tissue gene expression profile has led to draw key conclusions. There have been significant changes in the gene expression profiles in candidates with very low to low dietary calorie intake, with reduction in the level of metabolic genes in fat cells and increase or no changes in the expression of immunity-associated genes in macrophages (Capel et al. 2009). Dietary restriction with very low calorie diets, followed by weight maintenance diets, has shown opposite regulation of gene expression between the two phases (Viguerie et al. 2012). These findings suggest that in dietary intervention measures, there are differences in the adipose tissue gene expression and insulin sensitivity at different phases of diet intakes.

10.4.3 Cancer

Vast scientific literature cites the hidden therapeutic values of the herbs that could be panacea for treating number of diseases. Also, the natural products and the dietary constituents in them have been proven to possess preventive role in carcinogenesis. Recent advances demonstrate the role of phytochemicals in mediating gene expression regulation, whose impairment is the hallmark of cancer (Gonzalez-Vallinas et al. 2013; Hardy and Tollefsbol 2011). Nutrients and its role on cancer have been more comprehensively reviewed recently by Crujeiras and Lorenzo (2020). Gene expression during carcinogenesis and tumor suppression could be prevented by the effect of phytochemicals, some dietary nutrients through genetic or epigenetic means.

Extra virgin olive oil (EVOO), a Mediterranean source of lipids, is a classical example of dietary pattern that could have significant effect on cancer risk prevention, is worth mentioning in cancer therapy. The effect of EVOO has been demonstrated in animal models for regulating the genes in pathogenesis of colorectal cancer through epigenetic mechanisms (Di Francesco et al. 2015). Curcumin, a secondary metabolite of turmeric (*Curcuma longa*), has been associated with induction of methylation changes and regulates oncogenesis through modulation of miRNA expression patterns. Similarly, an isoflavone derived from soybean (*Glycine max*), genistein has active role in suppression of tumor and affecting the oncogenes by modulation of chromatin configuration and DNA methylation (Hardy and Tollefsbol 2011). Antiproliferative activity of resveratrol from grapes, by regulation of signaling pathways related to Akt, PI3K/Akt, and nuclear factor-kB, has been reported that is attributed to the expression of sirtuin (SIRT1) protein which regulates energy homeostasis (Gonzalez-Vallinas et al. 2013). Genome-wide transcriptomic analysis during the course of dietary intervention on individuals could possibly throw insights into therapeutic role of phytochemicals and helps identify biomarkers associated with the disease progression (van Breda et al. 2015).

10.5 Omic Approaches for Nutrigenomics and Precision Nutrition

Nutrigenomic methods warrant high-throughput techniques that analyze large datasets of genes, gene expression profiles, or proteins/molecules either in a single or as a combination of procedures. Recent developments in the field of bioinformatics and ever-increasing volume of data generated across labs have paved way for exploring the inter-individual differences as a result of genomic information and their relationship with nutrient-related metabolic variations (Camp and Trujillo, 2014). Precision nutrition is a consequence of this development which helps scientists understand the implications of dietary intake and prescribe personalized medication procedures (Kohlmeier and Kohlmeier 2013). Nutrigenomics deploys several methods, developed for nutritional and genomic sciences, including the multi-omics approaches from genomics to metabolomics (Fig. 10.3). The integration of omic data will definitely aid in designing the precision nutrition considering the anthropometric

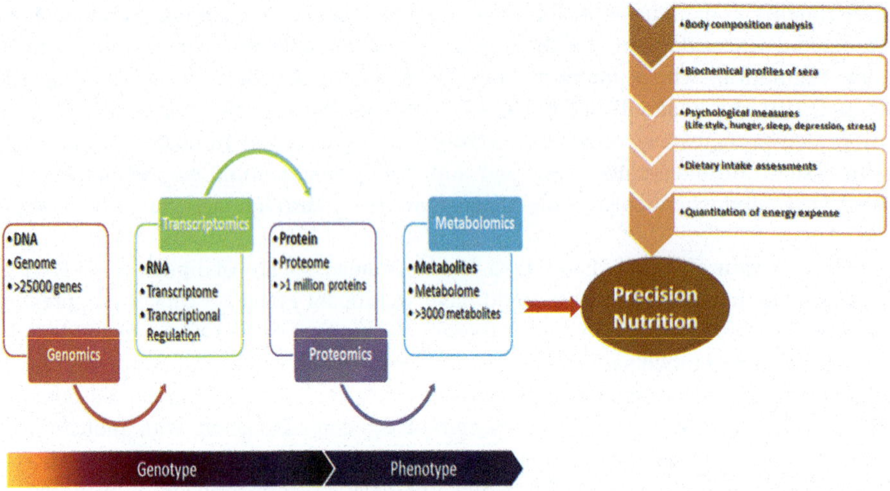

Fig. 10.3 Integration of Omics technologies as a measure of implementing precision nutrition. Based on Chirita-Emandi and Niculescu (2020), Omics landscape at various levels of gene expression influencing the metabolism is depicted

measurements and other dietary assessments and life considerations that shall optimize better response of individuals to dietary interventions.

Genomic science detect genetic variations due to change in chromosome structure and architecture (van Berkum et al. 2010); transcriptomic methods assess the levels of gene expression, i.e., mRNA and other small RNAs. The methods include microarrays, reverse-transcription polymerase chain reaction (RT-PCR), SAGE, RNA-sequencing, etc. Proteomic approaches measure the amount of specific proteins, protein-protein interactions and interactions among other structures like binding sites whereas the metabolomic approaches detect the level of known metabolites or identification of unknown metabolites, biomarkers, or targets that are of clinical significance. Epigenomic approaches focus on mechanisms that alter gene expression, by analyzing the gene expression rather than the changes in DNA sequence itself. These methods include analyses of methylation patterns of DNA and histone modifications by gene-specific analysis or genome-wide scans (Chirita-Emandi and Niculescu 2020).

The hypothesized changes in a biological system although analyzed by various omics approaches need the intervention of statistical methods that will imply the changes to be significant or not; thus, the biological data can be interpreted meaningfully. An offshoot of statistics is the bioinformatics that helps in analysis of biological data using informatics tools like sequence alignment of NGS data, annotation of the sequence, and also prediction of the biological implications as a result of identified changes in genes/proteins through metabolic pathway and gene ontology analysis. Despite the advantages and usage of bioinformatics, there are limitations with respect to introducing technical artifacts in the software and hardware that would most likely complicate the network. Further, normalization of data representations is always not adopted and data quality variations lead to complications in comparison of results from various experimental procedures (Mayer 2011).

Formulation of study designs in nutrigenomics should essentially consider methods for answering the hypothesized questions like sampling (number of samples, homogeneity), design to be chosen for identifying the thresholds, how cost-effective it would be, choice of tissues, and adequate use of bioinformatics tools to integrate data among various platforms.

With current advancements in sciences, nutrigenomic assessments can integrate the systems biology approach along with the high-throughput omics platforms for identification of nutrient-sensitive metabolic processes. These platforms would provide key information that can complement in understanding the mechanisms underlying nutritional disorders.

10.6 Nutrigenomics of Food Pesticides

The food that we consume nowadays contains a lot of non-nutritive compounds along with nutrients. These non-nutritive compounds include xenobiotics such as pesticide molecules, food additives, packaging, and processing compounds. Pesticides majorly can be divided into organochlorine, organophosphorus, and carbamate compounds. Pesticide toxicity mainly affect the central nervous system and cause psychomotor dysfunctions, mild cognitive dysfunctions, and neuro-degenerative and neurodevelopment effects (Kamel et al. 2004; Kori et al. 2018). In addition, these compounds are reported to affect the oxidation/detoxification enzymes such as paraoxonase (PON1), glutathione S transferase (GST), and a member of cytochrome P450 superfamily (CYP1A1) (Kaur et al. 2017). Individual's response to pesticide depends on their genetic difference in food tolerance, taste preference, nutrient absorption, and metabolism. The genetic difference in the gene structure along with the environmental exposure decides the individual variation risk to diseases.

The pesticide molecules modify the transcriptome of an individual by DNA methylation, histone modifications, and chromatin remodeling which in turn triggers the disease response (Bordoni et al. 2015; Shutoh et al. 2009; Song et al. 2011). Whenever exposure to pesticide dieldrin is prolonged, it induces histone hyperacetylation in the *corpus striatum* and *substantia nigra* in mice (Song et al. 2010; Bordoni and Gabbianelli 2020). Methylation in the DNA sequence of PON1 can lead to promoter polymorphism of PON1-108, suggesting its role in altered gene expression. It is also reported that exposure to these chemicals at an early state can trigger the onset of diseases at the later stage after a latency period. Pesticides such as dieldrin, paraquat, maneb, and permethrin were shown to cause Parkinson-like disease through dysfunction of the dopaminergic nigrostriatal neurons and/or abnormalities in motor response in animal studies, which prove that early-life exposure to these chemicals can exert adverse effects during later stage (Baltazar et al. 2014; Wang et al. 2020). Furthermore, Skinner (2016) demonstrated that exposure of gestating rats to methoxychlor increases the incidence of kidney disease, ovary disease, and obesity in offspring, spanning three generations. Pesticide toxicity also plays a key role in epigenome modulation since it can influence gene expression in a cell- and tissue-specific manner. As reported in mouse model system, epigenome modulation of xenobiotic detoxification pathways may control the xenobiotic-induced breast cancer susceptibility in mice (Mazambani et al. 2019).

Polymorphism in detoxification enzymes such as PON1, GST, and a member of cytochrome P450 superfamily (CYP1A1) is reported to increase the risk of xenobiotic toxicity in humans (Ginsberg et al. 2009; Araoud 2011; Kaur et al. 2017). Several studies suggest the association between CYP1A1-PON 1 polymorphism and occurrence of diseases in individuals exposed to organophosphates and polychlorinated biphenyls (Kaur et al. 2017). PON 1 polymorphism with low PON 1 protein levels is linked to adverse developmental and cognitive behavior in children. Prenatal mothers with PON1 and GST susceptible phenotypes, when exposed to organophosphates, possess a higher risk of toxicity in their children (Rossignol et al. 2014). Intake of cruciferous vegetables reduced the risk of cancer caused by GST polymorphism (Tse and Eslick 2014). These instances further emphasize the interactions between the xenobiotics and diet.

The consumption of organic food is associated with a lower occurrence of allergy and atopic disease in children and adults (Miyake et al. 2010; Eras et al. 2021). Organic food modulate gene expression favorably and also reduce the exposure to pesticides. Bioactive food supplements can be recommended as alternative strategy to surmount issues related to pesticidal exposure of foods. To partially counterbalance adverse effects caused by pesticides, dietary agents with antioxidant and anti-inflammatory properties and bioactive components which positively mediate epigenetic modifications might be useful. In the near future, detailed studies are warranted to address the pesticides/xenobiotic metabolism in biological system and individual genetic capacity to metabolize the toxic compounds. Along with this, the efficacy of organic food or diet supplements to protect the pesticide induced damage should also be investigated.

10.7 Ethical and Social Implications of Nutrigenomics

In recent years, advancement in genome sequencing techniques has made available 'big data' of several organisms on a larger scale including those of human genomic information. This raises few questions on whether this genetic information is anything to be considered unique or merely a piece of information communicated as a result of a routine bio-medical screening procedures. Considering the genetic information of an individual to be sensitive and more of a personal choice, disclose of it in public or too many data users in downstream pipeline who can access it for provision of insurance or employment formalities may have far-reaching societal implications due to in adequate data protection measures. Further, the disclosure of such sensitive information may be brought into the ambit of the legislations of a particular country, or under any other regulations involving international agreements or conventions and must be adhered to scrupulously (Görman et al. 2020; Castle and Ries 2007).

Results of the genetic tests normally performed for an individual may be routine and at times could be opening a Pandora's box where an individual's predisposition to future diseases and health complications is revealed. This also adds up the fact that the relatives of the tested individual may have similar complications owing to their common ancestry. Hence, disclosure of this information to the relatives as a measure of goodwill still is questionable considering the possibility of any misconception arising out of it, which may have far-reaching complications. Hence, an informed decision has to be taken about the disclosure of the issue to the relatives. The receiver's level of social awareness and mental health has to be ascertained and his concern, if any, has to be respected.

Genomics-based counseling suits well when there is scientific evidence for the interaction among genes-diet-health, which could categorically influence any diet-based intervention for human ailments. On this note, health complications like phenylketonuria, lactose intolerance for which genes linked to monogenic traits, are better choice for intervention than those governed by polygenes. Often the nutritional guidance for overcoming lifestyle disorders is cheaper alternative than genomics-based counseling, considering the cost effectiveness and better outreach to general public with lesser ethical implications.

Food, leave alone a source of nutrition, is a commodity that shapes the social, cultural, and personal identity of individual to the society. Nutritional advice based on provision of functional foods as a panacea for several problem has not been into fruition and hence personalized nutrition has to be focused which can integrate all the stigmas of cultural, emotional, ethical understandings of the food with the nutrigenetic approaches (Nordström et al. 2013). Any increased attention on healthy lifestyle as a result of personalized nutrition may have its own disadvantages due to limited reach of this personalized nutrition recommendations.

Nutrition recommendations as a measure of ensuring the public health, more particularly downscaling to the better health of individual patients, are often based on the outcome of the epidemiological studies and food policy taken at the administrative levels. Nutrigenomics research will serve as advisory of how diet and genomics are linked, and what a person could eat thus deciphering the implications of the food nutrients on the pattern of gene expression could influence individual health (McReynolds et al. 2022).

10.8 Perspectives and Concluding Remarks

Nutrients from plant or animal sources supply vital elements needed for daily routine of any organisms. These nutrients play various roles in regulating energy metabolism by modulating gene expression thus implicating the metabolic health of an individual. These changes have been studied at various levels using Omics landscape which provides comprehensive information of role played by individual nutrients and their interplay in general well-being of human health. These investigations help understand molecular mechanism behind the nutrient-regulated gene expression and can be useful to design new therapies for ameliorating metabolic pathologies. However, these dietary interventions have been limited and less appreciated due to ethical, legal, and social issues associated with genome-based nutrition guidance to individual and shall have far-reaching consequences on human health.

References

Alissa EM, Gordon AF (2012) Functional foods and nutraceuticals in the primary prevention of cardiovascular diseases. J Nutr Metab 2012:1–12

Araoud M (2011) Biological markers of human exposure to pesticides. In: Pesticides in the modern world-pests control and pesticides exposure and toxicity assessment, pp 191–212

Baltazar MT, Ricardo JD, Maria de Lourdes B, Aristidis MT, José AD, Félix C (2014) Pesticides exposure as etiological factors of Parkinson's disease and other neurodegenerative diseases-a mechanistic approach. Toxicol Lett 230(2):85–103

Barish GD, Narkar VA, Evans RM (2006) PPAR delta: a dagger in the heart of the metabolic syndrome. J Clin Investig 116:590–597

Barreca D, Domenico T, Antonella S, Giuseppina M, Orazio R, Maria RF, Giuseppe G, Nabavi SM (2021) Food flavonols: nutraceuticals with complex health benefits and functionalities. Trends Food Sci Technol 117:194–204

Bifari F, Nisoli E (2017) Branched-chain amino acids differently modulate catabolic and anabolic states in mammals: a pharmacological point of view. Br J Pharmacol 174(11):1366–1377

Bordoni L, Gabbianelli R (2020) Nutrigenomics of Food Pesticides. In: Caterin RDE, Martinez JA, Kohlmeier M (eds) Principles of nutrigenetics and nutrigenomics. Academic Press, Cambridge, MA, pp 513–518

Bordoni L, Cinzia N, Maria M, Fabio C, Gabbianelli R (2015) Intergenerational effect of early life exposure to permethrin: changes in global DNA methylation and in *Nurr1* gene expression. Toxics 3(4):451–461

Camp KM, Trujillo E (2014) Position of the academy of nutrition and dietetics: nutritional genomics. J Acad Nutr Diet 114:299–312

Capel F, Klimcakova E, Viguerie N, Roussel B, Vitkova M, Kovacikova M, Polak J, Kovacova Z, Galitzky J, Maoret JJ, Hanacek J, Pers TH, Bouloumie A, Stich V, Langin D (2009) Macrophages and adipocytes in human obesity: adipose tissue gene expression and insulin sensitivity during calorie restriction and weight stabilization. Diabetes 58:1558–1567

Caron S, Huaman SC, Dehondt H, Ploton M, Briand O, Lien F, Dorchies E, Dumont J, Postic C, Cariou B et al (2013) Farnesoid X receptor inhibits the transcriptional activity of carbohydrate response element binding protein in human hepatocytes. Mol Cell Biol 33:2202–2211

Castle D, Ries NM (2007) Ethical, legal and social issues in nutrigenomics: the challenges of regulating service delivery and building health professional capacity. Mutat Res Fundam Mol Mech Mutagen 622(1-2):138–143

Chirita-Emandi A, Niculescu M (2020) Methods for global nutrigenomics and precision nutrition. In: Caterin RDE, Martinez JA, Kohlmeier M (eds) Principles of nutrigenetics and nutrigenomics. Academic Press, Cambridge, MA, pp 49–58

Chou CJ, Affolter M, Kussmann M (2012) A nutrigenomics view of protein intake: Macronutrient, bioactive peptides, and protein turnover. Prog Mol Biol Transl Sci 108:51–74

Ciavarella C, Motta I, Valente S, Pasquinelli G (2020) Pharmacological (or synthetic) and nutritional agonists of PPAR-γ as candidates for cytokine storm modulation in COVID-19 disease. Molecules 25(9):2076

Crujeiras AB, de Lorenzo D (2020) Nutrients and gene expression in cancer. In: Caterin RDE, Martinez JA, Kohlmeier M (eds) Principles of nutrigenetics and nutrigenomics. Academic Press, Cambridge, MA, pp 483–488

De Sousa-Coelho AL, Marrero PF, Haro D (2012) Activating transcription factor 4-dependent induction of FGF21 during amino acid deprivation. Biochem J 443:165–171

Desvergne B, Michalik L, Wahli W (2006) Transcriptional regulation of metabolism. Physiol Rev 86:465–514

Di Francesco A, Falconi A, Di Germanio C et al (2015) Extravirgin olive oil up-regulates CB (1) tumor suppressor gene in human colon cancer cells and in rat colon *via* epigenetic mechanisms. J Nutr Biochem 26:250–258

Domouzoglou EM, Maratos-Flier E (2011) Fibroblast growth factor 21 is a metabolic regulator that plays a role in the adaptation to ketosis. Am J Clin Nutr 93:901S–905S

Düvel K, Yecies JL, Menon S, Raman P, Lipovsky AI, Souza AL, Triantafellow E, Ma Q, Gorski R, Cleaver S et al (2010) Activation of a metabolic gene regulatory network downstream of mTOR complex 1. Mol Cell 39:171–183

Elifani F, Amico E, Pepe G, Capocci L, Castaldo S, Rosa P, Montano E et al (2019) Curcumin dietary supplementation ameliorates disease phenotype in an animal model of Huntington's disease. Human Mol Genet 28(23):4012–4021

Ello-Martin JA, Liane SR, Jenny HL, Amanda MB, Barbara JR (2007) Dietary energy density in the treatment of obesity: a year-long trial comparing 2 weight-loss diets. Am J Clin Nutr 85(6): 1465–1477

Emilsson V, Thorleifsson G, Zhang B et al (2008) Genetics of gene expression and its effect on disease. Nature 452:423–428

Eras P, Ana PS, Carel T (2021) Influence of alternative lifestyles on antibiotic use during pregnancy, lactation and in children. Antibiotics 10(7):837

Erlich AT, Brownlee DM, Beyfuss K, Hood DA (2017) Exercise induces TFEB expression and activity in skeletal muscle in a PGC-1alpha-dependent manner. Am J Physiol Cell Physiol 314(1):C62–C72

Evangelakou Z, Maria M, Sentiljana G, Ioannis PT (2019) Nutrigenomics as a tool to study the impact of diet on aging and age-related diseases: the Drosophila approach. Genes Nutr 14(1): 1–18

Evans RM, Barish GD, Wang YX (2004) PPARs and the complex journey to obesity. Nat Med 10: 355–361

Feige JN, Gelman L, Michalik L, Desvergne B, Wahli W (2006) From molecular action to physiological outputs: Peroxisome proliferator-activated receptors are nuclear receptors at the crossroads of key cellular functions. Prog Lipid Res 45:120–159

Festuccia WT (2021) Regulation of adipocyte and macrophage functions by mTORC1 and 2 in metabolic diseases. Mol Nutr Food Res 65(1):1900768

Fuchsberger C, Flannick J, Teslovich TM et al (2016) The genetic architecture of type 2 diabetes. Nature 536:41–47

Ghanemi A, Yoshioka M, St-Amand J (2020) Will an obesity pandemic replace the coronavirus disease-2019 (COVID-19) pandemic? Med Hypotheses 144:110042

Ginsberg G, Susan S, Patricia N, Dale H, Katy W, Kathryn ZG, Douglas OJ, Babasaheb S (2009) The influence of genetic polymorphisms on population variability in six xenobiotic-metabolizing enzymes. J Toxicol Environ Health Part B 12(5-6):307–333

Glass CK, Olefsky JM (2012) Inflammation and lipid signaling in the etiology of insulin resistance. Cell Metab 15:635–645

Gonzalez-Vallinas M, Gonzalez-Castejon M, Rodriguez-Casado A, Ramirez de Molina A (2013) Dietary phytochemicals in cancer prevention and therapy: a complementary approach with promising perspectives. Nutr Rev 71:585–599

Görman U, Ahlgren J, Nordström K (2020) Ethical considerations in nutrigenetics and nutrigenomics. In: Caterin RDE, Martinez JA, Kohlmeier M (eds) Principles of nutrigenetics and nutrigenomics. Academic Press, Cambridge, MA, pp 543–548

Gross B, Pawlak M, Lefebvre P, Staels B (2017) PPARs in obesity induced T2DM, dyslipidaemia and NAFLD. Nat Rev Endocrinol 13:36–49

Hardy TM, Tollefsbol TO (2011) Epigenetic diet: impact on the epigenome and cancer. Epigenomics 3:503–518

Haro D, Marrero PF, Relat J (2019) Nutritional regulation of gene expression: carbohydrate-, fat-and amino acid-dependent modulation of transcriptional activity. Int J Mol Sci 20(6):1386

Hawley JA, Sassone-Corsi P, Zierath JR (2020) Chrono-nutrition for the prevention and treatment of obesity and type 2 diabetes: from mice to men. Diabetologia:1–7

He K, Hu FB, Colditz GA, Manson JE, Willett WC, Liu S (2004) Changes in intake of fruits and vegetables in relation to risk of obesity and weight gain among middle-aged women. Int J Obesity 28(12):1569–1574

Herman MA, Peroni OD, Villoria J, Schön MR, Abumrad NA, Blüher M, Klein S, Kahn BB (2012) A novel ChREBP isoform in adipose tissue regulates systemic glucose metabolism. Nature 484: 333–338

Herman MA, Samuel VT (2016) The sweet path to metabolic demise: fructose and lipid synthesis. Trends Endocrinol Metab 27:719–730

Hong F, Pan S, Guo Y, Xu P, Zhai Y (2019) PPARs as nuclear receptors for nutrient and energy metabolism. Molecules 24(14):2545

Hu Z, Zhou L, He T (2019) Potential effect of exercise in ameliorating insulin resistance at transcriptome level. J Sports Med Phys Fit 59(1):116–125

Huang L, Chengwei C, Xin Z, Xu L, Zupeng C, Chao Y, Xiaolong L, Guochong Z, Zhen X (2018) Neuroprotective effect of curcumin against cerebral ischemia-reperfusion via mediating autophagy and inflammation. J Mol Neuro Sci 64(1):129–139

Huang M, Jinqing L, Song Z, Xiaodeng M, Yang X (2011) Effects of bioactive extracts from four edible mushrooms on the lifespan of Drosophila melanogaster. Mycology 2(1):54–58

Jing G, Chen J, Xu G, Shalev A (2016) Islet ChREBP-β is increased in diabetes and controls ChREBP-α and glucose-induced gene expression via a negative feedback loop. Mol Metab 5: 1208–1215

Johnson CL, Weston JY, Chadi SA, Fazio EN, Huff MW, Kharitonenkov A, Köester A, Pin CL (2009) Fibroblast growth factor 21 reduces the severity of cerulein-induced pancreatitis in mice. Gastroenterology 137:1795–1804

Kabashima T, Kawaguchi T, Wadzinski BE, Uyeda K (2003) Xylulose 5-phosphate mediates glucose-induced lipogenesis by xylulose 5-phosphate-activated protein phosphatase in rat liver. Proc Natl Acad Sci U S A 100:5107–5112

Kamel F, Hoppin JA (2004) Association of pesticide exposure with neurologic dysfunction and disease. Environ Health Perspect 112(9):950–958

Katz LS, Baumel-Alterzon S, Scott DK, Herman MA (2021) Adaptive and maladaptive roles for ChREBP in the liver and pancreatic islets. J Biol Chem 296

Kaur G, Jain AK, Singh S (2017) CYP/PON genetic variations as determinant of organophosphate pesticides toxicity. J Genet 96(1):187–201

Kawaguchi T, Osatomi K, Yamashita H, Kabashima T, Uyeda K (2002) Mechanism for fatty acid "sparing" effect on glucose-induced transcription: regulation of carbohydrate-responsive element-binding protein by AMP-activated protein kinase. J Biol Chem 277:3829–3835

Kawaguchi T, Takenoshita M, Kabashima T, Uyeda K (2001) Glucose and cAMP regulate the L-type pyruvate kinase gene by phosphorylation/dephosphorylation of the carbohydrate response element binding protein. Proc Natl Acad Sci U S A 98:13710–13715

Kersten S, Seydoux J, Peters JM, Gonzalez FJ, Desvergne B, Wahli W (1999) Peroxisome proliferator-activated receptor alpha mediates the adaptive response to fasting. J Clin Investig 103:1489–1498

Kilberg MS, Shan J, Su N (2009) ATF4-dependent transcription mediates signaling of amino acid limitation. Trends Endocrinol Metab 20:436–443

Kim JH, Song J, Park KW (2015) The multifaceted factor peroxisome proliferator-activated receptor (PPAR) in metabolism, immunity, and cancer. Arch Pharm Res 38:302–312

Kohlmeier M, Kohlmeier GZ (2013) Nutrigenetics: applying the science of personal nutrition, 1st edn. Elsevier/Academic Press, Amsterdam, Boston, p 1

Kori RK, Manish KS, Abhishek KJ, Rajesh SY (2018) Neurochemical and behavioral dysfunctions in pesticide exposed farm workers: a clinical outcome. Ind J Clin Biochem 33(4):372–381

Kris-Etherton PM, Harris WS, Appel LJ (2002) Fish consumption, fish oil, omega-3 fatty acids, and cardiovascular disease. Circulation 106(21):2747–2757

Kumar PA, Reddy PY, Srinivas PNBS, Reddy GB (2009) Delay of diabetic cataract in rats by the antiglycating potential of cumin through modulation of α-crystallin chaperone activity. J Nutr Biochem 20(7):553–562

Lau FC, Bagchi M, Sen C, Roy S, Bagchi D (2008) Nutrigenomic analysis of diet-gene interactions on functional supplements for weight management. Curr Genom 9(4):239–251

Lee HJ, Cha JY (2018) Recent insights into the role of ChREBP in intestinal fructose absorption and metabolism. BMB Rep 51:429–436

Mayer B (2011) Bioinformatics for Omics data. Humana Press in Springer Science, pp 379–547

Mazambani S, Morris M, Cheriyath V (2019) Epigenome modulated xenobiotic detoxification pathways control DMBA-induced breast cancer in agouti Avy/a mice. Epigenetics 14(7): 708–720

McReynolds JG, Park NH, Wright M (2022) Nutrition food policy guidelines: what should patients eat? Physician Assist Clin 7(1):181–190

Meng J, Feng M, Dong W et al (2016) Identification of HNF-4α as a key transcription factor to promote ChREBP expression in response to glucose. Sci Rep 6:23944

Merla G, Howald C, Antonarakis SE, Reymond A (2004) The subcellular localization of the ChoRE-binding protein, encoded by the Williams-Beuren syndrome critical region gene 14, is regulated by 14-3-3. Hum Mol Genet 13:1505–1514

Milagro FI, Moreno-Aliaga MJ, Martínez JA (2020) Nutrients, obesity and gene expression. In: Caterin RDE, Martinez JA, Kohlmeier M (eds) Principles of nutrigenetics and nutrigenomics. Academic Press, Cambridge, MA, pp 431–440

Miyake Y, Sasaki S, Tanaka K, Hirota Y (2010) Consumption of vegetables, fruit, and antioxidants during pregnancy and wheeze and eczema in infants. Allergy 65(6):758–765

Monsalve FA, Pyarasani RD, Delgado-Lopez F, Moore-Carrasco R (2013) Peroxisome proliferator-activated receptor targets for the treatment of metabolic diseases. Mediat Inflamm 2013:549627

Mrudula T, Suryanarayana P, Srinivas PNBS, Reddy B (2007) Effect of curcumin on hyperglycemia-induced vascular endothelial growth factor expression in streptozotocin-induced diabetic rat retina. Biochem Biophy Res Comm 361:528–532

Napal L, Marrero PF, Haro D (2005) An intronic peroxisome proliferator-activated receptor-binding sequence mediates fatty acid induction of the human carnitine palmitoyltransferase 1A. J Mol Biol 354:751–759

Neeha VS, Kinth P (2013) Nutrigenomics research: a review. J Food Sci Tech 50(3):415–428

Nordström K, Coff C, Jönsson H, Nordenfelt L, Görman U (2013) Food and health: individual, cultural, or scientific matters? Genes Nutr 8(4):357–363

Ortega-Prieto P, Postic C (2019) Carbohydrate sensing through the transcription factor ChREBP. Front Genet 10:472
Poupeau A, Postic C (2011) Cross-regulation of hepatic glucose metabolism via ChREBP and nuclear receptors. Biochim Biophys Acta 1812:995–1006
Psota TL, Sarah KG, Penny KE (2006) Dietary omega-3 fatty acid intake and cardiovascular risk. Am J Cardiol 98(4):3–18
Qiu H, Dong J, Hu C, Francklyn CS, Hinnebusch AG (2001) The tRNA-binding moiety in GCN2 contains a dimerization domain that interacts with the kinase domain and is required for tRNA binding and kinase activation. EMBO J 20:1425–1438
Ramos-Lopez O, Fermín IM, Hooman A, Agata C, Myung SC, Rui C, De Caterina R et al (2017) Guide for current nutrigenetic, nutrigenomic, and nutriepigenetic approaches for precision nutrition involving the prevention and management of chronic diseases associated with obesity. Lifestyle Genom 10(1–2):43–62
Rodríguez JC, Gil-Gómez G, Hegardt FG, Haro D (1994) Peroxisome proliferator-activated receptor mediates induction of the mitochondrial 3-hydroxy-3-methylglutaryl-CoA synthase gene by fatty acids. J Biol Chem 269:18767–18772
Rossignol DA, Stephen JG, Frye RE (2014) Environmental toxicants and autism spectrum disorders: a systematic review. Transl Psychiatry 4(2):e360
Roy S, Cameron R, Savita K, Christina P, Bagchi D, Bagchi M, Sen CK (2003) Body weight and abdominal fat gene expression profile in response to a novel hydroxycitric acid-based dietary supplement. Gene Expression 11(5–6):251–262
Roy S, Hiral S, Cameron R, Savita K, Bagchi D, Bagchi M, Sen CK (2007) Transcriptome of primary adipocytes from obese women in response to a novel hydroxycitric acid–based dietary supplement. DNA Cell Biol 26(9):627–639
Sakiyama H, Wynn RM, Lee WR, Fukasawa M, Mizuguchi H, Gardner KH, Repa JJ, Uyeda K (2008) Regulation of nuclear import/export of carbohydrate response element-binding protein (ChREBP): Interaction of an alpha-helix of ChREBP with the 14-3-3 proteins and regulation by phosphorylation. J Biol Chem 283:24899–24908
Sancak Y, Bar-Peled L, Zoncu R, Markhard AL, Nada S, Sabatini DM (2010) Regulator-Rag complex targets mTORC1 to the lysosomal surface and is necessary for its activation by amino acids. Cell 141:290–303
Sancak Y, Peterson TR, Shaul YD, Lindquist RA, Thoreen CC, Bar-Peled L, Sabatini DM (2008) The Rag GTPases bind raptor and mediate amino acid signaling to mTORC1. Science 320: 1496–1501
Sanchez-Gurmaches J, Tang Y, Jespersen NZ, Wallace M, Martinez Calejman C, Gujja S, Li H, Edwards YJK, Wolfrum C, Metallo CM et al (2018) Brown Ffat AKT2 is a cold-induced kinase that stimulates ChREBP-mediated *de novo* lipogenesis to optimize fuel storage and thermogenesis. Cell Metab 27:195–209
Sever R, Glass CK (2013) Signaling by nuclear receptors. Cold Spring Harb Perspect Biol 5: a016709
Shan J, Ord D, Ord T, Kilberg MS (2009) Elevated ATF4 expression, in the absence of other signals, is sufficient for transcriptional induction via CCAAT enhancer-binding protein-activating transcription factor response elements. J Biol Chem 284:21241–21248
Sharma D, Sharma S, Chauhan P (2021) Acetylation of histone and modification of gene expression via HDAC inhibitors affects the obesity. Biomed Pharmacol J 14(1):153–161
Shutoh Y, Makio T, Ryoichi O, Atsuko H, Satoru Y, Hideaki F, Yutaka K, Keizo M, Takanori H (2009) Low dose effects of dichlorodiphenyltrichloroethane (DDT) on gene transcription and DNA methylation in the hypothalamus of young male rats: implication of hormesis-like effects. J Toxicol Sci 34(5):469–482
Singh RB, Mohammed AN, Ghosh S (1994) Effect on central obesity and associated disturbances of low-energy, fruit-and vegetable-enriched prudent diet in north Indians. Postgrad Med J 70(830):895–900
Skinner MK (2016) Epigenetic transgenerational inheritance. Nat Rev Endocrinol 12(2):68–70

Song C, Kanthasamy A, Jin H, Anantharam V, Kanthasamy AG (2011) Paraquat induces epigenetic changes by promoting histone acetylation in cell culture models of dopaminergic degeneration. Neurotoxicology 32(5):586–595

Song C, Arthi K, Vellareddy A, Faneng S, Anumantha GK (2010) Environmental neurotoxic pesticide increases histone acetylation to promote apoptosis in dopaminergic neuronal cells: relevance to epigenetic mechanisms of neurodegeneration. Mol Pharmacol 77(4):621–632

Thompkinson DK, Bhavana V, Kanika P (2014) Dietary approaches for management of cardio-vascular health: a review. J Food Sci Tech 51(10):2318–2330

Tsatsos NG, Davies MN, O'Callaghan BL, Towle HC (2008) Identification and function of phosphorylation in the glucose-regulated transcription factor ChREBP. Biochem J 411:261–270

Tse G, Eslick GD (2014) Cruciferous vegetables and risk of colorectal neoplasms: a systematic review and meta-analysis. Nutr Cancer 66(1):128–139

Vainshtein A, Tryon LD, Pauly M, Hood DA (2015) Role of PGC-1alpha during acute exercise-Induced autophagy and mitophagy in skeletal muscle. Am J Physiol Cell Physiol 308:C710–C719

van Berkum NL, Lieberman-Aiden E, Williams L, Imakaev M, Gnirke A, Mirny LA, Dekker J, Lander ES (2010) Hi-C: a method to study the three-dimensional architecture of genomes. J Vis Exp 39(e1869):1–7

van Breda SG, Wilms LC, Gaj S et al (2015) The exposome concept in a human nutrigenomics study: evaluating the impact of exposure to a complex mixture of phytochemicals using transcriptomics signatures. Mutagenesis 30:723–731

Vattem KM, Wek RC (2004) Reinitiation involving upstream ORFs regulates ATF4 mRNA translation in mammalian cells. Proc Natl Acad Sci USA 101:11269–11274

Viguerie N, Montastier E, Maoret JJ, Roussel B, Combes M, Valle C, Villa-Vialaneix N, Iacovoni JS, Martinez JA, Holst C, Astrup A, Vidal H, Clement K, Hager J, Saris WH, Langin D (2012) Determinants of human adipose tissue gene expression: impact of diet, sex, metabolic status, and cis genetic regulation. PLoS Genet 8:e1002959

Vijayakumar A, Aryal P, Wen J et al (2017) Absence of carbohydrate response element binding protein in adipocytes causes systemic insulin resistance and impairs glucose transport. Cell Rep 21:1021–1035

Vijayakumar MV, Pandey V, Mishra GC, Bhat MK (2010) Hypolipidemic effect of fenugreek seeds is mediated through inhibition of fat accumulation and upregulation of LDL receptor. Obesity 18(4):667–674

Vijayakumar MV, Bhat MK (2008) Hypoglycemic effect of a novel dialysed fenugreek seeds extract is sustainable and is mediated, in part, by the activation of hepatic enzymes. Phytother Res 22(4):500–505

Vijayakumar MV, Singh S, Chhipa RR, Bhat MK (2005) The hypoglycaemic activity of fenugreek seed extract is mediated through the stimulation of an insulin signalling pathway. Br J Pharmacol 146(1):41–48

Wagner AE, Stefanie P, Doerte R, Nieves B, Anke S, Manfred E, Achim S, Gerald R (2015) Epigallocatechin gallate affects glucose metabolism and increases fitness and lifespan in Drosophila melanogaster. Oncotarget 6(31):30568

Wanders D, Stone KP, Forney LA, Cortez CC, Dille KN, Simon J, Xu M, Hotard EC, Nikonorova IA, Pettit AP et al (2016) Role of GCN2-independent signaling through a noncanonical PERK/NRF2 pathway in the physiological responses to dietary methionine restriction. Diabetes 65: 1499–1510

Wang C, Charles TW, Thomas A, Xiaoping S, Jeanne S, Mara L, Edward S, Bradley K, De Cabo R, Zou S (2013) The effect of resveratrol on lifespan depends on both gender and dietary nutrient composition in *Drosophila melanogaster*. Age 35(1):69–81

Wang H, Zhen-ou S, Rizwan-ur R, Hong W, Yi-fei W, Hao W (2017) Rosemary extract-mediated lifespan extension and attenuated oxidative damage in drosophila melanogaster fed on high-fat diet. J Food Sci 82(4):1006–1011

Wang P, Li CG, Qi Z, Cui D, Ding S (2016) Acute exercise stress promotes Ref1/Nrf2 signalling and increases mitochondrial antioxidant activity in skeletal muscle. Exp Physiol 101:410–420

Wang R, Hongyang S, Guanghui W, Haigang R (2020) Imbalance of lysine acetylation contributes to the pathogenesis of Parkinson's disease. Intl J Mol Sci 21(19):7182

Xiang X, Han S, Xu D, Chen Q, Ji R, Zhao Z, Ai Q (2021) Oleic and palmitic acids induce hepatic angiopoietin-like 4 expression predominantly via PPAR-γ in *Larimichthys crocea*. Br J Nutr:1–27

Yue Y, Bin M, Jun Z, Ya-Jie Y, Lu L, Chang-Li Y, Wu L (2014) Neuroprotective effect of curcumin against oxidative damage in BV-2 microglia and high intraocular pressure animal model. J Ocul Pharmacol Ther 30(8):657–664

Zhou Y, Li-ying X, Li G, Xue-mei Q, Guan-hua D (2018) Ginger extract extends the lifespan of Drosophila melanogaster through antioxidation and ameliorating metabolic dysfunction. J Func Foods 49:295–305

Chapter 11
Next-Gen Biotech Crops for Human Nutrition

Kathleen L. Hefferon

Abstract The first and second generations of genetically modified crops have played a significant role in conferring biotic and abiotic stress tolerances to crops and thereby increased their yield levels to multiple fold. However, the present context warrants development of nutritionally superior plant phenotypes so as to alleviate nutrient deficiencies and to improve the nutritional security of many. Genetic engineering techniques utilizing multiple approaches such as protein overexpression, RNA-based gene silencing, and mutagenesis-based DNA modification techniques such as genome/gene editing have enabled the development of nutritionally superior plant types with a view to improve human health. This chapter describes the application of these technologies in developing next-gen biotech crops to address food and nutritional security of the world. The issues of consumer acceptance and the road ahead are also discussed.

Keywords Crop biotechnology · Genetic modification · Transgenics · Human nutrition

11.1 Introduction

Genetically modified (GM) organisms (GMOs) have been commercially made available for over two decades, yet they remain as controversial as ever. The data from the International Service for the Acquisition of Agri-biotech Applications (ISAAA) state that around 200 million hectares of land area of the world are currently occupied by crops that are generated through biotechnological approaches. Interestingly, over one half of this landholding belongs to smallholder farmers residing in developing nations (Fig. 11.1). The main aim of first-generation GM crops was to enhance economic yields and reduce cost of cultivation by incorporating traits such as resistance to biotic stresses namely insect infestation, weeds, and

K. L. Hefferon (✉)
Department of Microbiology, Cornell University, Ithaca, NY, USA
e-mail: klh22@cornell.edu

R. S. V., S. Praveen (eds.), *Conceptualizing Plant-Based Nutrition*,
https://doi.org/10.1007/978-981-19-4590-8_11

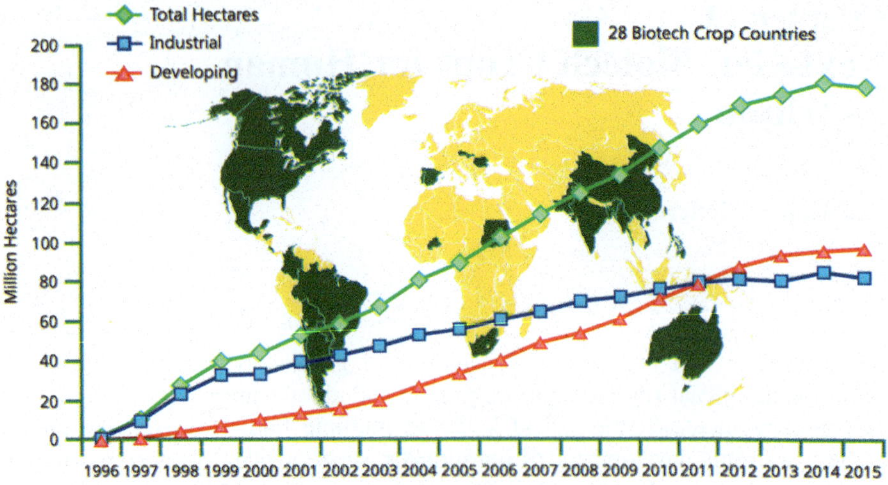

Fig. 11.1 Global area of biotech crops, 1996–2014

pathogen infections. As a follow-up, second-generation GM crops have focused on abiotic stresses namely drought, flooding, and elevated temperature in the wake of global climate change. The developments in the field of GM crops, improved comprehension of plant metabolism, and the significance of nutrition in human lives have led to the development of third-generation GM crops that value nutritional traits especially GM-based biofortification, enhancement in nutritional repertoire of food crops, etc. This set of GM crops is highly valued by the end user consumer and food processing industries owing to its advantages of nutritional value and reduction in food waste. Also, the number of poor across the globe, who experience chronic hunger, exceeds a billion. This situation warrants the development and adoption of radical approaches and GM crops for nutritional improvement which is a potential strategy to help alleviate hunger and malnutrition in the developing world.

This chapter discusses the importance of development of GM and genome-edited crops. The chapter then describes how these technologies have been used to address food security and human nutrition. The chapter ends with a discussion of the challenges that remain regarding consumer acceptance of these technologies.

11.2 Current Status of Agricultural Biotechnologies

The advancements in the field of conventional plant breeding techniques have led to the routine utilization of molecular marker-based approaches such as marker-assisted selection (MAS) in the development of improved phenotype of crops (Barabaschi et al. 2016). On the other end of the spectrum lies agricultural biotechnology that exploits the advancements in recombinant DNA technology to

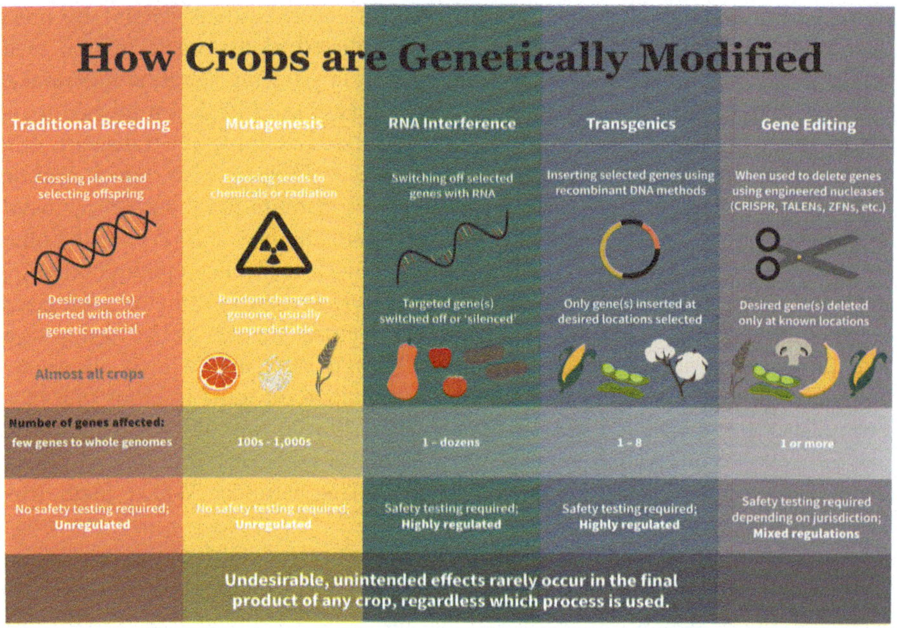

Fig. 11.2 Infographic depicting how crops are genetically modified. (Source: Genetic Literacy Project)

manipulate plant genome and incorporate a foreign trait of interest leading to the development of transgenic crops. The trait of interest varies from nutritional enhancement to imparting biotic or abiotic stress tolerance depending on the crops (Kamthan et al. 2016) (Fig. 11.2).

In this context, it is pertinent to acknowledge that development of crop varieties through alteration of genetic elements has existed long before the advent of recombinant DNA technology or genetic engineering. Many of the current crop varieties are the consequence of systematic breeding efforts wherein the genomes of the crops have been altered albeit without resorting to modern-day genetic modifications. For instance, crop mutation breeding originated from mutation research in the 1930s which entails the introduction of random mutations to plant genomes using chemical mutagens or in the process of irradiation-based mutagenesis. Mutations induced in seedlings or other propagules could be developed into novel crop varieties as the genetic changes made are heritable (Barabaschi et al. 2016). The Mutant Variety Database reveals that there are over 3000 different crop varieties, including the popular ruby red grapefruit, that have been generated through mutagenesis breeding (https://mvd.iaea.org).

Crop genetic engineering with an aim for enhanced nutritional and agronomic traits is indispensable and critical for modern plant science (Ricroch and Hénard-Damave 2015). These approaches may involve incorporation of a completely novel trait by introducing a gene or set of genes or making a little change in the gene(s) that forms part of genomic component of the crop. In general, novel gene(s) are introduced into the crop utilizing *Agrobacterium*-mediated plant transformation techniques aided with the developments in the field of in vitro regeneration potential of the crop. Alternatively, introduction of foreign genes could be accomplished using particle bombardment (gene gun). A well-characterized example of a transgenic crop having wider implications for nutrition of masses is Golden Rice, which harbors multiple genes derived from diverse species to reconstitute the β-carotene biosynthesis pathway so as to express β-carotene (Al-Babili and Beyer 2005). On the other hand, foreign genetic material could be derived from closely related plants belonging to same species and development of genetically modified crops utilizing such genes is called cisgenics. Cisgenics have advantages over transgenics as the former does not involve incorporation of a completely foreign gene and it also allows the cultivators to regain some of the agronomically important traits in crops that have been lost due to selective breeding approaches followed over the years. One successful example of cisgenic crop is wheat varieties harboring multiple resistance genes against the devastating fungal pathogen Ugg99 under Wheat Stem Rust Initiative (Singh et al. 2015).

Application of RNA biology in the development of GM crops has gained momentum with the advent of the phenomenon of RNA interference (RNAi). It is another form of genetic engineering which has gained popularity as it allows for suppression of gene expression so that an undesirable trait is eliminated. Plants are genetically engineered to express double-stranded RNA, either small or long enough to generate small non-coding RNAs (small interfering RNAs; siRNAs; microRNAs; miRNAs) which ultimately downregulate the cognate mRNA so that the trait expression is arrested. Small RNAs targeting genes of pest or pathogen-origin cause failed establishment of pest or pathogen in plant system thereby enhancing resistant status of the crops (Ramesh et al. 2007; Praveen et al. 2010; Ramesh 2013). For example, GM papaya grown in Hawaii confers resistance to the viral pathogen papaya ring spot virus by expressing an antisense RNA that targets the incoming viral RNA molecule (Gonsalves 1998).

One of the most recent and potent additions to crop biotechnology is genome editing approach. It does not warrant incorporation of novel gene sequences; rather, it works to effect one or few nucleotide changes in the plant gene or specific genomic region (Rani et al. 2016; Mao et al. 2016). Genome editing technologies exploit the evolutionarily conserved cellular machinery comprising clustered regularly interspaced short palindromic repeats (CRISPR) and Cas9, an RNA-guided nuclease of bacteria, to target specific sequences of DNA and cleave them at these sites. Following the site-specific cleavage, the inherent DNA repair mechanisms in the cells of all organisms are utilized to repair the sites of cleavage to effect specialized changes. The changes will then be carried forward to subsequent generations through the genome of the 'edited' organism. Also, genome editing is more precise than conventional crop breeding or other genetic engineering methodologies in vogue. Hence, it is considered a powerful technology not only for the development of nutritionally superior phenotypes but also in modifying complex traits such as yield, tolerance to abiotic stresses, and traits that are governed by multiple genes (Abdallah et al. 2015).

Taken together, these technologies can advance agriculture in ways that were never believed possible, and at speeds unheard of a few decades ago. The following section describes some recent innovations in genetic engineering to improve crops.

11.3 Resistance to Biotic Stresses

Application of GM crop technology was exemplified by the development of insect-resistant crops that express Bt, a bacterial toxin from *Bacillus thuringiensis*. Bt toxin is safe for mammals but creates pores in the alkaline digestive tract of insects, making them susceptible to the protein if the insects feed on plants expressing the toxin. Adoption of crops expressing Bt toxin in field conditions (cotton, maize, etc.,) has significantly reduced (around 30%) pesticide consumption throughout the world and offers improved health benefits for the farm workers. As a consequence of insect resistance, the secondary microbial infections following the insect attacks in crops have been reduced leading to the decreased levels of cancer-causing mycotoxins from those secondary fungal infections. This in turn provides health and economic benefits to farmers (Gressel and Polturak 2018). Another widely adopted GM technology is incorporation of herbicide tolerance trait in crops. Cultivation of herbicide tolerant GM crops (maize, canola, soybean, etc.) has not only helped farmers manage weeds but the technology is also compatible with no-till methods (Lombardo et al. 2016). For example, glyphosate is a broad-spectrum weed killer that acts by inhibiting the synthesis of three amino acids in plants yet breaks down easily and is less toxic than most previously used herbicides (Duke et al. 2012). Development of glyphosate-resistant GM crops have greatly aided in the large-scale cultivation of crops like soybean and maize.

Interestingly, traits herbicide and insect resistance constitute over 90% of GM crops that are cultivated. The reasons underlying high adoption of these technologies include the fact that farmers can practice conservation tillage, use considerably less (up to 37%) plant protection chemicals, and that there are potential implications for improving biodiversity by converting less wild space into farmland (James 2019). Furthermore, adoption of GM crops in the lower income households of developing nations, where the weed and insect pressure are high, will soon surpass the number of adoptions in developed and industrialized nations (Qaim 2020). Transgenic plants have been developed which exhibit resistance against a variety of other pathogens, including fungi, bacteria, and viruses.

Another viable approach for developing disease-resistant plants is the application of CRISPR–CAS9-based genome editing technology. There are ample opportunities to develop pathogen-resistant genome-edited crops via altering the target–effector interactions, downregulating the plant susceptibility factors, or suppressing the protein factors that are involved in the uncoupling of defense hormones, etc.

Genome editing may become the method of choice in the future due to its ease of use, among other things.

11.4 Tolerance to Abiotic Stresses

Climate change has made farming more difficult and yield or production less stable. For example, in the case of cereals such as wheat and barley, both drought and heat stress have been found to reduce grain size and expression of genes involved in starch production are downregulated (Thomas 2015). There are many reports of transgenic approaches to improve drought tolerance. For example, expression of dehydrins can have positive influences on plant various abiotic stresses such as tolerance toward drought, salinity, and cold. Similarly, expression of transcription factors (TFs) such as the dehydration responsive element binding (DREB) proteins could confer multiple stress tolerance (Campbell and Close 1997). The overexpression of DREB proteins can improve the survival of wheat and barley under drought conditions. Besides, TFs such as *WRKY*2, HDG11 (of HDZip IV TF subfamily), NAC, bZIP, etc., have been known to confer drought or abiotic stress tolerance in wheat (Khan et al. 2019). Unfortunately, current restrictions on growing transgenic plants in the field generally limit a test of the effectiveness of transgenic approaches to improve drought tolerance (Agarwal et al. 2006).

Transgenic rice has also been developed for drought tolerance using a number of strategies. For example, the TF *OsERF71* was overexpressed in rice. The underlying mechanism of tolerance toward drought suggests that these transgenics suppressed the essential process of photosynthesis but diverted the internal energy for those physiological mechanisms which ensured survival of the rice plants (Ahn et al. 2017). Alternatively, Gaudin et al. (2013) identified maize TF *ZmPIF*3 that has an important role in stomatal closure and prevents the excess water loss. Ectopic expression of *ZnPIF*3 in rice plants have demonstrated the utility of the gene in providing improved drought tolerance to rice through reducing the size of the stomatal aperture. Extensive field trials have not been completed for drought-tolerant rice due to the lack of regulatory structure available. In maize, OSCA family is comprised of hyperosmolality-gated calcium-permeable channel proteins, whose promoter regions harbor the genetic elements that are responsive to abiotic stresses. These gene families are up-regulated over 200-fold under drought conditions, and transgenic plants exhibited improved resistance to drought. The authors speculated that one of these genes, *ZmOSCA2.4*, was regulated by the microRNA miR5054. These results could also be used to generate drought-resistant crops in the future.

Soil salinity and flooding due to climate change can seriously reduce the crop productivity. Regulatory and transporter proteins can be used to enhance salt tolerance in crop plants. Salt tolerance can also be regulated through the overexpression of specific TFs or ion transporters. For example, Sun et al. (2020) discovered that the brassinazole-resistant 1 (BZR1) family of TFs, which control plant growth and development, improved the salt and drought tolerance. The authors found, using RNA-seq analysis, that this TF regulated salt tolerance by inducing the expression of 84 downstream stress-related genes (Sun et al. 2020)

Genetic engineering can be used to make plants more productive, under heat stress situations anticipated by climate change and especially since improvements using traditional breeding methods have reached their limits (Nowicka et al. 2018). Photosynthesis is an important determinant of crop yield. A number of approaches have been taken to increase the rate of photosynthesis in plants. These include using the enzymes from cyanobacteria or green algae to increase carbon sequestration and introducing the C4 pathway into C3 plants. Simkin et al. 2019) have found that photosynthesis may be improved over 40% using genetic engineering approaches. Overexpression of enzymes involved in photosynthesis, such as SBPase (sedoheptulose-1,7-bisphosphatase), can increase both photosynthetic carbon assimilation and biomass yield.

11.5 Improved Yield and Nutrition Using Genetic Modification

Genetically engineered plants have been developed to improve crop yield. One avenue to improve yield has been to make use of miRNAs, TFs, and proteins involved in signaling cascades (Garcia 2008). Most miRNAs control TF expression (Fu et al. 2012). Pan et al. (2018) showed that overexpression of the precursor of miR408, one of the most conserved plant miRNAs, caused the induction of photosynthetic genes, an increase in grain yield, and higher vegetative growth in *Arabidopsis*, tobacco, and rice. Other ways to increase grain width also exist. For example, Shi et al. (2019) identified a ubiquitin-specific protease to increase rice grain size.

Another way to improve plant yield is to increase levels of plant proteins responsible for stimulating cell proliferation or expansion. Some of these result in larger leaf size for biomass. Manipulating the levels of phytohormones, especially cytokinins, auxins, and gibberellins, can improve plant growth (Ciura and Kruk 2018). For example, transgenic crops that express the *iaaM* gene encoding tryptophan monooxidase, derived from bacteria and involved in auxin synthesis, have been developed to increase fruit size in berries (Mezzetti et al. 2004). Other approaches have involved the regulation of senescence and thus cell proliferation in plants, using changes in cytokinin metabolism (Kolachevskaya et al. 2015). For example, Swartzberg et al. (2006) found that tomato, canola, and maize with increased cytokinin synthesis through biotechnology resulted in greater fruit weight.

Improvements in nitrogen use efficiency in crops can be found in Good et al. (2004), Li et al. (2017), and McAllister et al. (2012). One achievement would be to generate microbial nitrogenase into higher plants to allow atmospheric nitrogen to be fixed within the plants themselves. To this end, an active Fe subunit of nitrogenase has been expressed in tobacco (Ivleva et al. 2016). Phosphorus is also critical for plant growth. Overexpression of phosphatases has brought about faster growth in plants and increased seed yield (Sun et al. 2012). Similar results were found for *Camelina sativa* plants which overexpressed a phosphatase from Arabidopsis (Chhikara et al. 2018). The authors were able to increase oil yield up to 13% higher seed oil content and up to a 52% increase in seed mass in comparison with wild-type plants.

Improvements in yield have also been explored using CRISPR-Cas9 technologies by selecting a variety of target genes (Ricroch 2019). Li et al. (2014) edited rice (Zhonghua 11) genes responsible for grain number, panicle shape, grain size, and plant architecture (Gn1a, DEP1, GS3, and IPA1). The first exon of Gn1a and GS3 and the third exon of DEP1 and IPA1 were chosen as targets for the sgRNAs because mutations within these regions have been proven to result in higher yield. The DEP1 mutants increased the number of flowers per panicle (about 50% more than the control). IPA1 mutations result in improved yield phenotypes as well.

Another way that yield can be increased is by reducing crop waste due to browning. For example, the polyphenol oxidase (PPO) gene is responsible for oxidative browning of a number of fruits and vegetables including potatoes and apples. Genome editing has been used to block oxidation by polyphenols and reduce browning in both of these crops (Waltz 2015; Mellidou et al. 2014).

11.6 Potential to Improve Human Health Via the Biofortification and Nutritional Enhancement of Food Crops

Micronutrient deficiencies in crops can be addressed through the direct fortification of crops in the form of fertilizers and foliar sprays by the addition of dietary supplements containing vitamins and minerals such as vitamin A, iron, zinc, and folate, or via the biofortification of plant varieties using modern breeding techniques (Ricroch and Hénard-Damave 2015). The production of genetically modified, biofortified food crops is potentially advantageous for populations who find it difficult to change their dietary habits or who lack access to nutritional programs. Staple crops such as rice, banana, cassava, and maize are low in micronutrients and sufficient quantities of each must also be bioavailable in order to contribute to a healthy diet. In many cases, the rural poor have little access to the rich source of micronutrients found in fresh fruits and vegetables and cannot afford to diversify their diets. Biofortification using technology could represent a facile answer to their challenges. Here are several examples of crops which have been biofortified by genetic engineering.

11.6.1 Golden Rice

Golden Rice is a biofortified carotenoid-rich variety developed with an aim to improve the dietary value of this major food crop. Carotenoids are plant pigments that also have cancer-fighting and anti-inflammatory properties. The carotenoids, beta-carotene, is converted in the body to vitamin A, which is essential to vision, normal growth, and development (Bollineni et al. 2014). Golden Rice is thus a well-known example of using genetic engineering to address a public health problem. Death and blindness of young children due to vitamin A deficiency (VAD) are widespread in economically challenged populations where rice is a primary food source. Natural rice does not express beta-carotene in the endosperm yet is the primary staple of rural poor populations of Southeast Asia.

Primarily, Golden Rice was developed through the insertion of multiple transgenes *psy* (phytoene synthase) derived from daffodil (*Narcissus pseudonarcissus*) and the *crtI* (phytoene desaturase) from bacteria (*Erwinia uredovora*) into the nuclei of rice variety BR29 under the transcriptional control of the glutelin 1 (*Gt*1) promoter. Later, Golden Rice 2 was developed using *psy* gene derived from maize. Golden Rice 2 produces significantly high amount of β-carotene compared to the original Golden Rice. Bioavailability of carotene from Golden Rice was confirmed in human trials, and the genetically modified rice variety Golden Rice has now been approved for human food use in the United States, Canada, Australia, and New Zealand (Coghlan 2018).

11.6.2 'Golden' Bananas to Combat Vitamin A Deficiency

Banana, which is one of the world's most important fruit crops, is a major staple in many African countries, where vitamin A deficiency tends to be the greatest (Amah et al. 2018). The inherent characteristic features of bananas, that they are slow growers, and low fertility rates along with the hurdles encountered in fast breeding of bananas, have made the improvement of its nutritional features a challenging task. However, prospecting for variability in vitamin A levels in banana species has made it amenable for biofortification through the application of GM technologies. The East African highland banana (EAHB) (*M. acuminata*), that is consumed after cooking in Uganda, is high in starch but has very low vitamin A levels, with serious nutritional implications for both the infants as well as women of childbearing age. It has led to the development of transgenic EAHB rich in vitamin A (20 μg/g dry weight) by incorporating the gene phytoene synthase 2a (*MtPsy2a*) derived from Fe′i banana (Paul et al. 2017). Thus, pro-vitamin A (PVA) biofortified Cavendish bananas were generated and field trials have been conducted in Australia. Biofortified Super bananas will improve the vitamin A status to some of the poorest subsistence farmers of Africa (Waltz 2014).

11.6.3 Biofortified Maize and Cassava

Maize germplasm has very wide variability for the production of β-carotene levels. Both the conventional breeding and transgenic strategies are being employed to increase the β-carotene content. Clinical trials conducted in North America and Africa showed that genetically modified maize, biofortified with β-carotene, remarkably improved the health of the subjects (Li et al. 2010; Mugode et al. 2014). Nevertheless, the modified maize, which is biofortified with β-carotene, is orange in color warranting immense efforts to change the perception of public Africans toward this product. Orange maize is traditionally associated with animal feed and white maize is considered to be used for human consumption.

Cassava is a staple food crop of millions of sub-Saharan Africans; however, the crop is deficient in iron and β-carotene (Sayre et al. 2011). In a randomized control trial, consumption of biofortified yellow cassava, allocated to the children, significantly enhanced the serum retinol and β-carotene contents (Talsma et al. 2016). It thus suggests that enhancement in the vitamin A levels of masses, especially of sub-Saharan Africa and Asia, where Cassava is consumed, is a viable strategy by developing GM cassava with pro-vitamin A factors as demonstrated in other food crops namely rice and maize (Talsma et al. 2016).

11.6.4 Nutritionally Enhanced Tomatoes

In addition to biofortification with vitamins and minerals, crops have also been engineered with enhanced nutritional properties. Tomatoes can be grown worldwide; they are also easily amenable for metabolic engineering for improved nutritional properties as well as decrease the risk of chronic diseases, such as hypertension, diabetes, and cancer. Many studies have been conducted to improve the nutritional content of tomato through transgenic approaches. For instance, suppression of fruit-specific gene *DET*1 (*DE-ETIOLATED 1*) has improved the biochemicals carotenoids, tocopherols, flavonoids, phenylpropanoids, and anthocyanidins. Elevated levels of β-carotene content via overexpression of *CYC-B/LCY-B/LCY-1* in tomato have been performed (Apel and Bock 2009). Similarly, tomatoes with high β-carotene and xanthophylls contents, astaxanthin, etc., were developed (Huang et al. 2013). Transcription factors derived from snapdragon have been shown to increase anthocyanin content in tomato (Tohge et al. 2015). The health benefits of plant-derived anthocyanins in suppressing the cancer pathways are demonstrated in clinical trials. Another important biochemical compound whose production in tomato plants is worth exploring is resveratrol. It is a plant bioactive, found in red grapes and wine, with ample beneficial health effects. GM tomatoes that express stilbene synthase gene derived from *Vitis vinifera* L. accumulated appreciable quantities of resveratrol (D'Introno et al. 2009; Giovinazzo et al. 2005).

Application of metabolic engineering tools to produce resveratrol in tomatoes would go long way in supplying this bioactive compound to masses.

11.6.5 Designer Oilseed Crops

Nutritional significance of long-chain polyunsaturated fatty acids, such as eicosapentaenoic acid (EPA) and docosahexaenoic acid (DHA) (which are omega-3 fatty acids) especially for dietary requirements and brain health, is recognized. However, the rich sources of omega-3 fatty acids are fishes and marine sources which cannot be made available for all in sufficient quantities. Hence, plant-derived omega-3 fatty acid via the process of metabolic engineering has gained momentum. Several 'proof-of-concept' studies and developments in the field of transgenic plants yielding omega-3 fatty acids have been compiled (Napier et al. 2015; Haslam et al. 2016). In this context, development of 'designer oilseed' plants such as (*Camelina sativa* L.) to synthesize omega-3 fatty acids (Ruiz-Lopez et al. 2014; Betancor et al. 2015) and its field testing will provide an alternative source of nutritionally important omega-3 fish oils for the end users (Yuan and Li 2020). More such instances of designer oil seed crops include the enhanced production of acetyl glyceride and glucoraphanin contents (Liu et al. 2015; Augustine and Bisht 2015). Thus, metabolic engineering of *Brassica juncea*-derived GSL-ALK gene family, which is involved in the production of glucoraphanin, is a valuable strategy for the production of anticancerous metabolites (Augustine and Bisht 2015).

11.7 Plant-Made Pharmaceuticals

Plants have also been designed as production platforms for vaccines, antibodies, and therapeutic agents. Vaccines derived from plant sources could be effortlessly scaled up, economical, secure, and remain effective. Initially, plant-derived vaccines have targeted infectious diseases, viz., enterotoxigenic *E. coli*, rotavirus, and cholera which remain the major reasons of infant mortality observed in developing countries (Yu and Langridge 2001). Of late, plant-based vaccines are developed and stockpiled to prepare for potential pandemics. The monoclonal antibody developed by Mapp Pharmaceuticals using tobacco is meant for neutralizing the Ebola virus. The clinical efficacy of this tobacco-derived anti-Ebola cocktail was demonstrated in the USA during the Ebola outbreak of 2015 (Budzianowski 2015). Another model of a plant-made vaccine, quadrivalent influenza vaccine (QIV) produced by the Quebec-based company Medicago, is to neutralize the influenza virus (Chen and Davis 2016; Lindsay et al. 2018). This model of vaccine production has several advantages as it does not require long incubation in eggs as performed in conventional vaccine production process. Along these lines, plant-based vaccine for the management of current pandemic COVID-19 produced by Medicago has been approved for use in Canada by Health Canada (https://www.reuters.com/business/healthcare-pharmaceuticals/canada-approves-medicagos-plant-based-covid-19-vaccine-adults-2022-02-24/). Furthermore, plant-derived vaccines have superior efficacy over conventional vaccines developed from mammalian systems. For instance, plant-made vaccine against Dengue fever virus did not evince any antibody-dependent adverse effects (Chen 2015). The efficacy of plant-based microbicide (a combination of monoclonal antibodies and plant-derived lectins) against the transmission of HIV was demonstrated (Seber Kasinger et al. 2019). In addition, plant-derived extraneous compounds could be employed in the treatment of rare genetic diseases in a cost-effective manner. An example is the plant-made version of glucocerebrosidase, made in carrot suspension cells by the Israeli company Protalix (Shaaltiel et al. 2015). This plant-made version, known as Taliglucerase alfa, is under one hundredth the cost of the conventional version of the drug.

11.8 Consumer Acceptance of Plant Biotechnology

Concerns have been expressed regarding GM crops, both in industrialized and in developing countries (Paarlberg 2008; Wesseler et al. 2017). Several of these apprehensions focus on the potentially harmful effects of GM crops to human health and/or the environment, as well as various ethical issues regarding the definition of the terms 'natural' or 'unnatural'. Also, global-scale application of intellectual property rights (IPRs) concerned with the GM crops and the involvement of multinational corporations are the worries in adoption of transgenic technology. It is pertinent to consider that technologies derived from conventional plant breeding approaches also entail IPRs. The imbalance of GM crops commercialized by large corporations is the end product of multiple regulations that many smaller corporate entities and 'not-for-profit' institutes find impossible to overcome (Wesseler and Zilberman 2014; Smyth 2017).

These problems facing the use of plant biotechnology in the food space continue to impact policy, regulation, and development (Adenle et al. 2017). For example, mandatory labeling practices now exist for GMOs in a number of countries. In the USA, a 'GMO-free' label has been exploited to entice consumers to pay higher prices for foods from which there is in reality no GMO equivalent.

The USA follows a 'substantial equivalence' policy toward regulating innovations in crop biotechnology, whereas the EU follows the 'precautionary principle', initially designed by the United Nations of the Convention on Biological Diversity (CBD) under the Cartagena Protocol on Biosafety. These differences in regulatory framework concerning 'product' vs 'process' have led to serious obstacles in terms of food trade, particularly for those in developing countries. NGOs have collectively spent over $10 billion USD in 2015 in an attempt to prevent the spread of use of GM crops around the globe (Byrne 2015). This can be compared to $8.5 billion spent by multinational companies on crop biotechnology. The result of this incentive has been bleak for post-colonial Africa and Southeast Asia, where regulation of crops such as BT cotton, GM eggplant, and Golden Rice has been prohibitively restrictive.

In the case of Golden Rice, for example, release has been hindered in countries such as Bangladesh and the Philippines with field trials destroyed by anti-GMO activists on more than one occasion in both countries (Potrykus 2010). Golden Rice could make a world of difference by contributing to the reduction of malnutrition in the developing world. After 20 years, Golden Rice has finally been approved in several countries (Wesseler and Zilberman 2017). However, 1.4 billion life years have been lost over the past 10 years in India, due to vitamin A deficiency. More recently, a genome-edited version of Golden Rice has also been developed (Dong et al. 2020). Whether anti-GM activists will block its release as well remains to be seen.

11.9 Conclusion

Agricultural biotechnology can improve the yield and nutritional quality of crops. Although GM and genome-edited plants can supply limited gene pools of a particular crop species with novel traits, policy controversies will remain a significant hurdle to overcome. In spite of this, the acreage of GM crops continues to increase with every new year, illustrating that farmers wish to take advantage of the new traits that are offered. A study determined that 124 out of 168 farmers chose to adapt GM. The fact that most of the farmers were from developing countries is consistent with the data collected by ISAAA (Fig. 11.1). Agricultural biotechnology can address hunger, nutrition, biodiversity, increase yield, and reduce the amount of farmland required. GM and genome-edited crops can improve economic outcomes for the rural poor, as well as environmental outcomes through decreased agricultural inputs. These technologies will continue to improve over the years to come.

References

Abdallah NA, Prakash CS, McHughen AG (2015) Genome editing for crop improvement: challenges and opportunities. GM Crops Food 6(4):183–205

Adenle AA, Morris EJ, Murphy DJ (2017) Genetically modified organisms in developing countries: risk analysis and governance. Cambridge University Press, Cambridge

Agarwal PK, Agarwal P, Reddy MK, Sopory SK (2006) Role of DREB transcription factors in abiotic and biotic stress tolerance in plants. Plant Cell Rep 25(12):1263–1274

Ahn H, Jung I, Shin SJ, Park J, Rhee S, Kim JK, Jung W, Kwon HB, Kim S (2017) Transcriptional network analysis reveals drought resistance mechanisms of AP2/ERF transgenic rice. Front Plant Sci 8:1044. https://doi.org/10.3389/fpls.2017.01044

Al-Babili S, Beyer P (2005) Golden Rice—five years on the road—five years to go? Trends Plant Sci 10(12):565–573

Amah D, van Biljon A, Brown A, Perkins-Veazie P, Swennen R, Labuschagne M (2018) Recent advances in banana (*Musa* spp.) biofortification to alleviate vitamin A deficiency. Crit Rev Food Sci Nutr 59(21):3498–3510

Apel W, Bock R (2009) Enhancement of carotenoid biosynthesis in transplastomic tomatoes by induced lycopene-to-provitamin A conversion. Plant Physiol 151(1):59–66

Augustine R, Bisht NC (2015) Biofortification of oilseed *Brassica juncea* with the anti-cancer compound glucoraphanin by suppressing GSL-ALK gene family. Sci Rep 10(5):18005. https://doi.org/10.1038/srep18005

Barabaschi D, Tondelli A, Desiderio F, Volante A, Vaccino P, Valè G, Cattivelli L (2016) Next generation breeding. Plant Sci 242:3–13

Betancor MB, Sprague M, Sayanova O, Usher S, Campbell PJ, Napier JA, Caballero MJ, Tocher DR (2015) Evaluation of a high-EPA oil from transgenic *Camelina sativa* in feeds for Atlantic salmon (*Salmo salar* L.): effects on tissue fatty acid composition, histology and gene expression. Aquaculture 444:1–12

Bollineni H, Gopala KS, Sundaram RM, Sudhakar D, Prabhu KV, Singh NK et al (2014) Marker assisted biofortification of rice with pro-vitamin A using transgenic Golden Rice lines: progress and prospects. Indian J Genet 74(4):624–630

Budzianowski J (2015) Tobacco against Ebola virus disease. Przegladlekarski 72(10):567–571

Byrne J (2015) Presentation by president of v-Fluence interactive at the Agricultural Bioscience International Conference, Melbourne

Campbell SA, Close TJ (1997) Dehydrins: genes, proteins, and associations with phenotypic traits. New Phytol 137:61–74

Chen Q (2015) Plant-made vaccines against West Nile virus are potent, safe, and economically feasible. Biotechnol J 10(5):671–680. https://doi.org/10.1002/biot.201400428

Chen Q, Davis KR (2016) The potential of plants as a system for the development and production of human biologics. F1000Res 19:5. https://doi.org/10.12688/f1000research.8010.1

Chhikara S, Abdullah HM, Akbari P, Schnell D, Dhankher OP (2018) Engineering *Camelina sativa* (L.) Crantz for enhanced oil and seed yields by combining diacylglycerol acyltransferase 1 and glycerol-3-phosphate dehydrogenase expression. Plant Biotechnol J 16(5):1034–1045. https://doi.org/10.1111/pbi.12847

Ciura J, Kruk J (2018) Phytohormones as targets for improving plant productivity and stress tolerance. J Plant Physiol 229:32–40

Coghlan A (2018) GM golden rice gets approval from food regulators in the US. New Scientist Retrieved 2018-06-07

D'Introno A, Paradiso A, Scoditti E, D'Amico L, De Paolis A, Carluccio MA, Nicoletti I, DeGara L, Santino A, Giovinazzo G (2009) Antioxidant and anti-inflammatory properties of tomato fruits synthesizing different amounts of stilbenes. Plant Biotechnol J 7(5):422–429

Dong OX, Yu S, Jain R, Zhang N, Duong PQ, Butler C, Li Y, Lipzen A, Martin JA, Barry KW, Schmutz J (2020) Marker-free carotenoid-enriched rice generated through targeted gene insertion using CRISPR-Cas9. Nat Commun 11:1178. https://doi.org/10.1038/s41467-020-14981-y

Duke SO, Lydon J, Koskinen WC, Moorman TB, Chaney RL, Hammerschmidt R (2012) Glyphosate effects on plant mineral nutrition, crop rhizosphere microbiota, and plant disease in glyphosate-resistant crops. J Agric Food Chem 60(42):10375–10397

Fu LL, Zhao X, Xu HL, Wen X, Wang SY, Liu B, Bao JK, Wei YQ (2012) Identification of microRNA-regulated autophagic pathways in plant lectin-induced cancer cell death. Cell Prolif 45(5):477–485. https://doi.org/10.1111/j.1365-2184.2012.00840.x

Garcia D (2008) A miracle in plant development: role of microRNAs in cell differentiation and patterning. Semin Cell Dev Biol 19(6):586–595. https://doi.org/10.1016/j.semcdb.2008.07.013

Gaudin AC, Henry A, Sparks AH, Slamet-Loedin IH (2013) Taking transgenic rice drought screening to the field. J Exp Bot 64(1):109–117. https://doi.org/10.1093/jxb/ers313

Giovinazzo G, D'Amico L, Paradiso A, Bollini R, Sparvoli F, DeGara L (2005) Antioxidant metabolite profiles in tomato fruit constitutively expressing the grapevine stilbene synthase gene. Plant Biotechnol J 3(1):57–69

Gonsalves D (1998) Control of papaya ringspot virus in papaya: a case study. Annu Rev Phytopathol 36:415–437

Good AG, Shrawat AK, Muench DG (2004) Can less yield more? Is reducing nutrient input into the environment compatible with maintaining crop production? Trends Plant Sci 9(12):597–605

Gressel J, Polturak G (2018) Suppressing aflatoxin biosynthesis is not a breakthrough if not useful. Pest Manag Sci 74(1):17–21

Haslam RP, Sayanova O, Kim HJ, Cahoon EB, Napier JA (2016) Synthetic redesign of plant lipid metabolism. Plant J 87(1):76–86. https://doi.org/10.1111/tpj.13172

Huang J-C, Zhong Y-J, Liu J, Sandmann G, Chen F (2013) Metabolic engineering of tomato for high-yield production of astaxanthin. Metab Eng 17:59–67

Ivleva NB, Groat J, Staub JM, Stephens M (2016) Expression of active subunit of nitrogenase via integration into plant organelle genome. PLoS One 11:e0160951

James C (2019) ISAAA Brief 46 Executive Summary Global status of commercialized biotech/GM crops. In: The international service for the acquisition of Agri-biotech applications

Kamthan A, Chaudhuri A, Kamthan M, Datta A (2016) Genetically modified (GM) crops: milestones and new advances in crop improvement. Theor Appl Genet 129(9):1639–1655

Khan S, Anwar S, Yu S, Sun M, Yang Z, Gao ZQ (2019) Development of drought-tolerant transgenic wheat: achievements and limitations. Int J Mol Sci 20(13):3350. https://doi.org/10.3390/ijms20133350

Kolachevskaya OO, Alekseeva VV, Sergeeva LI, Rukavtsova EB, Getman IA, Vreugdenhil D, Buryanov YI, Romanov GA (2015) Expression of auxin synthesis gene tms1 under control of the tuber-specific promoter enhances potato tuberization in vitro. J Integr Plant Biol 57:734–744

Li S, Nugroho A, Rocheford T, White WS (2010) Vitamin A equivalence of the β-carotene in β-carotene—biofortified maize porridge consumed by women. Am J Clin Nutr 92(5):1105–1112

Li Q, Song J, Peng S, Wang JP, Qu GZ, Sederoff RR, Chiang VL (2014) Plant biotechnology for lignocellulosic biofuel production. Plant Biotechnol J 12(9):1174–1192. https://doi.org/10.1111/pbi.12273

Li X, Zhou W, Ren Y, Tian X, Lv T, Wang Z, Fang J, Chu C, Yang J, Bu Q (2017) High-efficiency breeding of early-maturing rice cultivars via CRISPR/Cas9-mediated genome editing. J Genet Genom 44(3):175–178. https://doi.org/10.1016/j.jgg.2017.02.001

Lindsay BJ, Bonar MM, Costas-Cancelas IN, Hunt K, Makarkov AI, Chierzi S, Krawczyk CM, Landry N, Ward BJ, Rouiller I (2018) Morphological characterization of a plant-made virus-like particle vaccine bearing influenza virus hemagglutinins by electron microscopy. Vaccine 36:2147–2154

Liu Y, Zhang YX, Song SQ, Li J, Neal Stewart C Jr, Wei W, Zhao Y, Wang WQ (2015) A proteomic analysis of seeds from Bt-transgenic *Brassica napus* and hybrids with wild *B. juncea*. Sci Rep 5:15480. https://doi.org/10.1038/srep15480

Lombardo L, Coppola G, Zelasco S (2016) New technologies for insect-resistant and herbicide-tolerant plants. Trends Biotechnol 34(1):49–57

Mao Y, Botella JR, Zhu JK (2016) Heritability of targeted gene modifications induced by plant-optimized CRISPR systems. Cell Mol Life Sci 74(6):1075–1093

McAllister CH, Beatty PH, Good AG (2012) Engineering nitrogen use efficient crop plants: the current status. Plant Biotechnol J 10(9):1011–1025. https://doi.org/10.1111/j.1467-7652.2012.00700.x

Mellidou I, Buts K, Hatoum D, Ho QT, Johnston JW, Watkins CB, Schaffer RJ, Gapper NE, Giovannoni JJ, Rudell DR, Hertog ML, Nicolai BM (2014) Transcriptomic events associated with internal browning of apple during postharvest storage. BMC Plant Biol 14:328. https://doi.org/10.1186/s12870-014-0328-x

Mezzetti B, Landi L, Pandolfini T, Spena A (2004) The defH9-iaaM auxin-synthesizing gene increases plant fecundity and fruit production in strawberry and raspberry. BMC Biotechnol 4(1):1–10

Mugode L, Ha B, Kaunda A, Sikombe T, Phiri S, Mutale R, Davis C, Tanumihardjo S, De Moura FF (2014) Carotenoid retention of biofortified provitamin A maize (*Zea mays* L.) after Zambian traditional methods of milling, cooking and storage. J Agric Food Chem 62(27):6317–6325

Napier JA, Usher S, Haslam RP, Ruiz-Lopez N, Sayanova O (2015) Transgenic plants as a sustainable, terrestrial source of fish oils. Eur J Lipid Sci 117:1317–1324. https://doi.org/10.1002/ejlt.201400452

Nowicka B, Ciura J, Szymańska R, Kruk J (2018) Improving photosynthesis, plant productivity and abiotic stress tolerance—current trends and future perspectives. J Plant Physiol 231:415–433. https://doi.org/10.1016/j.jplph.2018.10.022

Paarlberg R (2008) Africa's organic farms. The New York Times. http://www.nytimes.com/2008/02/29/opinion/29iht-edpaarlberg.1.10576543.html

Pan J, Huang D, Guo Z, Kuang Z, Zhang H, Xie X, Ma Z, Gao S, Lerdau MT, Chu C, Li L (2018) Overexpression of microRNA408 enhances photosynthesis, growth, and seed yield in diverse plants. J Integr Plant Biol 60(4):323–340. https://doi.org/10.1111/jipb.12634

Paul JY, Khanna H, Kleidon J, Hoang P, Geijskes J, Daniells J, Zaplin E, Rosenberg Y, James A, Mlalazi B, Deo P (2017) Golden bananas in the field: elevated fruit pro-vitamin A from the expression of a single banana transgene. Plant Biotechnol J 15(4):520–532

Potrykus I (2010) Lessons from the 'Humanitarian Golden Rice' project: regulation prevents development of public good genetically engineered crop products. New Biotechnol 27(5): 466–472

Praveen S, Ramesh SV, Mishra AK, Koundal V, Palukaitis P (2010) Silencing potential of viral derived RNAi constructs in tomato leaf curl virus-AC4 gene suppression in tomato. Transgenic Res 19(1):45–55

Qaim M (2020) Role of new plant breeding technologies for food security and sustainable agricultural development. Appl Econ Perspect Policy 42(2):129–150. https://doi.org/10.1002/aepp.13044

Ramesh SV (2013) Non-coding RNAs in crop genetic modification: considerations and predictable environmental risk assessments (ERA). Mol Biotechnol 55(1):87–100

Ramesh SV, Mishra AK, Praveen S (2007) Hairpin RNA-mediated strategies for silencing of tomato leaf curl virus AC1 and AC4 genes for effective resistance in plants. Oligonucleotides 17(2):251–257

Rani R, Yadav P, Barbadikar KM, Baliyan N, Malhotra EV, Singh BK, Kumar A, Singh D (2016) CRISPR/Cas9: a promising way to exploit genetic variation in plants. Biotechnol Lett 38(12): 1991–2006

Ricroch A (2019) Global developments of genome editing in agriculture. Transgenic Res 28(Suppl 2):45–52. https://doi.org/10.1007/s11248-019-00133-6

Ricroch AE, Hénard-Damave MC (2015) Next biotech plants: new traits, crops, developers and technologies for addressing global challenges. Crit Rev Biotechnol 36(4):675–690

Ruiz-Lopez N, Haslam RP, Napier JA, Sayanova O (2014) Successful high-level accumulation of fish oil omega-3 long-chain polyunsaturated fatty acids in a transgenic oilseed crop. Plant J 77(2):198–208. https://doi.org/10.1111/tpj.12378

Sayre R, Beeching JR, Cahoon EB, Egesi C, Fauquet C, Fellman J, Fregene M, Gruissem W, Mallowa S, Manary M, Maziya-Dixon B, Mbanaso A, Schachtman DP, Siritunga D, Taylor N, Vanderschuren H, Zhang P (2011) The BioCassava plus program: biofortification of cassava for sub-Saharan Africa. Annu Rev Plant Biol 62:251–272

Seber Kasinger LE, Dent MW, Mahajan G, Hamorsky KT, Matoba N (2019) A novel anti-HIV-1 bispecific bNAb-lectin fusion protein engineered in a plant-based transient expression system. Plant Biotechnol J 17(8):1646–1656. https://doi.org/10.1111/pbi.13090

Shaaltiel Y, Gingis-Velitski S, Tzaban S, Fiks N, Tekoah Y, Aviezer D (2015) Plant-based oral delivery of β-glucocerebrosidase as an enzyme replacement therapy for Gaucher's disease. Plant Biotechnol J 13(8):1033–1040. https://doi.org/10.1111/pbi.12366

Shi C, Ren Y, Liu L, Wang F, Zhang H, Tian P, Pan T, Wang Y, Jing R, Liu T, Wu F, Lin Q, Lei C, Zhang X, Zhu S, Guo X, Wang J, Zhao Z, Wang J, Zhai H, Cheng Z, Wan J (2019) Ubiquitin specific protease 15 has an important role in regulating grain width and size in rice. Plant Physiol 180(1):381–391. https://doi.org/10.1104/pp.19.00065

Simkin AJ, López-Calcagno PE, Raines CA (2019) Feeding the world: improving photosynthetic efficiency for sustainable crop production. J Exp Bot 70(4):1119–1140. https://doi.org/10.1093/jxb/ery445

Singh RP, Hodson DP, Jin Y, Lagudah ES, Ayliffe MA, Bhavani S, Rouse MN, Pretorius ZA, Szabo LJ, Huerta-Espino J, Basnet BR, Lan C, Hovmøller MS (2015) Emergence and spread of new races of wheat stem rust fungus: continued threat to food security and prospects of genetic control. Phytopathology 105(7):872–884. https://doi.org/10.1094/PHYTO-01-15-0030-FI

Smyth SJ (2017) Genetically modified crops, regulatory delays, and international trade. Food Energy Secur 6(2):78–86

Sun F, Suen PK, Zhang Y, Liang C, Carrie C, Whelan J, Ward JL, Hawkins ND, Jiang L, Lim BL (2012) A dual-targeted purple acid phosphatase in *Arabidopsis thaliana* moderates carbon metabolism and its over-expression leads to faster plant growth and higher seed yield. New Phytol 194:206–219

Sun F, Yu H, Qu J, Cao Y, Ding L, Feng W, Khalid MHB, Li W, Fu F (2020) Maize ZmBES1/BZR1-5 decreases ABA sensitivity and confers tolerance to osmotic stress in transgenic *Arabidopsis*. Int J Mol Sci 21(3):E996. https://doi.org/10.3390/ijms21030996

Swartzberg D, Dai N, Gan S, Amasino RM, Granot D (2006) Effects of cytokinin production under two SAG promoters on senescence and development of tomato plants. Plant Biol 8:579–586

Talsma EF, Brouwer ID, Verhoef H, Mbera GN, Mwangi AM, Demir AY, Maziya-Dixon B, Boy E, Zimmermann MB, Melse-Boonstra A (2016) Biofortified yellow cassava and vitamin A status of Kenyan children: a randomized controlled trial. Am J Clin Nutr 103(1):258–267

Thomas WT (2015) Drought-resistant cereals: impact on water sustainability and nutritional quality. Proc Nutr Soc 74(3):191–197

Tohge T, Zhang Y, Peterek S, Matros A, Rallapalli G, Tandrón YA, Butelli E, Kallam K, Hertkorn N, Mock HP, Martin C, Fernie AR (2015) Ectopic expression of snapdragon transcription factors facilitates the identification of genes encoding enzymes of anthocyanin decoration in tomato. Plant J 83(4):686–704

Waltz E (2014) Vitamin A super banana in human trials. Nat Biotechnol 32(9):857

Waltz E (2015) USDA approves next-generation GM potato. Nat Biotechnol 33(1):12–13. https://doi.org/10.1038/nbt0115-12

Wesseler J, Zilberman D (2014) The economic power of the Golden Rice opposition. Environ Dev Econ 19(06):724–742

Wesseler J, Zilberman D (2017) Golden Rice: no progress to be seen. Do we still need it? Environ Dev Econ 22(2):107–109

Wesseler J, Smart RD, Thomson J, Zilberman D (2017) Foregone benefits of important food crop improvements in sub-Saharan Africa. PLoS One 12(7):e0181353. https://doi.org/10.1371/journal.pone.0181353

Yu J, Langridge WH (2001) A plant-based multicomponent vaccine protects mice from enteric diseases. Nat Biotechnol 19(6):548–552

Yuan L, Li R (2020) Metabolic engineering a model oilseed *Camelina sativa* for the sustainable production of high-value designed oils. Front Plant Sci 11:11. https://doi.org/10.3389/fpls.2020.00011

Chapter 12
Food Safety: A Multidimensional Concept

Vinod Kotwal

Abstract Food is an indispensable part of daily life, and therefore, food safety is of paramount importance. Food safety affects people across the globe as millions around the world are severely affected and many lose their life due to consumption of unsafe food. Besides the well-known microbial or chemical challenges of food safety, personal and environmental hygiene also form an important constituent of challenges in ensuring food safety worldwide. As standard and quality of living improve, food safety concerns and potential health hazards continue to be an important public health issue worldwide. Further, safe food warrants sound scientific principles and equitable legislative enforcements. Safe food not only supports nutrition security of the masses, but also helps the national economy to grow and achieve sustainable development goals. This chapter discusses the concept of food safety, multidimensionality of food safety, various sources of risks to food, working principles of risk analysis, operationalizing the risk analysis, and appropriate standards to mitigate the food risks. It also presents view on international perspective in food safety and holistic approaches to food safety.

Keywords Food security · Food trade · Foodborne disease · Codex Alimentarius · Risk analysis

12.1 Introduction

In recent years, food safety has become one of the core issues in the domain of public health. The concept of food safety is closely interlinked to food and nutritional security too. Poverty and inadequate diet cause chronic food insecurity whereas transient food insecurity is the result of risks associated with food availability and the issue of safety of food (Vemula et al. 2012). WHO report delineates that foodborne diseases (FBDs) are a major reason of morbidity and mortality, and FBDs are a

V. Kotwal (✉)
National Pharmaceutical Pricing Authority (NPPA), Government of India, New Delhi, India
e-mail: vinod.kotwal@gov.in

R. S. V., S. Praveen (eds.), *Conceptualizing Plant-Based Nutrition*,
https://doi.org/10.1007/978-981-19-4590-8_12

serious hindrance to the socio-economic development (WHO 2015). FBD can be defined as "any disease usually either infectious or toxic in nature, caused by agents that enter the body through ingestion of food" (Adams and Moss 2003). The FBD could be attributed to the microbes, toxins produced by the microbial agents or any other chemicals that might have gained entry into the food supply chain (Hall et al. 2008; Hui et al. 2001). Thus, the presence of disease-causing agents such as bacteria, viruses, parasites, microbial toxins, or chemicals is responsible for more than 200 human diseases ranging from diarrhea to cancers. An estimate reveals that around 600 million are affected due to FBDs and around 420,000 die annually causing an irreparable loss of around 33 million healthy life years. This burden of illness or disease on the lifespan is calculated based on disability-adjusted life years (DALYs) (Cissé 2019). Furthermore, unsafe food is a contributory agent to the vicious cycle of human disease and malnutrition, critically affecting the infants, and the elderly alike.

In view of some global changes, like rapid urbanization, relentless modifications in microbial and other ecological systems and reduced supplies of food, feed, and fresh water, food safety assumes important position in the twenty-first century (Käferstein and Abdussalam 1999). The Second International Conference on Nutrition (ICN2), held in Rome in November 2014, emphasized the significance of food safety in providing improved human nutrition through healthy diets (Food and Agriculture Organization 2014). It also reiterated the need to launch, implement, and support appropriate food control systems, including the suitable national-level food safety legislation and regulations so as to ensure that all the players of the food chain right from producers and suppliers operate conscientiously. The critical components of a food control system (FCS) are as follows: setting and maintaining science-based standards; robust enforcement and surveillance mechanisms; ensuring proper food safety management systems; and regular, transparent communications to the stakeholders.

Food safety is a key principle to achieve United Nations Sustainable Development Goals (SDGs). SDG 2, 3, 12, and 17 are closely linked to food safety (UN 2020) (Table 12.1) and safe food is an important ingredient for improved economic conditions, public prosperity, development in the field of agriculture, improving the market access, and it ultimately aids tourism and sustainable development. Today food safety is not only a public health priority (WHO 2020) but food safety warranty forms a fundamental tenet of international trade (Carneiro and Kaneene 2017) to guarantee that imported foods conform to prescribed national guidelines (FAO and WHO 2003).

12.2 Multidimensionality of Food Safety

Food Safety and Standards Act of India (FSSAI) (2006) defines food safety as "assurance that food is acceptable for human consumption according to its intended use." This is consistent with the Codex Alimentarius Commission (CAC), joint

Table 12.1 Food safety and linkage to UN Sustainable Development Goals (SDGs)

Sustainable development goal (SDG)	Linkage to food safety
SDG 2: zero hunger	Food security cannot be achieved without food safety. Hence zero hunger refers access to safe, nutritious, and sufficient food to all people and all year round
SDG 3: healthy lives and promotion of well-being all at all stages	People's health and nutritional intake are directly linked to the food safety further FBDs are avertable
SDG 12: ensure sustainable consumption and production patterns	In order to achieve the sustainable food production and consumption by a country, it is imperative to fortify the science and technology-based regulatory regimen to ensure safe and quality food throughout the food chain
SDG 17: rejuvenate the international partnership for sustainable development	In an era of globalized food supply (food exports valued at over USD 1.6 trillion), international cooperation is imperative. Also, food safety is a shared responsibility of all the stakeholders

FAO-WHO Food Standards program framework (Kotwal 2016). CAC, set-up in 1963, is the intergovernmental body mandated to develop code of food and related texts that are part of the Codex Alimentarius, the Food Code.

Food safety and health are measurable indices of the incidence of foodborne illnesses and quality of life or the alleviation from communicable (food poisoning, acute diarrhea, etc.) and non-communicable (obesity, diabetes, hypertension, etc.) diseases. Considering the impact of FBDs on the overall human health, it is important that National Governments initiate public policy interventions and put in place regulatory systems to coordinate effective food safety protocols so that the entire food chains operate responsibly to ensure safe supply of food to the end users. The food safety management protocols at international level have witnessed a shift toward risk-based approach wherein the regulators are adopting risk analysis framework as a major instrument for decision-making (Koutsoumanis and Aspridou 2016).

12.3 Risks from Various Sources to Food

A number of hazards have been associated with food and the process of food consumption. Biological contaminants such as bacteria, viruses, and parasites are a significant source of FBDs. Also, physical hazards like pieces of glass in pulses and chemical hazards related to food that may either be natural chemical components of food (Lathyrus toxin in *Lathyrus sativus*) or human-made (e.g., chemical preservatives added to food) or residues of pesticides/insecticides/veterinary drugs or natural toxins in food, etc., are documented. Food regulatory systems all over the world therefore strive to manage the risk, i.e., the probability of something going wrong.

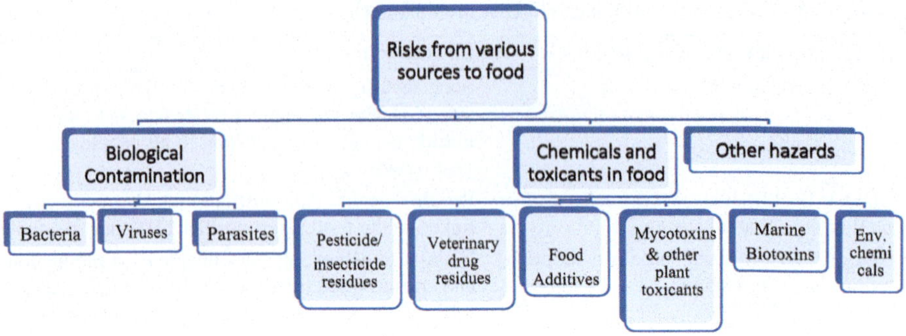

Fig. 12.1 Risks from various sources to food

Various types of risks associated with food are from different sources (Fig. 12.1). The details of common causes of biological contamination, chemicals and other toxicants, and other hazards are presented in Table 12.2.

12.4 Principles of Risk Analysis

To determine the risk of a particular situation, one must know the hazard and measure the exposure to it. Therefore, risk is represented as:

$$\text{Risk} = \text{Hazard} \times \text{Exposure}.$$

CAC has defined the concept of risk as "a function of the probability of an adverse health effect and the severity of that effect, consequential to a hazard(s) in food." Hazard is defined as any agent (biological, chemical, or physical) or condition of food that could potentially cause an ill health. Hence, risk analysis, with reference to food, comprises three main activities such as risk assessment, risk management, and risk communication. Based on the working principles for risk analysis adopted by CAC in the year 2003, these activities are distinct, nevertheless closely interlinked (Fig. 12.2). The main objectives of these principles are to serve as a guide for the activities of CAC, the Joint FAO/WHO expert bodies, and other consultations so that risk analysis forms the basis for food safety and health-related operations of Codex. The characteristic feature of risk analysis used in Codex suggests that the analysis has to be consistent, transparent with appropriate documentation, conducted in accordance with scientific principles governing Codex decision-making process among others. Also, it should be amenable for modification in light of future scientific discoveries.

Table 12.2 Common causes of biological contamination, chemicals, other toxicants, and other hazards

Risks	Source		
Biological contamination	Bacteria	*Bacillus cereus, Campylobacter jejuni, Clostridium perfringens, Escherichia coli, Listeria* spp., *Salmonella, Shigella* spp., *Staphylococcus aureus, Vibrio* spp., *Yersinia enterocolitica*	
	Viruses	Norovirus, Hepatitis A virus, Rotaviruses	
	Parasites	Protozoa	*Entamoeba histolytica, Cryptosporidium parvum, Giardia lamblia, Toxoplasma gondii*
		Roundworms, nematodes	*Anisakis simplex, Pseudoterranova decipiens, Ascaris lumbricoides, Trichinella spiralis*
		Tapeworms, Cestodes	*Taenia saginata, Diphyllobothrium latum, Taenia solium*
Chemicals and toxicants in food	Pesticides/insecticides		
	Veterinary drug residues		
	Food additives		
	Natural toxins	Mycotoxins (secondary metabolites of fungi) *Aflatoxins* from *Aspergillus parasiticus* and *A. flavus* *Ochratoxins* produced by *Aspergillus* and *Penicillium* species *Trichothecenes* are mainly produced by *Fusarium* species but *Trichoderma, Trichothecium, Myrothecium, Calonectria,* and *Stachybotrys* are also known as trichothecene producers *Ergot alkaloids* from fungus *Claviceps purpurea* growing parasitically on some grasses and several cereal crops such as wheat, barley, and rye *Fumonisins* mainly produced by *Fusarium moniliforme,* plant pathogen growing on maize	
	Inherent plant toxins	*Glycoalkaloids*: α-solanine and α-chaconine in potatoes *Glucosinolates*: Occur mainly in family Cruciferae *Cyanogens*: Occur widely in plants including cassava, sorghum, almonds, bamboo, and legume seeds *Hydrazines*: Mushroom hydrazines are considered plant toxins *Pyrrolizidine alkaloids*: Occur in herbs, herbal teas, and comfrey *Antinutrients*: Components of plants that interfere with metabolic processes *Other plant toxins*: Coumarins, furocoumarins, saponins, vicine, lupin alkaloids, etc.	
	Marine phycotoxins or marine biotoxins: Shellfish poisons (produced by dinoflagellates belonging to genus *Alexandrium*) and the ciguatera toxins (harbored by finfish and toxins originate from benthic dinoflagellates *Gambierdiscus toxicus*)		
	Environmental chemicals: Heavy metals like lead, calcium, mercury entering the food chain		
Other hazards	Diets deficient in micronutrients like iodine, iron, niacin, vitamin A, niacin		

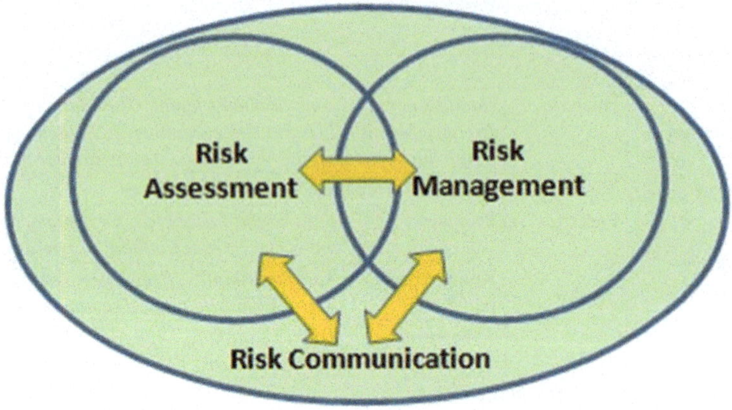

Fig. 12.2 Process of risk analysis

12.5 Operationalization of Risk Analysis Framework

Classical hazard-based approach of food safety relies heavily on the frequent regulatory inspections followed by food sampling, which may not yield considerable consumer protection. Moreover, in the classical hazard-based strategy, presence of a potentially harmful agent at a detectable level warrants risk management activities. Of late, regulatory bodies around the globe are moving toward establishing risk-based approaches to food safety control wherein the criteria are to assess whether any unacceptable risks to health exist or not (Barlow et al. 2015; Koutsoumanis and Aspridou 2016).

A generic framework of a risk-based food safety management system comprises four distinct stages (FAO 2006). First stage involves preliminary risk management activities such as (1) food safety issue identification, (2) developing a risk profile, (3) establishing risk management goals, (4) decision regarding the requirement for the risk assessment, (5) establishing suitable policy, (6) developing risk ranking, and (7) analysis of the results. In the second stage, various risk management options are evaluated and suitable one is selected. Third stage comprises implementation of measures to manage the risk. The measures could be mandatory through legislation or voluntary followed by codes of practice and defined guidelines. In this step, role of communication tools is also very crucial in order to implement consumer-related risk management decisions. In the final stage, effective monitoring activities have to be undertaken to ascertain the efficient implementation of risk management measures. Hence, activities such as surveillance of public health and collection of data related to changes in rates of foodborne illness are conducted. Also, revamp of food safety controls is required when the intended goals of food safety are not achieved

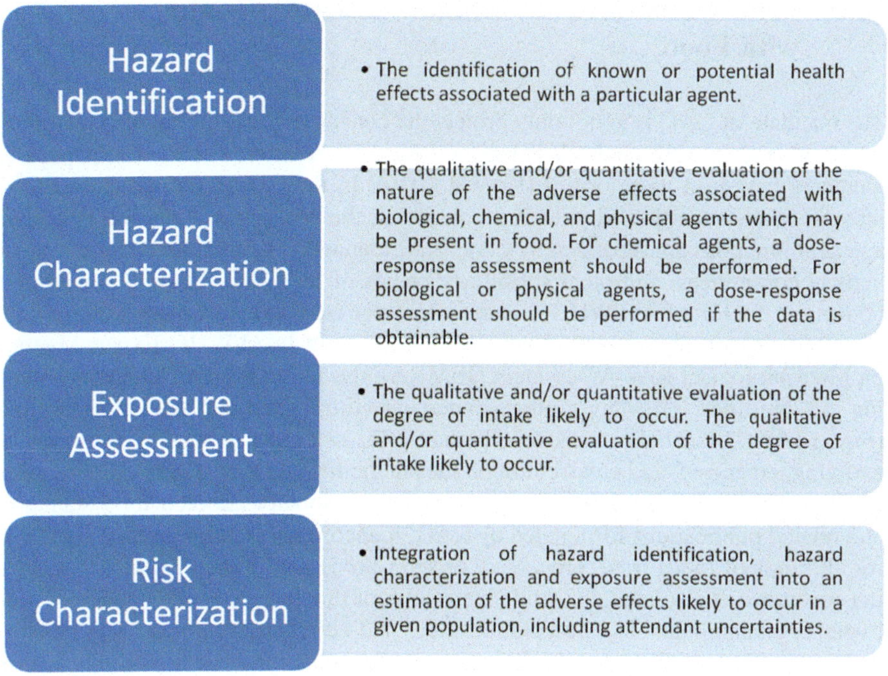

Fig. 12.3 Steps involved in risk assessment

and this iterative process can be repeated depending upon the necessity (Koutsoumanis and Aspridou 2016)

Thus, risk analysis has emerged as the cornerstone for developing food safety systems and policies (Buchanan 2010) as a systematic approach for making decisions related to food safety. It consists of a three-stage process as follows (FAO/WHO 1995, 1997) (1) *risk assessment*: any risk posed by the foodborne hazard to human health is ascertained. Thus, risk assessment involves (a) identification of hazard; (b) characterization of hazard; (c) assessment of exposure to hazard; and (d) characterization of risk (Fig. 12.3); (2) *risk management*: appropriate decisions are made with respect to the threshold level of risk that is acceptable and effective risk control measures that are required to be implemented; and (3) *risk communication*: a major component wherein risk information and selected control methods are communicated among the stakeholders. Though it is recognized that risk analysis is an iterative process that warrants effective interaction between the risk assessors and risk managers, a functional separation among these two entities is obligatory to avoid conflict of interest and to uphold scientific integrity.

12.6 Setting Standards to Mitigate Risks Associated with Food

The mandate of CAC is to not only protect the consumers' health but also guarantee fair food trade practices. It shall prepare the draft standards with the help of its members based on its priorities (Kotwal 2016). In the process of development of international standards and guidelines on foods, the risk assessment and risk management functions are separated by CAC. Risk managers include the general subject, vertical committees, and other subsidiary bodies of the CAC. The risk assessment bodies are the Joint FAO/WHO Expert Committee on Food Additives (JECFA), the Joint Meeting on pesticide residues (JMPR), the Joint FAO/WHO Expert Meeting on Microbiological Risk Assessment (JEMRA), the Joint FAO/WHO Expert Meeting on Nutrition (JEMNU) other expert meetings, and ad hoc consultations (Fig. 12.4). These risk assessment bodies offer scientific advice with regard to evolving, emerging, and cross-cutting issues in the field of food safety upon request.

Thus, Codex Alimentarius is a compilation of globally adopted food standards and related publications formulated by CAC. It encompasses international standards for all kinds of foods (raw, processed, or semi-processed) meant for distribution to the consumer. It also contains guidelines/codes of practices for food additives, food hygiene, contaminants like pesticide residues and veterinary drugs in food, labeling and presentation of food commodities, appropriate food analytical methods, export import inspection, and certification. Codex standards are not alternatives for national legislation; however, national legislations have freedom to include the Codex standards in their respective legislations/regulations.

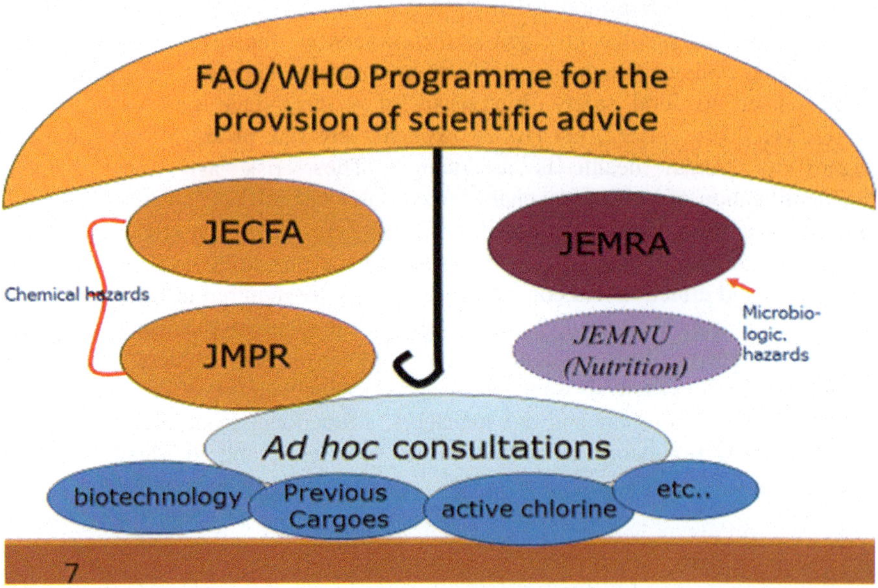

Fig. 12.4 FAO/WHO framework for provision of scientific advice

The General and Vertical Codex Committees are the risk managers. General Subject Committees work is applicable to all the Commodity Committees and hence is also referred to as "horizontal committees." These Committees are involved in developing appropriate concepts and principles applicable for foods in general. On the other hand, Commodity Committees are responsible for formulating specific food standards often called as "vertical standards." As on February 2022, there are ten and four active General subject and Vertical committees, respectively.

In addition, Commission may establish an Ad hoc Intergovernmental Task Force (TF) for a *specific purpose* and *specified period*. Currently, only Task Force on Antimicrobial Resistance (TFAM) remains active. The details of different risks associated with food and the committee handling are given in Table 12.3. The horizontal standards can be divided into broad three categories namely standards, guidelines, and recommended codes of practices while vertical standards are primarily standards.

12.7 Prevention and Control of Various Hazards

As elaborated in Sect. 12.1, foodborne diseases are caused by a wide range of agents (Table 12.2) and three hazards associated with them are microbiological, chemical, and physical. These hazards can be introduced in the supply chain during production, harvesting, processing operations, storage and transportation, preparation of food, and while serving of food. Biological contamination caused by bacteria, viruses, and parasites is a major source of FBDs and a major source of microbiological hazards. Similarly, it is important to ensure the chemical safety of food supplies as chemicals and toxicants originate from residues of pesticides/insecticides/veterinary drugs, food additives, environmental chemicals, or natural sources (natural toxins, inherent plant toxins, and marine phycotoxins), which are major chemical hazards. Physical hazards can result from accidental contamination/poor food handling practices, and/or adulteration.

12.8 Microbiological Hazards

Depending upon geo-climate, type of crops produced, socio-economic development, the health problems related to food contamination vary across the globe. However, the basic principles for prevention and control of microbiological hazards are available (Käferstein et al. 2019). Adoption of good agricultural practices and animal husbandry activities including the appropriate environmental conditions, where animals are reared, would result in hygienic quality raw food. The control of hazards pertaining to contamination, recontamination, or continued existence of microbial hazards during processing can be restricted by following strategies such as good manufacturing practice (GMP), good hygiene practice (GHP), and hazard analysis and critical control points (HACCP) program (Huss et al. 2000).

Table 12.3 Codex Committees and their role in food safety

S. no.	Subsidiary body	Remarks
General subject committees		
1.	Codex Committee on contaminants in foods	Responsible for establishment or endorsing permitted maximum levels (MLs) or guideline levels for contaminants and naturally occurring toxicants in food and feed
2.	Codex Committee on food additives	Responsible for establishment or endorsing permitted MLs for individual food additives
3.	Codex Committee on food hygiene	Responsible for drafting basic provisions on food hygiene applicable to all food
4.	Codex Committee on food import and export certification and inspection systems	To develop principles and guidelines for food import and export inspection and certification systems
5.	Codex Committee on food labelling	To draft provisions on labeling applicable to all food
6.	Codex Committee on general principles	Deals with procedural and general matters referred to it by CAC
7.	Codex Committee on methods of analysis and sampling	To define the criteria appropriate to Codex methods of analysis and sampling
8.	Codex Committee on nutrition and foods for special dietary uses	Looking at general nutritional issues
9.	Codex Committee on pesticide residues	To establish MLs for pesticide residues in specific food or groups of food or animal feed
10.	Codex Committee on residues of veterinary drugs in foods	To recommend MLs of residues of veterinary drugs in food and feed
Commodity Committees[a]		
1.	Codex Committee on fish and fishery products	To elaborate worldwide standards for fresh, frozen (including quick frozen), or otherwise processed fish, crustaceans, and mollusks
2.	Codex Committee on fresh fruits and vegetables	To elaborate worldwide standards and codes of practices as may be appropriate for fresh fruits and vegetables
3.	Codex Committee on spices and culinary herbs	To elaborate worldwide standards for fats and oils of animal, vegetable, and marine origin including margarine and olive oil
4.	Codex Committee on fats and oils	To elaborate worldwide standards for spices and culinary herbs in their dried and dehydrated state in whole, ground, cracked, or crushed form

[a]Five committees were abolished and eight adjourned sine die

The Codex Committee on Food Hygiene (CCFH) had developed the first Recommended Code of Practice (RCP) under Codex Alimentarius on the *General Principles of Food Hygiene* in 1969. It was amended in 1999 and was further revised in the years 1997, 2003, and 2020. These General Principles form a strong foundation to ensure food hygiene. It traverses the entire food chain right from primary production through final consumption, highlighting the salient hygiene controls at each stage. It also recommended HACCP-based approach wherever possible to enhance food safety including the seven principles of HACCP (Box 12.1) to be followed. In addition, there are other RCPs too that recommend code of hygienic practices for meat, milk and milk products, eggs and egg products, tree nuts, canned fruits, vegetable products, etc. There are a number of guidelines established by CCFH too that focus on various aspects of food safety (Table 12.4).

Box 12.1: Seven principles of the HACCP system

Principle 1: Conduct hazard analysis.

Principle 2: Determine the critical control points (CCPs).

Principle 3: Establish critical limit(s).

Principle 4: Establish a system to monitor control of the CCP.

Principle 5: Establish the corrective action to be taken when monitoring indicates that a particular CCP is not under control.

Principle 6: Establish procedures for verification to confirm that the HACCP system is working effectively

Principle 7: Establish documentation concerning all procedures and records appropriate to these principles and their application.

Table 12.4 Guidelines formulated by Codex Committee on Food Hygiene (CCFH)

S. no.	Name of the guideline	Year of adoption
1.	Principles and guidelines for the establishment and application of microbiological criteria related to foods	2013
2.	Principles and guidelines for the conduct of microbiological risk assessment	2014
3.	Guidelines on the application of general principles of food hygiene to the control of *Listeria monocytogenes* in ready-to-eat foods	2009
4.	Principles and guidelines for the conduct of microbiological risk management	2008
5.	Guideline for the validation of food safety control measures	2008
6.	Guidelines on the application of general principles of food hygiene to the control of pathogenic vibrio species in seafood	2010
7.	Guidelines for the control of *Campylobacter* and *Salmonella* in chicken meat	2011
8.	Guidelines on the application of general principles of food hygiene to the control of viruses in food	2012
9.	Guidelines for the control of *Taenia saginata* in meat of domestic cattle	2014
10.	Guidelines for the control of *Trichinella* spp. in meat of Suidae	
11.	Guidelines on the application of general principles of food hygiene to the control of foodborne parasites	2016
12.	Guidelines for the control of non typhoidal *Salmonella* spp. in beef and pork meat	2016

Second, application of processing technologies not only extends the shelf life of the food and food products but also enhances their safety by decreasing or eliminating the pathogenic microorganisms. Pasteurization, sterilization, fermentation, irradiation, or thermal heating not only extends the shelf life of foods but also increases their safety levels. However, consumers have started demanding fresh foods packed with dense nutrients and antioxidants besides the appropriate food safety. Technological advancements in the field of food processing and application of thermal sterilization/pasteurization approaches significantly reduce the content of microorganisms; however, it also causes loss of thermo-labile nutrients and severely impairs the food sensory and nutritional properties. Therefore, advancements and adoption of many non-thermal treatments such as high hydrostatic pressure, pulsed electric fields, pulsed light, ultraviolet light, and cold plasma have gained prominence (Morales-de la Peña et al. 2019; Prithviraj et al. 2021; Kaavya et al. 2021). Application of nanotechnology in the field of food safety is also increasing (Alfadul and Elneshwy 2010).

Poor hygiene standards, while preparing the food and the lack of trained food handlers in the field of food safety, are important causes of FBD (Greig et al. 2007). Food handlers can transmit pathogens actively or passively (Fig. 12.5). To overcome these problems, not only food handlers need to be trained in maintaining personal hygiene and good hygienic practices at work, but attention also needs to be paid to the occupational hazards and measures to prevent those (Dudeja and Singh 2017). Codex Alimentarius also has a number of RCPs and GLs focusing on these aspects of food safety. For example, *Codex Code of Hygienic Practice for Precooked and Cooked Foods in Mass Catering* deals with the hygienic requirements for foods meant for large masses of public including school children and elderly.

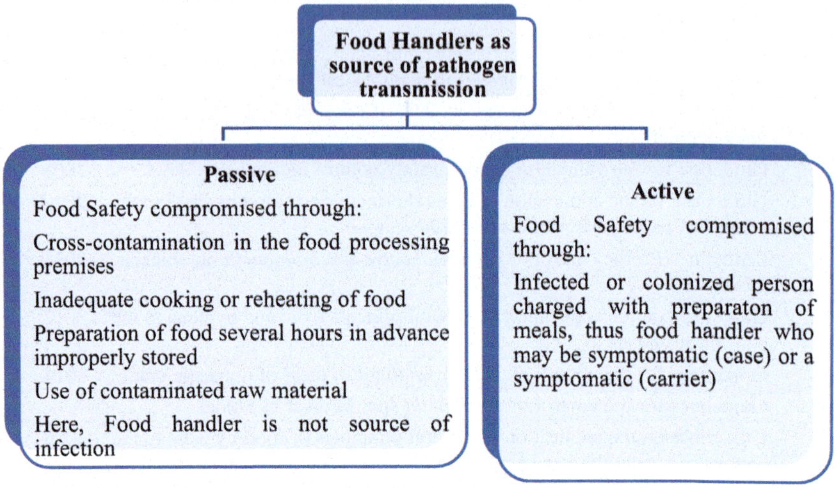

Fig. 12.5 Food handlers as source of pathogen transmission

12.9 Chemical Hazards

Wide range of health risks are posed by chemical hazards in food varying from irritation to chronic diseases and cancer as certain chemicals are proven carcinogenic. Chemical hazards can be prevented and controlled following a multi-pronged approach. To begin with, during production of food, quantities of chemicals added should lie within the limits prescribed by legislation. At the international level, CAC has established these through its various committees. For example, Codex Committee on Food Additives (CCFA) establishes permissible MLs for individual food additives. Codex Committee on Pesticide Residues (CCPR) establishes MLs for pesticide residues in food items and for animal feeds. Similarly, Codex Committee on Residues of Veterinary Drugs in Foods (CCRVDF) is involved in prioritizing the deliberations on veterinary drugs-related residues in foods and fixes a maximum permissible limit for the same. Codex Alimentarius has also laid down *General Standards for Contaminants and Toxins in food and feed.* The Codex has defined the maximum level (ML) for a chemical contaminant in a food or feed. It refers to the highest permissible concentration of that contaminant in food as recommended by the CAC that could be lawfully acceptable. For example, ML of total aflatoxins in peanuts and hazelnuts is 15 μg/kg while it is 10 μg/kg for almonds, pistachios, and dried figs. Similarly, ML of ochratoxin A allowed in wheat, barley, and rye is 5 μg/kg. These limits are laid down based on the risk assessment done by JECFA.

Likewise, countries through legislations have prescribed limits for these chemicals. For example, in India Food Safety and Standards (Contaminants, Toxins and Residues) Regulation, 2011 lays down the limits for various types of contaminants, toxins, and residues allowed in foods. Apart from laying down standards for various food products, Food Safety and Standards (Food Products Standards and Food Additives) Regulation, 2011, also prescribes the list of permitted additives in food along with their limits. However, adherence to these limits would require implementation of good agricultural and animal husbandry practices along with good manufacturing practices.

Another approach to prevent and control chemical hazards is to adopt technology. For instance, application of suitable drying technology could avert the growth of mold and mycotoxins production during storage. For instance, *Codex Code of Practice for the Prevention and Reduction of Mycotoxins Contamination in Cereals* provides recent updates regarding the prevention and reduction of contamination of mycotoxin in foods derived from cereals and animal feeds. The Code clearly lays down the importance of adoption of GAP (especially during post-harvest handling, and storage) by the primary producers to avoid contamination due to mycotoxins followed by implementation of GMP (during handling, grain sorting, cleaning, etc.) by processing industries. *Codex Code of Practice for the Prevention and Reduction of Aflatoxin contamination in Tree nuts* enumerates common principles for aflatoxins reduction in tree nuts. It is mandatory for the National Authorities to instruct all the stakeholders, viz., producers, transporters, and storage personnel in the processing chain about the measures and environmental factors that hasten the process of fungal infections in tree nuts leading to the production of aflatoxin. Food irradiation can be used for insect disinfestations and also inhibits spoilage losses due to sprouting (Loaharanu and Ahmed 1991).

Monitoring, inspection, and surveillance activities of domestic as well as imported foods through an efficient National Food Control System (NFCS) entail the incorporation of regulatory approaches along with sound preventive and educational strategies to ensure safety of food from farm to table (FAO and WHO 2003). Codex Alimentarius guidelines (CAC/GL 82-2013) on principles governing NFCS have articulated 13 principles that are: Protection of consumers; Whole food chain approach; Transparency, Defining specific roles and responsibilities in NFCS; Consistency and impartiality; Risk-based, science-based and evidence-based decision making; Cooperation and coordination between multiple competent authorities; Preventive measures; Self-assessment and review procedure; Recognition of other systems (including equivalence); Legal foundation; Harmonisation; and Sufficient resources to meet the objectives of NFCS (Table 12.5). Thus, there is a need to

Table 12.5 Principles governing national food control system

S. no.	Principles
1.	Protection of consumers
2.	*Whole food chain approach*: Should cover the entire food chain from production to consumption
3.	*Transparency*: All aspects of NFCS should be transparent and open to scrutiny by all stakeholders while respecting legal requirement to protect confidentiality, wherever applicable
4.	*Roles and responsibilities*: Specific roles and responsibilities of participants in NFCS should be clearly defined
5.	*Consistency and impartiality*: All aspects of NFCS should be applied consistently and impartially, free of improper or undue influence, or conflict of interest
6.	*Risk-based, science-based, and evidence-based decision-making*: Decisions within NFCS should be based on scientific information, evidence, and/or risk analysis principles as appropriate
7.	*Cooperation and coordination between multiple competent authorities*: Competent authorities in NFCS should operate in a cooperative and coordinated manner
8.	*Preventive measures*: To prevent and when necessary to respond to food safety incidents
9.	*Self-assessment and review procedures*: NFCS should possess the capacity and capability to undergo continuous improvement and review of its objectives
10.	*Recognition of other systems (including equivalence)*: Concept of recognition of systems, including equivalence should be provided for in the NFCS
11.	*Legal foundation*: Fundamental legal structures should be in place
12.	*Harmonization*: Codex standards including international intergovernmental organizations to be considered
13.	*Resources*: NFCS should have sufficient resources to meet its objectives

articulate a comprehensive, integrated approach for food safety in any country with public health as an integral part.

12.10 International Perspective in Food Safety

The large-scale integration of global food industry, spread beyond the traditional national boundaries, catering to food availability and food diversification at the global level also raises concerns of food safety. In this context, measures to tackle food safety concerns and nutritional measures for diverse geographical regions, institutions, and development of international food standards based on sound scientific principles are all the more important.[1] Every year, millions of people suffer from FBD causing great socio-economic loss to the society (WHO 2015) and this has prompted countries across the globe to strengthen their food regulatory systems. The attributes of latest food regulatory systems are based on the strong foundations of responsiveness, being outcome oriented, predictability, proportionality, and independence (Committee on Strengthening Core Elements of Regulatory Systems in Developing Countries; Board on Global Health; Board on Health Sciences Policy; Institute of Medicine, et al. 2012).

The Codex Standards, Guidelines, and Codes of practices formed the reference for Agreement on Sanitary and Phytosanitary Measures (SPS agreement) under WTO in 1995. Thus, Codex Alimentarius along with World Organization for Animal Health (OIE) and the International Plant Protection Convention (IPPC) is one of "the three sisters" for human, animal, and plant health, respectively. Consequently, the Standards of Codex are considered as an international criterion for the evaluation of national legislative measures with reference to food safety. Further, these standards are evaluated for implementation under WTO Agreements and are consistent with the WTO Technical barriers to trade.

Adoption of new regulations, such as WTO agreement on SPS, involves applications of risk analysis principles which warrant regulatory actions strictly based on scientific risk assessment. Further, countries are expected to associate their targeted level of protection with its regulatory goals which in turn are linked to the extant systems of standards and inspection. All these measures are to be undertaken with minimal possible restrictions on the international trade on food.[2]

12.11 Holistic Approach to Ensure Food Safety

Any country implementing risk analysis framework needs to put in place three essential building blocks as given below:

[1] http://www.who.int/bulletin/volumes/91/7/13-125518/en/

[2] http://ageconsearch.umn.edu/bitstream/16567/1/fo031004.pdf

12.11.1 Science-Based Food Quality and Safety Standards

Standards and regulations based on science and also to harmonize the domestic food Standards with international Standards including the Codex Alimentarius Standards.

12.11.2 Food Safety Regulation, Quality Testing, and Risk-Based Surveillance

Laboratories are an integral part of the food safety system. For efficient food safety management, the food testing laboratories need to be strengthened; new ones' set-up, if required; and most importantly networked for the flow of information. These then have to be integrated with a robust surveillance network active as well as passive, which in turn will handshake with all the ports of entry of food into the country. This will lead to the creation of integrated food risk assessment and surveillance network.

12.11.3 Support Services and Communication

An increasingly important role is the delivery of information; education, and advice to the stakeholders across the value chain particularly the consumers. This would involve undertaking mass awareness programs, conducting capacity-building activities and regular communication with all the stakeholders.

Many types of information are required to implement a modern, science-based risk approach to food safety to prevent FBDs and assure the consumers about the safety of the food they are consuming. The wide range of information that a modern food safety regulatory system requires is illustrated in Table 12.6. The wide range of information illustrated above comes from a wide range of sources, and there are multiple users of this information, thus adding to the complexity.

12.12 Conclusion

It is apparent that adoption of food safety measures is a mutual responsibility of multiple players (Jen 2017). Moreover, the industry, academia, government, consumers, and media constitute the five pillars of food safety. The shared responsibilities among these entities are imperative for successful implementation of food safety programs. Nevertheless, broadening of stakeholder base and inducting food testing laboratories within the fold would be quite valuable in the long run as they play a significant role in risk analysis framework. Analysis and prevention of untoward incidents with respect to food safety require a large quantum of

Table 12.6 Categories and types of food safety information

Category	Type of information	
Human health	Illness surveillance	Attribution Health valuation
	Medical/clinical	
	Host factors	
Measurement of contamination	Microbiological contamination	Other contamination
	Chemical contamination	Contamination of imports
Indicators of contamination	Animal health/disposition	Sanitation and inspection
	Recalls and violations	
Hazard identification	Pathogen subtyping	Food toxicology
	Pathogen biology	
Modeling	Predictive microbiology	Risk assessment
Total diet study	Hazard characterization based on food consumed	Exposure assessment
Trade and industry	Facilities and processes	Intervention cost
	FSMS	Economic impacts
	Trace back	International trade
	Intervention efficacy	
Consumers and workers	Food consumption	Risk perception/ communication
	Consumer and worker behavior	Population and demographics
Food and environment	Food composition and characteristics	Environmental characteristics

Source: Modified from "Harnessing knowledge to ensure Food Safety: Opportunities to Improve the Nation's Food Safety Information Infrastructure"

information regarding detection, regulation, supervision, and information on prior cases. In addition, a common platform for discussion among the stakeholders such as public health, veterinary and food safe experts, experts in epidemiology is warranted to assess the trends in the established diseases and to detect novel emerging pathogens. Also, it is pertinent to comprehend the relationship between these pathogens and their respective environments in the process of transmission to formulate prevention and control strategies in a proactive manner.

References

Adams MR, Moss MO (2003) Significance of foodborne diseases. In: Food microbiology, 2nd edn. RSC Publishing, Cambridge, pp 160–164

Alfadul SM, Elneshwy AA (2010) Use of nanotechnology in food processing, packaging and safety—review. Afr J Food Agric Nutr Dev 10(6):58068. https://doi.org/10.4314/ajfand.v10i6.58068

Barlow SM, Boobis AR, Bridges J, Cockburn A, Dekant W, Hepburn P, Houben GF, König J, Nauta MJ, Schuermans J, Bánáti D (2015) The role of hazard- and risk-based approaches in ensuring food safety. Trends Food Sci Technol 46(2, Part A):176–188

Buchanan RL (2010) Understanding and managing food safety risks. Food Safety Magazine, Troy, pp 25–31

Carneiro P, Kaneene JB (2017) Food inspection services: a comparison of programs in the US and Brazil. Food Control 80(Supplement C):314–318

Cissé G (2019) Food-borne and water-borne diseases under climate change in low-and middle-income countries: further efforts needed for reducing environmental health exposure risks. Acta Trop 194:181–188

Committee on Strengthening Core Elements of Regulatory Systems in Developing Countries; Board on Global Health; Board on Health Sciences Policy; Institute of Medicine (2012) In: Riviere JE, Buckley GJ (eds) Ensuring safe foods and medical products through stronger regulatory systems abroad. National Academies Press (US), Washington, DC

Dudeja P, Singh A (2017) Food handlers. In: Gupta RK, Dudeja P, Minhas AS (eds) Food safety in the 21st century. Academic Press, Amsterdam, pp 269–280

FAO (2006) Food safety risk analysis: a guide for national food safety authorities. FAO Food and Nutrition Paper

FAO/WHO (1995) Application of risk analysis to food standards issues: report of the Joint FAO/WHO expert consultation, Geneva, Switzerland, 17 March 1995

FAO/WHO (1997) Risk management and food safety. Report of Joint FAO/WHO consultation, Rome, Italy, 27 to 31 January 1997. United Nations, FAO Food Nutr. Paper

FAO and WHO (2003) Assuring food safety and quality: guidelines for strengthening national food control systems. FAO, Rome. https://www.fao.org/3/y8705e/y8705e.pdf. Accessed 27 Dec 2021

Food and Agriculture Organization (2014) Rome declaration on nutrition. https://www.fao.org/3/ml542e/ml542e.pdf. Accessed 9 Jan 2022

Greig JD, Todd EC, Bartleson CA, Michaels BS (2007) Outbreaks where food workers have been implicated in the spread of foodborne disease. Part 1. Description of the problem, methods, and agents involved. J Food Prot 70(7):1752–1761

Hall G, Vall H, Kirk M (2008) Foodborne illness: overview. International Encyclopedia of public health. Elsevier, Amsterdam, pp 638–653

Hui YH, Merle D, Pierson J, Gorham R (2001) Surveillance of foodborne diseases. Foodborne Dis Handb 1:541–543

Huss HH, Reilly A, Embarek PKB (2000) Prevention and control of hazards in seafood. Food Control 11(2):149–156

Jen JJ (2017) Shared responsibility of food safety. In: Jen JJ, Chen J (eds) Food safety in China: science, technology, management and regulation. Wiley, New York, pp 1–14

Kaavya R, Pandiselvam R, Abdullah S, Sruthi NU, Jayanath Y, Ashokkumar C, Khanashyam AC, Kothakota A, Ramesh SV (2021) Emerging non-thermal technologies for decontamination of *Salmonella* in food. Trends Food Sci Technol 112:400–418

Käferstein F, Abdussalam M (1999) Food safety in the 21st century. Bull World Health Organ 77(4):347

Käferstein FK, Motarjemi Y, Moy GG, Quevado F (2019) Food safety: a worldwide public issue. In: International food safety handbook. Routledge, New York, pp 1–20

Kotwal V (2016) Codex Alimentarius Commission: role in international food standards setting. In: Caballero B, Finglas PM, Toldrá F (eds) Encyclopedia of food and health. Academic Press, Oxford, pp 197–205

Koutsoumanis KP, Aspridou Z (2016) Moving towards a risk-based food safety management. Curr Opin Food Sci 12:36–41

Loaharanu P, Ahmed M (1991) Advantages and disadvantages of the use of irradiation for food preservation. J Agric Environ Ethics 4(1):14–30

Morales-de la Peña M, Welti-Chanes J, Martín-Belloso O (2019) Novel technologies to improve food safety and quality. Curr Opin Food Sci 30:1–7. https://doi.org/10.1016/j.cofs.2018.10.009

Prithviraj V, Pandiselvam R, Babu AC, Kothakota A, Manikantan MR, Ramesh SV, Beegum PS, Mathew AC, Hebbar KB (2021) Emerging non-thermal processing techniques for preservation of tender coconut water. LWT 149:111850

United Nations (2020) Food safety and sustainable development goals. https://www.un.org/en/observances/food-safety-day/background. Accessed 9 Jan 2022

Vemula SR, Kumar RN, Polasa K (2012) Foodborne diseases in India—a review. Br Food J 114(5): 661–680. https://doi.org/10.1108/00070701211229954

World Health Organization (2015) WHO estimates of the global burden of foodborne diseases: foodborne disease burden epidemiology reference group 2007–2015. World Health Organization, Geneva

World Health Organization (2020) Food safety. Key facts. http://www.who.int/mediacentre/factsheets/fs399/en/. Accessed 30 Dec 2021

Chapter 13
Future Perspectives: Plant-Based Nutrition

Ramesh S. V. and Shelly Praveen

Abstract The concept of plant-based human nutrition deserves a major shift in planning dietary requirements, identification of potential sources of nutrients, and to unravel its impending effects on human health. It also requires collaborative research approaches in the field of nutrition science, sociology, human medicine, plant breeding among others. A glance at the huge leap of scientific literature in the field of plant-based nutrition suggests that this concept has gained the status of 'next-big thing' in the field of nutrition science. This chapter discusses the prospects and future course of action in the context of wide acceptance and adoption of plant-based human nutrition for the wellness of personal, societal, and planetary health.

Keywords Antioxidants · Human health · Metabolic fate · Nutrigenomics · Plant-based diet · Plant-based meat substitutes

Accumulating scientific evidences have supported the concept of plant-based nutrition and its health advantages. The whole food, plant-based nutrition, comprise a wide repertoire of ingredients such as whole grains (brown rice, oats, quinoa, etc.), fruits, vegetables, legumes (beans, lentils, soy-based), nuts (of both seed and tree), seeds (flax, chia, hemp, etc.), herbs, leafy green vegetables (lettuce, cabbage, broccoli, etc.), fortified plant milks (soybean, almond, coconut, rice), and spices, individually or their infinite combinations. Further, advances in preventive medicine, meta-analysis, cohort studies, and nutrition interventions have categorically proved the convenience of plant-based nutrition in decreasing the overall mortality and mortality linked to heart diseases, severe reduction in the medication needs, help in

R. S. V. (✉)
Physiology, Biochemistry and Post-Harvest Technology Division, ICAR-Central Plantation Crops Research Institute, Kasaragod, Kerala, India
e-mail: ramesh.sv@icar.gov.in

S. Praveen
Division of Biochemistry, ICAR-Indian Agricultural Research Institute, New Delhi, Delhi, India
e-mail: shellyparveen@icar.gov.in

R. S. V., S. Praveen (eds.), *Conceptualizing Plant-Based Nutrition*,
https://doi.org/10.1007/978-981-19-4590-8_13

weight management, and in greatly reducing the high-risk situations namely obesity, hyperglycemia, hyperlipidemia, hypertension, and even in the reversion of non-communicable diseases such as cardiovascular complications and type 2 diabetes (Hever and Cronise 2017).

Plant-based diets are substantial sources of antioxidants including polyphenols (phenolic acids, flavonoids, proanthocyanins, lignans, stilbenes), carotenoids (carotenes and xanthophylls), co-enzymes (vitamin E, vitamin C), etc. Consumption of antioxidant-rich diets lowers the risk of cancer, neurodegenerative, and cardiovascular diseases and is known for reducing inflammation and improvement in cognitive functions. Antioxidant-rich foods, as in plant-based, negate the ill effects of reactive oxygen species and consequently arrests the process of cellular aging, etc. (Loi and Paciolla 2021). Furthermore, consumption of plant-derived biochemicals either raw or in concentrated forms provides immuno-modulatory effects and anti-tumor benefits (Rodriguez-Casado 2016). It is pertinent to devise suitable and highly efficient extraction procedures so that antioxidants and immunity conferring phytochemicals could be exploited for greater health benefits of human.

Finding right combination of plant-based diet which mimics nutritional profile of animal food for western countries not only requires nutritional intervention but also development of legumes which can withstand cooler climates (Aschemann-Witzel et al. 2021). Therefore, the opportunities for plant biochemists, nutritionists, and breeders to devise suitable cereal–legume nutritional complementation strategies are enormous. Consumer trends have highlighted the preference for 'freedom foods' (plant-based protein is considered 'freedom foods' since it does not carry environmental concerns associated with animal foods) and 'clean label' foods-the tag plant-based foods generally fulfill (Aschemann-Witzel et al. 2021).

Besides the perceived importance of protein quantity and quality in assessing the appropriateness of alternative diet plans, nutritional shift in inorganic nutrient contents also necessitates a thorough investigation. The case in point was exemplified in comparative nutritive profiling study of novel plant-based diets and a reference omnivore diet which revealed that the former was below daily requirements for inorganic nutrients such as Ca, Mg, Zn, and vitamin B12 however showed excessive in saturated fat, sugar, and Na contents (Tso and Forde 2021). This nutritional imbalance encountered due to the shift from animal diet to plant-based nutrition offers massive prospects for designing novel, superior plant-based alternative diets (Tso and Forde 2021).

A comprehensive review on the adoption of plant-based diet clearly points out the objective and perceived barriers such as risk of low protein intake, excessive commitment to consuming meat, the risk of low ingestion of essential micronutrients (vitamin B12, vitamin D, riboflavin, iron, calcium, zinc, etc.), boring and tasteless, among others to switch in to this endeavor (Fehér et al. 2020). Nevertheless, complementation strategies to develop wholesome nutritious food, plant-based meat alternatives (Estell et al. 2021), fermentation techniques to add flavor and acceptability are suggested to overcome these barriers (Tangyu et al. 2019). In this regard, application of advanced and innovative food processing techniques to enhance the nutritional and functional properties of non-dairy, plant-based beverages is also warranted (Munekata et al. 2020). Further, the state-of-the-art metabolomics approaches offer opportunities to continue the process of food innovation, enhancing the sensorial and nutritional attributes of plant-based food and would greatly aid even in climate-smart food production processes (Jacobs et al. 2021).

Multiple studies on human gut microbiota, gut–brain health axis, its role in absorption of essential nutrients, and the microbiota dysbiosis-induced impact on overall human health have necessitated further exploration of influence of individual plant diet-derived components (polyphenols, fibers, etc.) on the gut microbiome composition and their potential health effects. The functional significance of gut microbiota in modulating the bioactivity and bioavailability of dietary components and the microbial enzyme repertoire involved in these processes requires thorough investigation (Marchesi et al. 2016). Even though the influence of vegan diet on the microbial population and their metabolic pathways have been positive by enhancing the beneficial microorganism, further studies are imperative to discover their individualistic effect and devise suitable nutrition plan backed by medicinal science (Sakkas et al. 2020).

Moving forward, the concept of precision nutrition is garnering more attention which tailors the diet depending on the individual's genome, microbiome, metabolome, and epigenome in order to achieve the goal of personalized disease management and prevention. Nevertheless, this arena of precision nutrition is still in its infancy. It is also pertinent to scrutinize and document the local knowledge of plant-based nutrition sources from the traditional foods. The role of relevant disciplines such as ethnobotany and social science techniques is crucial in this endeavor to unearth the nutritional repertoire of forgotten foods (Afrianto et al. 2021). In this framework, it is fundamental to incorporate the concepts of plant-based nutrition in nutrition education in medical curriculum in those regions of the world where animal nutrition is predominant (Mulpuri et al. 2021).

Adoption of novel biotechnological approaches such as 'nutrigenomics' is of paramount importance in order to decipher the impact of diet-derived nutrients in the expression of human genes especially when the diet is primarily derived from non-conventional, neglected, and under-utilized plant sources such as buckwheat (*Fagopyrum esculentum* Moench.), amaranth (*Amaranthus* spp.), quinoa (*Chenopodium quinoa* Wild), and chia (*Salvia hispanica* L.) (Mir et al. 2022). It not only aids in ascertaining the genetic basis of metabolic fate of food but also helps in designing novel super foods to combat lifestyle-induced diseased conditions (Mir et al. 2022). In addition, application of novel biotechnological tool—genome editing—is expected to improve the nutritional and functional quality of cereals, horticultural crops, and other non-conventional crops (Ku and Ha 2020).

Public health nutrition strategies have to be streamlined with renewed interventions and policy framework to improve the overall health of population and the larger goal of sustainable planetary health. The recent developments in the public policy notifications emphasize the concept that healthy food is also more sustainable and vice versa underscores the relevance of plant-based food over animal food (BCFN Foundation 2020; FAO 2020). Food industry and entrepreneurs are required to be aware of the road ahead and the challenges posed due to the increasing trend of plant-based food.

References

Afrianto WF, Tamnge F, Hidayatullah T, Hasanah LN (2021) Local knowledge of plant-based nutrition sources from forgotten foods in Datengan Village, East Java, Indonesia. Asian J Ethnobiol 4(1):106. https://doi.org/10.13057/asianjethnobiol/y040106

Aschemann-Witzel J, Gantriis RF, Fraga P, Perez-Cueto FJ (2021) Plant-based food and protein trend from a business perspective: markets, consumers, and the challenges and opportunities in the future. Crit Rev Food Sci Nutr 61(18):3119–3128

BCFN Foundation (2020) Double Pyramid: a diet which is healthy for people and sustainable for the planet. https://www.barillacfn.com/en/dissemination/double_pyramid/. Accessed 5 July 2020

Estell M, Hughes J, Grafenauer S (2021) Plant protein and plant-based meat alternatives: consumer and nutrition professional attitudes and perceptions. Sustainability 13(3):1478. https://doi.org/10.3390/su13031478

FAO (2020) Food-based dietary guidelines—Sweden. http://www.fao.org/nutrition/education/food-dietary-guidelines/regions/sweden/en/. Accessed 5 Jul 2020

Fehér A, Gazdecki M, Véha M, Szakály M, Szakály Z (2020) A comprehensive review of the benefits of and the barriers to the switch to a plant-based diet. Sustainability 12(10):4136. https://doi.org/10.3390/su12104136

Hever J, Cronise RJ (2017) Plant-based nutrition for healthcare professionals: implementing diet as a primary modality in the prevention and treatment of chronic disease. J Geriatr Cardiol 14(5):355–368. https://doi.org/10.11909/j.issn.1671-5411.2017.05.012

Jacobs DM, Van Den Berg MA, Hall RD (2021) Towards superior plant-based foods using metabolomics. Curr Opin Biotechnol 70:23–28

Ku HK, Ha SH (2020) Improving nutritional and functional quality by genome editing of crops: status and perspectives. Front Plant Sci 11:577313. https://doi.org/10.3389/fpls.2020.577313

Loi M, Paciolla C (2021) Plant antioxidants for food safety and quality: exploring new trends of research. Antioxidants 10:972. https://doi.org/10.3390/antiox10060972

Marchesi JR, Adams DH, Fava F, Hermes GD, Hirschfield GM, Hold G, Quraishi MN, Kinross J, Smidt H, Tuohy KM, Thomas LV (2016) The gut microbiota and host health: a new clinical frontier. Gut 65(2):330–339

Mir RA, Nazir M, Naik S, Mukhtar S, Ganai BA, Zargar SM (2022) Utilizing the underutilized plant resources for development of life style foods: putting nutrigenomics to use. Plant Physiol Biochem 171:128–138

Mulpuri L, Allen N, Lunde A, Thomas S, Ray M, Polanco E, Cret N, Molinari J, Dowell L (2021) Rooting for wellness: an initiative introducing plant-based nutrition to first year medical students. Int J Dis Reversal Prev 3(2):12. https://doi.org/10.22230/ijdrp.2021v3n2a283

Munekata PES, Domínguez R, Budaraju S, Roselló-Soto E, Barba FJ, Mallikarjunan K, Roohinejad S, Lorenzo JM (2020) Effect of innovative food processing technologies on the physicochemical and nutritional properties and quality of non-dairy plant-based beverages. Foods 9(3):288. https://doi.org/10.3390/foods9030288

Rodriguez-Casado A (2016) The health potential of fruits and vegetables phytochemicals: notable examples. Crit Rev Food Sci Nutr 56(7):1097–1107

Sakkas H, Bozidis P, Touzios C, Kolios D, Athanasiou G, Athanasopoulou E, Gerou I, Gartzonika C (2020) Nutritional status and the influence of the vegan diet on the gut microbiota and human health. Medicina 56(2):88. https://doi.org/10.3390/medicina56020088

Tangyu M, Muller J, Bolten CJ, Wittmann C (2019) Fermentation of plant-based milk alternatives for improved flavour and nutritional value. Appl Microbiol Biotechnol 103:9263–9275. https://doi.org/10.1007/s00253-019-10175-9

Tso R, Forde CG (2021) Unintended consequences: nutritional impact and potential pitfalls of switching from animal-to plant-based foods. Nutrients 13(8):2527. https://doi.org/10.3390/nu13082527

The manufacturer's authorised representative in the EU is Springer Nature Customer Service Centre GmbH, Europaplatz 3, 69115 Heidelberg, Germany. If you have any concerns regarding our products, please contact ProductSafety@springernature.com

Printed and bound by CPI Group (UK) Ltd, Croydon, CR0 4YY
01/10/2026
02225869-0001